AF767596

BEHAVIORAL MEDICINE

International Perspectives

Volume 2

Development in Clinical Psychology

Glen R. Caddy, series editor
Nova University

MMPI-168 Codebook, by Ken R. Vincent, Iliana Castillo, Robert I. Hauser, H. James Stuart, Javier A. Zapata, Cal K. Cohn, and Gregory O'Shanick, 1984

Integrated Clinical and Fiscal Management in Mental Health: A Guidebook, by Fred Newman and James Sorensen, 1986

The Professional Practice of Psychology, edited by Georgiana Shick Tryon, 1986

Clinical Applications of Hypnosis, edited by Frank A. DePiano and Herman C. Salzberg, 1986

Full Battery Codebook, by Ken R. Vincent, 1987

Developments in the Assessment and Treatment of Addictive Behaviors, edited by Ted D. Nirenberg, 1987

Feminist Psychotherapies, edited by Mary Ann Douglas and Lenore E. Walker, 1988

Child Multimodal Therapy, by Donald B. Keat II, 1990

Psychophysiology for Clinical Psychologists, by Walter W. Surwillo, 1990

Strategic Health Planning: Methods and Techniques Applied to Marketing and Management, by Allen D. Spiegel and Herbert H. Hyman, 1991

Behavioral Medicine: International Perspectives (Vol. 1–3), edited by D.G. Byrne and Glenn R. Caddy, 1992

The MMPI: A Contemporary Normative Study of Adolescents, by Robert L. Colligan and Kenneth P. Offord, 1992

In Preparation:

Language and Psychopathology, by Stephen Schwartz

BEHAVIORAL MEDICINE

International Perspectives

Volume 2

Edited by

Glenn R. Caddy, Ph.D., ABPP, AABM,
Academy of Medicine and Psychology
and Nova University
Ft. Lauderdale, FL

D.G. Byrne, Ph.D., M.A.Ps.S., F.I.C.P.M.
Department of Psychology
Australian National University
Canberra, A.C.T.

ABLEX PUBLISHING CORPORATION
NORWOOD, NEW JERSEY

Printed in the United States of America.

Library of Congress Cataloging-in-Publication Data

Behavioral medicine : international perspectives / edited by D.G. Byrne, Glenn R. Caddy.
p. cm. — (Developments in clinical psychology)
Includes bibliographical references and index.
ISBN 089391-680–3 (v. 2)
1. Medicine and psychology. 2. Medicine, Psychosomatic.
I. Byrne, D.G. (Donald Glenn) II. Caddy, Glenn R. III. Series.
[DNLM: 1. Behavioral Medicine. 2. Psychology, Medical.
3. Psychophysiologic Disorders. WM 90 B4194]
R726.5.B4256 1991
616′.001′9—dc20
DNLM/DLC
for Library of Congress 91-26136
CIP

Ablex Publishing Corporation
355 Chestnut Street
Norwood, New Jersey 07648

To Gavin David and Janice Lynn,
with love, always.

G.R.C.

To Annie

D.G.B.

Table of Contents

Preface *ix*

I Foundations of Behavioral Medicine

1 Health Promotion and Preventive Behavioral Medicine *3*
Alan L. Peterson and Glenn R. Caddy

2 Program Development Research for Public Health: The Example of Smoking *31*
J. Allan Best, Edward A. Smith, and Deborah J. Ossip-Klein

3 Policy Issues Influencing Behavioral Medicine: An International Analysis *65*
Jonathan S. Raymond, Patrick H. DeLeon, Gary R. VandenBos, and Jerrold M. Michael

II The Musculoskeletal System

4 The Pathophysiology of Musculoskeletal Pain and Dysfunction *91*
Rene Cailliet

5 Functional Assessment of the Musculoskeletally Impaired Patient *103*
Cynthia C. Smith, Frances Oakley, Gloria Furst, and Lynn Gerber

6 Behavioral Approaches in the Treatment of Inflammatory Arthritis Disability–A Selected Review *127*
Matthew H. Liang, Alison Partridge, and Raymond Partridge

7 Electromyographic Biofeedback and Musculoskeletal Disorders *149*
Glenn R. Caddy and Trudy Block

III Pain

8 Psychological Assessment of Chronic Pain *175*
Stanley L. Chapman

9 Psychological Responses to Chronic Pain *211*
Neil Spence

10 The Behavioral Management and Prevention of Chronic Pain *253*
Steven J. Linton

IV Behavioral Neurology

11 Behavioral Causes and Management of Tension Headaches *297*
Paul R. Martin

12 Behavioral Aspects of Seizure Disorders *331*
Bjorn Ellersten, Hallgrim Klöve, and David I. Mostofsky

13 Sleep Disorders: Their Prevalence and Behavioral Treatment *347*
Leon C. Lack and Steven J. Thorn

V Other Issues in Behavioral Medicine

14 Behavioral Approaches to Exercise and Health *399*
Christina Lee and Neville Owen

Author Index *429*

Subject Index *452*

Preface

There have been many landmarks in the history of clinical psychology. In the late 1950s and the 1960s, great progress in the theories and applications of behavior therapy signalled an inevitable but much welcomed shift in orientation from that of counselor and psychometrician to that of independent psychotherapist. The advent of behavior therapy gave the clinical psychologist, at last, a basis for the treatment of behavioral disorders and personal distress which was theoretically unique to the science of psychology. If there has been a professional landmark in the last decade, however, it must surely be seen in the arrival of behavioral medicine.

Behavioral medicine, as a distinct discipline, has existed for not much longer than 10 years, yet in that time it has made a considerable impact both on clinical psychology and on the practice of medicine. The course and magnitude of this impact are obvious in the amount of written material, both empirical and speculative, which has been generated in the past decade. In addition to a large array of text documenting important areas of behavioral medicine, the area has given rise to its own specialized journal (the *Journal of Behavioral Medicine*) and several complete issues of other clinical and research journals (see, for example, *British Journal of Clinical Psychology,* No. 4, 1982, and *Journal of Psychosomatic Research,* No. 5, 1982). The sheer prominence of material emerging in the area provides adequate testimony to the seriousness and interest with which the formative years of behavioral medicine have been greeted.

In the early years of any field, definitions are often rather diverse, and those attached to behavioral medicine are no different. Schwartz and Weiss (1978) defined it as:

> The interdisciplinary field concerned with the development and integration of behavioral and biomedical science, knowledge and techniques relevant to health and illness and the application of this knowledge and these techniques to prevention, diagnosis, treatment and rehabilitation.

Somewhat more succinctly, Surwit, Williams, and Shapiro (1981) wrote:

> Behavioral medicine is broadly defined to encompass the application of principles from all behavioral sciences to medical problems.

Along more rigidly behavioral lines, Pomerleau and Brady (1979) claimed behavioral medicine to be:

> The clinical use of techniques derived from the experimental analysis of behavior—behavior therapy and behavior modification—for the evaluation, prevention, management or treatment of physical disease or physiological dysfunction.

Whichever position one takes, whether it be rigidly behavioral or more flexibly biopsychosocial, the essence of these definitions is clear. Behavioral medicine concerns the use of psychological evidence and techniques, typically but not exclusively those deriving from behavior therapy, in the diagnosis, prevention, and management of physically manifest illness.

Behavioral medicine is frequently confused with its close cousin, psychosomatic medicine, and the practitioner of the former is often asked to distinguish between the two. Surwit et al. (1981) argued that, whereas psychosomatic medicine placed its emphasis on the pathogenic influence of personality traits leading, through neurotic conflicts, to physical illness, behavioral medicine was concerned with physiological responses arising initially through maladaptive environmental interactions, becoming established or learned by means of objectively testable chains of causal influence, and leading ultimately to physical pathology. In practice, behavioral medicine rejected psychodynamic labelling, emphasized the experimental principles of learning in treatment, and confirmed the importance of evaluation and replicability of treatment procedures.

If psychosomatic medicine takes its theoretical beginnings from the psychodynamic movement of Freud and his successors, behavioral medicine is firmly rooted in the stress theories of Selye and those who followed him, the learning theories of Skinner and those coming after, and the integrative work on biopsychosocial approaches to illness beginning with Levi and his colleagues.

Just as clinical psychology had developed scientifically to the point where it could legitimately give rise to a new area of practice, medicine too was demonstrating, by and large, a readiness to accept approaches more broadly based than those concerned with the strict application of technology. The recognition by both professions that the treatment of human disease required attention to the *environment* and the *psyche,* as well as the *soma,* created a fertile ground for the integration of knowledge and practice. This promise of growth, and the considerable body of evidence it had already produced, prompted the development of this series of books.

The intention of *Behavioral Medicine: International Perspectives* is not to supplant any of a number of excellent works in the field, but to provide, as far as possible, a total overview of contemporary thought and clinical wisdom. In doing so, it draws widely and diversely, mixing contributory chapters from North American, European, and Australasian authors, with invitations to contribute being dependent only upon the judgment of the editors that individual authors would produce the best possible overviews of the area. The deliberate diversity of sources is reflected in the title of the volumes. Any exercise involving such judgment is bound to attract disagreement; in recognizing this, the editors are aware that many who are eminent in their own areas are not represented in these volumes. Nevertheless, we are confident that the breadth of authorship of each of the volumes in this series more than adequately compensates for individual omissions.

Uppermost in our minds in the early stages of planning was the need for comprehensiveness within a systematic organization of material. Consequently, as the project progressed, it grew from one to two and then three volumes. The sheer wealth of material in the area demanded that size could only be reduced by sacrificing whole sections crucial to a complete overview of behavioral medicine. In the final construction, it was decided that breadth of coverage overrode other considerations.

The organization of the three volumes is traditional, and follows an "organ/system" approach. Importantly, however, we have attempted to preface each section with a chapter outlining the anatomy, physiology, pathology, and epidemiology of the set of medical conditions under consideration. While the set of volumes will have a wide application across professional boundaries, the essentially interdisciplinary nature of behavioral medicine means that many readers will not have a background in the medical sciences. For them, it is important that concepts and terminologies in the substantive chapters are understood, and quick reference to an introductory summary seemed the best way of achieving this. Similarly, in the opening section of each volume, certain key issues in the clinical psychology of assessment and intervention have been discussed in summary chapters designed to acquaint the reader not trained in psychology with the unique contributions of this science to behavioral medicine. These additions, while somewhat increasing the length of the works, seek to establish the utility of these works across professional boundaries.

It is our hope that this series of books will serve a wide audience. In guiding our large group of excellent contributors, we have attempted to encourage chapters encompassing the inextricably joined areas of empirical evidence and clinical skill and practice. It was our hope from the beginning that the series would be as useful to the clinical practitioner grappling with the problems of single patients as it would be to the researcher requiring contemporary and comprehensive reviews of the available evidence needed to guide further studies. In principle, we hold the view that the two areas cannot be separated; if this comes across in individual chapters, it is a tribute to the subject grasp and clear thinking of the many eminent scientists and practitioners who have contributed so ably to the series.

Enterprises such as these owe much to many people. In this respect, the contributing authors are most immediately deserving of our thanks. In spite of heavy teaching and research loads, and overwhelming clinical commitments, such contributor worked to the difficult deadlines imposed to produce chapters of both breadth and depth. To our contributors, then, we are inestimably grateful. The editing of a series of works, when editors themselves are separated by some thousands of kilometers of land and ocean, produces its own particular difficulties. One is inclined to thank the systems of international postage, but at times these have not proven the most reliable means of communication. Colleagues on both sides of the Pacific have, however, helped our task very considerably. Of course, families tolerate much from members who pursue such ephemeral activities as editing books, and for this tolerance we are distinctly grateful.

The task of putting this work together has brought to each of us unique rewards. If we share one, however, it is the feeling that the series will have contributed palpably to the promotion of behavioral medicine as an area so new but with so much promise for the future.

D. G. Byrne
G. R. Caddy

REFERENCES

Pomerleau, O. F., & Brady, J. P. (Eds.). (1979). *Behavioral medicine: Theory and practice*. Baltimore: Williams & Wilkins.

Schwartz, G. E., & Weiss, S. M. (1978). Behavioral medicine revisited: An amended definition. *Journal of Behavioral Medicine, 1,* 249–251.

Surwitt, R. S., Williams, R. B., & Shapiro, D. (1981). *Behavioral approaches to cardiovascular disease*. New York: Academic Press.

I

FOUNDATIONS OF BEHAVIORAL MEDICINE

1

Health Promotion and Preventive Behavioral Medicine

Alan L. Peterson
Glenn R. Caddy
Nova University
Fort Lauderdale, Florida

INTRODUCTION

Health promotion and the *prevention of disease* has become one of the greatest challenges for the behavioral sciences during this second half of the 20th century. Widespread health promotion practices started slowly in the 1960s, began to receive experimental confirmation of their effectiveness in disease prevention in the early 1970s—especially in the United States—and burgeoned into a full-fledged revolution with attendant "hype" in the late 1970s and early 1980s. More than ever before, individuals are being exposed to the view that lifestyle has a direct impact on health and well being. However, changing one's life-style—decreasing health risk factors and increasing health promotion practices—is a formidable task, and one which many a citizen will resist. This chapter reviews the changing perspectives of health and disease, the assessment of health status, health epidemiology, health risk factors, risk factor intervention, arenas for promoting health and preventing disease, and problems encountered in the implementation of health promotion practices.

DEFINITIONS OF HEALTH

"Health" is a term frequently used and easily understood colloquially. Attempting to define health operationally, however, can be somewhat more difficult. *Webster's Ninth New Collegiate Dictionary* (1984) defines health as "the condition of being sound in body, mind, or spirit; freedom from physical disease or pain." Such a definition notwithstanding, it remains unclear if health is an actual positive quality or condition of an individual or merely the absence of illness or disease. Improved health can be defined in terms of improvements in mortality and morbidity patterns; however, good health is more than simply the absence of pathology. Health may best be viewed unidimensionally from disease and illness on one end, through the absence of disease or illness, and to a state of optimal health at the other end of the continuum. Dorland's Medical Dictionary (Saunders, 1974) provides an excellent definition of health: "a state of optimal physical, mental, and social well-being, and not merely the absence of disease or infirmity." Important factors to consider regarding optimal health include factors such as drug, alcohol, and tobacco use, nutrition, safety, exercise and activity, and rest and relaxation.

CHANGING PERSPECTIVES IN HEALTH AND DISEASE

Throughout history acute infectious diseases and starvation have been the leading causes of death. Throughout the Middle Ages, bubonic plague alone decimated some 150 million people. Other acute diseases that have been leading causes of death include cholera, diphtheria, malaria, poliomyelitis, smallpox, and typhoid.

In the 20th century, advances in society's general knowledge about disease prevention, improved sanitation, the development of vaccines and antibiotics, and the implementation of inoculation programs have almost eradicated acute infectious diseases in the developed countries. And, even in the case of the more recently identified and disquieting diseases such as Acquired Immune Deficiency Syndrome (AIDS), substantial research currently is being directed to an understanding of the nature and etiology of the condition. The presumption of such research is that it will result in a treatment option which will extend the already existing options for prevention. The social concern regarding AIDS notwithstanding, it is nevertheless the case that the acute diseases of yesteryear have been replaced as leading causes of death, primarily by cardiovascular disease and cancer. Recently, for example, the percentage of all deaths due to cardiovascular diseases and malignancies was about 70 percent in the United States, 72 percent in the United Kingdom, 67 percent in Australia, and 54 percent in Japan (United Nations, 1986).

The decrease in acute infectious diseases is largely due to the identification of specific disease-causing microorganisms. Most recently—in the case of AIDS, for example—even though the precise etiological basis of the condition has yet to be established, within four years of commencing the research for a test to detect AIDS such a test was developed and is now widely available throughout the developed countries (Weiss, Goedert, Sarngadharan, & Bodner, 1985). The identification of specific biological pathogens as causes for the chronic degenerative disorders, however, has been less successful. These disorders, by and large, are the products of various lifestyle events interacting with the biological dispositions of a progressively aging organism.

The treatment strategies also are different for patients suffering the acute vs. chronic diseases. Drugs are used to treat acute infections and diseases. The outcome of such treatment is usually determined in the short term and it has been generally held that the treatment requires little active cooperation on the part of the patient beyond, of course, compliance with the medication regimen. The treatment of chronic disorders, on the other hand, commonly requires drug therapy, surgery, and changes in lifestyle. The payoffs on such therapy are usually long-term, and the patient commonly is required to be quite actively involved in his or her convalescence. Unfortunately, compliance with such prescriptions of involvement is all too often poor (Sackett & Haynes, 1976).

Trite as it might be to again present the assertion, it is nevertheless the case that "diseases of lifestyle" appear to be the big killers of today. Poor eating behaviors, drug, alcohol, and tobacco use, stress and anxiety, lack of exercise, and poor safety habits contribute to and exacerbate the chronic disease processes. The 10 leading causes of death in the United States are: (a) heart diseases, (b) malignant neoplasms, (c) cerebrovascular diseases, (d) accidents, (e) chronic destructive pulmonary disease, (f) influenza and pneumonia, (g) diabetes mellitus, (h) cirrhosis of the liver, (i) atherosclerosis, and (j) suicide (United States Bureau of the Census, 1985). Other developed countries such as Canada, the United Kingdom, Switzerland, Australia, and Japan report similar causes of mortality (United Nations, 1986). To varying degrees, all of these causes of death involve behavioral factors. It is little wonder, therefore, that the field of behavioral medicine is in such a state of expansion. Professionals in the behavioral sciences, trained to change the behaviors and lifestyles of individuals, offer an ever-increasing contribution to the reduction of morbidity and mortality related to the chronic degenerative disorders which present the greatest health risk to human beings today.

ASSESSMENT OF HEALTH STATUS

While the assessment of health status clearly is critical in evaluating the efficacy of health promotion programs, the value of specific health promotion practices can be assessed only within the limits of the validity of the instruments or methods used to measure health status. Davies (1975) identified five features to be considered in the assessment of health status: (a) freedom from symptoms; (b) physical health; (c) functional capacity; (d) mental and emotional health; and (e) well-being. He used four instruments to obtain estimates of the status of current health as well as to gain prognostic estimates of health status. The instruments employed included a test profile, a health history, a mental health history, and a health hazard appraisal. Physical health was assessed via a physician's physical examination including measures of chemical, physiological, and anatomical states. A self-administered history form was used to help assess symptoms that are more difficult to quantify. Mental and emotional health were assessed from a shortened version of the Minnesota Multiphasic Personality Inventory. Well-being was derived from the mental health history data and from self-reports of well-being. Davies' health status profile approach to the assessment of health is very comprehensive, but it requires considerable time and trained professionals to complete it.

Self-administered health status questionnaires are less comprehensive, and perhaps less accurate, but they can be completed in a shorter period of time. Sintonen (1981) developed a battery of self-administered questionnaires in an attempt to measure and value health status. He included 12 dimensions of health: perceived health, breathing, seeing, sleeping, communicating, eating, incontinence, hearing, moving, intellectual or mental functioning, working, and social participation. Sintonen's initial results indicated his approach to the measurement and evaluation of health status to be a viable one and worthy of further development. This health status classification system is somewhat limited, however, in that it is disease-independent.

The Health Habits Questionnaire (Tapp, 1978) is a 44-item self-administered questionnaire designed to provide information for primary care physicians and other health care professionals on the extent to which individuals engage in health habits. Items are clustered into the following eight categories: nutrition, tobacco use, alcohol use, drug use, road and water safety, exercise and activity, rest and relaxation, and personal health care. The questionnaire is easy to administer and score, can be completed in less than 5 minutes, and has been shown to be a good measure of health behaviors.

HEALTH EPIDEMIOLOGY AND RISK FACTORS

Biological, environmental, and behavioral factors all interact in determining health problems. The susceptibility for certain illnesses and diseases such as Huntington's chorea or sickle cell anemia have strong biological and hereditary components. Other health problems such as cancer and cardiovascular disorders also show a biologically based etiology but have added environmental and behavioral concomitants as well. Many factors in the physical environment such as infectious diseases, toxic substances in the food, water, and air, exposure to radiation, and safety hazards all increase health risks. Influences in the socioeconomic environment such as financial status and geographic location, and factors in the family environment such as divorce or separation also affect health. Behavioral factors also are inextricably tied to the etiology of certain disabilities, diseases, and illnesses. Certain behaviors, such as careless driving, drinking, smoking, and eating patterns, are all clearly related to health.

Many studies of health epidemiology have been conducted (Belloc, Breslow, & Hochstim, 1971; Haynes, Levine, Scotch, Feinleib, and Kannell, 1978; Metzner, Carman, & House, 1983; Multiple Risk Factor Intervention Trial Research Group, 1982; Rosenman, Friedman & Strauss, 1964). One of the better epidemiological studies is the Alameda County study (Belloc et al., 1971). This study analyzed the physical health status in an adult population and examined the possible relationship between health status and a number of independent variables. Data for the study were gathered via questionnaires completed by a sample of 6,928 adult residents of Alameda County, California, in 1965. Initial results (Belloc & Breslow, 1972) indicated that common health practices, including hours of sleep, regularity of meals (eating breakfast; snacking between meals), physical activity, smoking, drinking, and weight in relation to desirable standards for height were related to physical health status. Good practices were found to be associated with positive health. The relationship between these activities was cumulative with those who followed all of the good practices being in better health, even though older, than those who failed to do so. Age, sex, and economic factors were found to be independent of this association.

Personal health practices were also shown to be related to mortality (Belloc, 1973). When the health practices were combined to form a health practice score from 0 to 7, the number of health practices showed a striking inverse relationship, especially for men. Income level and physical health status were independent of this relationship. In fact, mortality was more strongly associated with poor health practices than with current physical health status. At a nine-year follow-up (Wingard, Berkman, & Brand, 1982), five of the health practices were found to be associated with lower mortality from all causes. Neither eating breakfast nor snacking were associated with lower mortality.

In addition to the findings of the Alameda County study, much more evidence is available identifying specific risk factors. Other known risk factors include the use of tobacco, alcohol, and drugs, appropriate nutrition practices, lack of the use of safety practices, and the presence of stress.

Tobacco

Numerous studies have demonstrated quite clearly that smoking is indeed hazardous to one's health (see Califano, 1979; National Cancer Institute, 1984). It is associated with heart and blood vessel diseases; chronic bronchitis and emphysema; and cancer of the lung, larynx, pharynx, oral cavity, esophagus, pancreas, and urinary bladder. The mortality rate for smokers is about 70 percent greater from all causes. In the United States, smoking is related to 85–90 percent of all lung cancer, 40 percent of all cancers in males, and 25 percent of all cancers in females. In many of the European countries the cancer rates from smoking are even higher than the United States, whereas in other countries such as Canada, Australia, and Japan the cancer rates are significantly less (National Cancer Institute, 1985). The mortality rate from coronary heart disease is 60 percent higher in male smokers (Kannel & Lerner, 1984). The mechanisms involved in bringing about disease from tobacco-related cancer are not fully understood, but probably involve the tars absorbed into the body and the inhalation of carbon monoxide and nicotine (Brady, 1983). Radioactive material in tobacco also may be involved. And, of course, elements in the functioning of smokers other than their use of tobacco also may be implicated in the health prognosis of this population.

The toxicity of active smoking is well established, but the health problems associated with passive smoking are just now coming to light. Nicotine has been shown to cross the placental barrier resulting in changes in fetal heart rate, temperature, and oxygen consumption. Smoking has been shown to be correlated with decreased birthweight, length, head circumference, and chest circumference (Anderson, Blidner, & McClemont, 1984; Sausa & Azevedo, 1984). It increases the risk of spontaneous abortion, fetal death, neonatal death, abruptio placentae, placenta previa, bleeding and membrane rupture during pregnancy, and premature delivery (Dwyer, 1984). Parental side-stream smoke has been shown to be significantly associated with digestive symptoms and postprandial colic in 253 three-month old infants (Said, Patois, & Lellouch, 1984). Recent studies have shown that passive smoking by nonsmokers may acutely aggravate angina pectoris (Aronow, 1978), induce small airway dysfunction (Tager, Weiss, Rosner, & Speizer, 1979; White & Froeb, 1980), and increase the risk of lung cancer (Correa, Pickle, Fontham, Lin, & Haenszel, 1983; Trichopoulos, Kalandidi, Sparros, & MacMahon, 1981).

The use of smokeless tobacco, a current fad among many teenagers, also has been implicated in the development of certain oral cancers (Massey, Moore, & Yonkers, 1984). The occurrence of lesions is related to total contact time and total years of use. Persons using smokeless tobacco for 50 or more years increase the risk of oral cancer almost 50 times. Other problems can include habituation, peridontal destruction, and increases in blood pressure and heart rate.

Alcohol and Drugs

Alcohol and other drug abuse has the potential to lead to long-term chronic diseases. Cirrhosis is largely attributable to a combination of alcohol abuse and poor dietary practices and ranks among the top 10 leading causes of death in the United States. Alcohol use also is associated with cancer of the liver, esophagus, and mouth and with increased myocardial infarct occurrence (Deutscher, Rockette, & Krishnaswami, 1984). Long-term heavy alcohol consumption also has been related to the Wernicke-Korsakoff constellation (Victor, Adams, & Collins, 1971). Excessive drinking during pregnancy can lead to severe abnormalities in infants, the so called fetal alcohol syndrome (Jones & Smith, 1973; Mills, Braubard, Harley, Rhodes, & Berendes, 1984; Wilson, 1981). Alcohol use also leads to increased risk of suicide, homicide, and is implicated in about half of all vehicular fatalities (DeLuca, 1981).

Other drug abuse also represents a serious health hazard. The health effects of the myriad of potentially abused drugs are too many to elaborate here. Hallucinogens, stimulants, sedatives, opiates, marijuana, and even a range of prescription drugs have been implicated in increased rates of morbidity and mortality. Of substantial significance is the fact that the extent of the harmful effects of the experimentation and use of drugs may be difficult to determine for an individual case. The psychological and physical effects of drugs, of course, are highly variable from one individual to another.

Nutrition

Nutrition is another important factor in health epidemiology. High blood pressure may result from high dietary salt intake and cardiovascular disease has been shown to be related to the high intake of cholesterol and saturated fat (Public Health Service, 1985). A more tenuous relationship exists between diet and cancer. High consumption of animal protein, low consumption of fiber from plant sources, and high consumption of both saturated and unsaturated fats may all be related to colon, ovary, and prostate cancer; however, further research in these areas is clearly needed.

Obesity also increases the risk factors for disease. Diabetes, high blood pressure, heart disease, neoplasms, and digestive diseases have all been shown to be related to obesity (Bray, 1984). The degree of excess morbidity and mortality increases as the degree of excess weight rises.

Safety

Morbidity and mortality rates are directly related to safety practices. During 1981, the following number of Americans died in accidents: 53, 172 in motor vehicle accidents; 13,294 from accidental falls; 5,233 from accidental drownings; 5,697 from burns; 4,523 from accidental poisonings; and 1,871 from firearms (United States Bureau of the Census, 1985).

Environmentally-related safety practices determine the health risks from toxic chemicals. Industrial and agricultural chemicals have found their way into our water and food supplies. In developed nations, air pollution is also hazardous with toxic gases or matter from automobiles or industries polluting the atmosphere. Another environmental hazard is radiation. The full effects of potentially hazardous radioactive materials in our food, water, air, and environment are difficult to measure. Toxic chemicals in food and water supplies have been associated with cancer and severe neurological and reproductive defects in animals and humans. Air pollution has been associated with cancer and debilitating respiratory disorders. Radiation can cause cancer, genetic defects, and tissue injury. The toxic chemical accident in Bhopal, India in 1984 killed some 2,300 people and injured 200,000. The long-term effects of the Chernobyl radiation leak in the U.S.S.R. in 1986 may never fully be known.

Exercise

While it has become a truism that exercise and health go together, some researchers have questioned whether the long-term benefits of vigorous exercise outweigh the risks. Physical fitness has become a passion pursued at times to the point of injury and even death. Myocardial ischemia, cardiac arrhythmias, and even sudden death seem to occur with unusually high frequency during vigorous exercise (Jackson, Beaglehole, & Sharpe, 1983; Thompson, 1982; Thompson, Funk, Carleton, & Sturner, 1982; Waller & Roberts, 1980). Conversely, other epidemiological evidence suggests that habitual vigorous exercise is associated with an overall reduction in the risk of sudden cardiac insult (Garcia-Palmieri, Costas, Cruz-Vidal, Sortic, & Havlik, 1982; Morris, Everitt, Pollard, & Chave, 1980; Paffenberger & Hale, 1975; Siscovick, Weiss, Hallstrom, Invi, & Peterson, 1982; Siscovick & Weiss, 1984).

Overall, the research indicates that strenuous activities can sometimes precipitate a heart attack, increasing by perhaps sevenfold a person's chances of dying suddenly during or just after exercising. Although the overall risk of dying is low, it is nonetheless higher than the estimate for the same amount of time spent quietly. The "weekend athlete" is particularly at risk. Over one's lifetime, however, vigorous exercise far outweighs the risks and can directly reduce the chances of heart attack and premature death, even after myocardial infarction.

Stress

Stress is another health hazard that everyone experiences in their lives to some extent. Very high levels of stress that continue for long periods of time have been shown to be deleterious to one's health. Most standard medical textbooks attribute anywhere from 50 to 80 percent of all diseases to stress-related or psychosomatic origins. Research is accumulating to support two main physiological effects of stress: (a) disruption of a particular neurophysiological or organ system in and of itself, and (b) suppression of normal immunological functions, leading to increased susceptibility to viral or aberrant cell disorders (Pelletier, 1977). Some physical disorders in which stress has been implicated include hypertension, arteriosclerosis, cancer, arthritis, respiratory disease, and gastrointestinal disorders. Stress is also implicated as a factor in virtually every type of mental illness and effects other hazardous behaviors such as smoking, excess alcohol and other drug use, and disordered eating.

HEALTH PROMOTION AND RISK FACTOR INTERVENTION

There are several models on which to base a strategy for risk factor intervention. Bland (1982) reviewed three basic approaches that have been employed: the medical model, the public health model, and the ecological model. The medical model is interruptive and somewhat ex post facto. When an individual is diagnosed as having specific signs of potential health problems, (e.g., high blood pressure, angina) he or she is treated with the appropriate medication.

Education and behavior modification are the primary foci of the public health model of risk factor intervention. This is not a diagnostic approach based on treating disease; rather, it is a prognostic approach designed to modify certain aspects of a person's lifestyle that are potential health risks.

The ecological model focuses on broader social questions. This model examines how to reduce risk by changing occupational hazards, by improving the quality of the air, water, and food, and by the implementation of regulations addressing concerns such as highway speed and seat belt use, and so on.

All three of these models of risk factor intervention involve a strategy of prognostic screening followed by some form of intervention. Most intervention programs are based on the results derived from large-scale epidemiological studies. The factors most frequently intervened against are tobacco, drug and alcohol use, dietary practices, safety practices, physical exercise, and rest and relaxation.

To improve health, both passive and active measures can be employed (Williams, 1982). This passive-active dimension is defined in terms of the amount of action required of an individual to maintain his or her protection. At one end of the dimension are passive measures which automatically protect individuals without their action or cooperation. Passive measures include the pasteurization of milk, the iodination of salt, the child proofing of caps on medicine bottles, and the introduction of air bags and automatic restraints in automobiles. Active measures require individual action (though often minimal) for the person to be protected. Such measures include fastening seat belts or taking vitamins on a daily basis. Active measures also may require certain action (though often minimal) for the person to be protected. Such measures include fastening seat belts or taking vitamins on a daily basis. Active measures also may require certain actions to be performed infrequently (e.g., immunizations), occasionally (e.g., dental exams), or frequently (e.g., vigorous exercise). Active measures may require increasing or decreasing the frequency of behaviors. As the following review of the primary risk factors will indicate, most health risk factors can be reduced significantly by using a combination of both active and passive measures.

Smoking Cessation

Cigarette smoking is the largest single preventable cause of morbidity and mortality in our society. Smoking cessation, however, is no easy task. In the United States about 90 percent of all current smokers have expressed a desire to quit, but only about 10 percent of those people manage to succeed by quitting each year (Ockene & Camic, 1985). Increasing public knowledge of the health risks of smoking can significantly reduce smoking. A massive national educational campaign following the U.S. Surgeon General's first report on smoking and health in 1964 (U.S. Public Health Service, 1964) led to a significant decrease in the percentage of smokers in the United States. Apparently, simply imparting knowledge on the health hazards of smoking was sufficient enough for thousands of individuals to quit the habit.

Most individuals are now aware of the link between smoking and lung cancer—few are aware of the numerous other problems related to smoking. Much more should be done to increase public knowledge of the hazards of smoking. Physicians and other health professionals should serve as role models and actively encourage smoking cessation in their patients. Children and adolescents should be better educated and encouraged to make intelligent decisions regarding smoking.

Education has been the most effective method of reducing smoking. It has been reported that 95 percent of smokers who quit do so on their own (Califano, 1979). Knowledge of the health consequences of smoking undoubtedly is of primary importance in an individual's decisions to stop the habit. Myriad smoking cessation programs have been developed to help the millions of individuals who continue to smoke, despite being bombarded by information of its health hazards. Hypnosis, acupuncture, psychotherapy, behavior modification, and psychopharmacological agents have all been used with varying degrees of success with about 15–20 percent of the participants remaining abstinent after 1 year (Lichtenstein & Brown, 1982).

During the past several years, many methodological improvements have been made. Such improvements include more intensive follow-up, biological verification of self-reports, the provision of information regarding sample characteristics, and attrition rates. Multicomponent behavioral, self-management, and aversive packages have produced the most consistent results and report 40–50 percent abstinence 6 months to 1 year after treatment is over (Kamarck & Lichtenstein, 1985). Most programs still have a substantially high relapse rate and relapse prevention should be an important focus for future studies. Continued research on the biological mechanisms underlying smoking should suggest new treatment strategies including a combination of biological, behavioral, and psychological components.

Reducing Alcohol and Drug Use

The prevention and treatment of alcohol and other drug problems is a difficult task—psychological, physical, and social concomitants are inextricably intertwined in the etiology of addictive behaviors. Education regarding the potentially harmful effects of drugs and alcohol is of paramount importance but has only achieved limited success. Parental role models, peer pressure, and commercial advertisement are but a few of the many factors that can counteract education programs. Nevertheless education programs have undoubtedly helped countless youth and adults avoid the health-related problems inherent in drug and alcohol misuse and abuse. Public education programs should certainly be continued and even expanded along with other deterrents such as stringent legislation and law enforcement.

Myriad programs have been developed for the treatment of alcoholism. Treatment goals may focus on complete abstinence or restricted drinking (Miller & Caddy, 1977). Alcoholics Anonymous (AA) is the oldest and best known program for alcoholism treatment and includes well over a million members worldwide. AA promotes total abstinence and their statement "For an alcoholic, one drink is too many and a thousand not enough" summarizes their belief. However, the experimental evidence in support of the disease notion of alcoholism, which is a conceptual foundation of the AA model, has been demonstrated to be deficient for some time (see Sobell & Sobell, 1975; Caddy & Gottheil, 1982). Further, while there can be little question that the fellowship has been of great significance to many an alcoholic, there is little research supporting the relative efficacy of the AA approach across the diversity of drinking difficulties. Only two controlled studies of AA have been conducted (Brandsma, Maultsby, & Welsh, 1980; Ditman, Crawford, Forgy, Moskowitz, & MacAndrew, 1967): both studies found AA to be no more effective than a no-treatment control group.

Traditional treatment programs other than AA (but often including AA participation as a component) typically have aimed at total abstinence. Other approaches in which controlled drinking training was evaluated, as well as the more traditional approaches, have all reported improvement at the end of treatment for about two-thirds of the alcoholics who completed their treatment (Armor, Polich, & Stambul, 1976). The U.S. National Institute on Alcohol Abuse and Alcoholism conducted a review in 1976 of the treatment effectiveness of eight large treatment centers. The results indicated that some 70 percent of the alcoholics were abstinent at the end of treatment, and at a 4-year follow-up, 28 percent were abstaining and 18 percent were drinking "socially." Emrick (1975) reviewed 384 studies of psychologically oriented alcoholism treatment and found that differences in treatment methods did not significantly affect long-term outcome. In formal treatment programs, 25 percent of the subjects were abstinent compared to 16 percent of subjects not in a formal treatment program. Total improvement (including both abstinence and controlled drinking was 64 percent for patients in formal treatment versus 42 percent for those not in a formal treatment program. A recent review of 26 controlled studies (Miller & Hester, 1986) showed no overall advantage for inpatient versus outpatient or for longer over shorter inpatient programs for treating alcohol abuse. In summary, existing treatment programs do not appear to differ in treatment effectiveness, but most are more effective than no formal treatment in the management of alcoholism. Adequate experimentally controlled treatment outcome studies are basically very few and should be pursued.

In the United States, in particular, the relative political influence of the predominant (disease) perspective, with its attendant assertions for abstinence, appears to have substantially curtailed much of the behavioral work looking at a range of possible outcomes in the management of the alcohol abuser.

With the increasing recognition of the continued expansion of drug abuse in our society, a further expansion of the development of drug treatment programs also is occurring. One of the older programs, Synanon, has claimed the highest success rate in any program to date. Synanon, however, requires addicts to continue forever to live in the Synanon Center, or, after being clearly stabilized, to move into nearby living quarters and thereby stay affiliated and involved with the Synanon program (Ray, 1983). Synanon involves cold-turkey withdrawal by ex-addicts, it provides jobs and money, and works, in part, through encounter groups called Synanons.

In another approach, in Britain, opiate addicts receive doses of opiates free or at minimal cost under the supervision of knowledgeable physicians. The drug culture remains stable in Britain, and little crime is attributed to opiate addicts. In the United States, methadone maintenance is used in a similar fashion. Although drug abuse is a severe problem worldwide and many treatment programs have been developed, there exists little empirical data verifying the effectiveness of drug treatment programming. Research in this area clearly is needed.

Improved Nutritional Habits

Changes in nutritional habits and the reduction of obesity can improve health and reduce disease in many ways. The consumption of fat, sugar, cholesterol, salt, and alcohol has been related to 6 out of 10 of the leading causes of death in the United States. Increased consumption of fiber and decreased consumption of animal protein has been shown to be related to decreased levels of colon cancer. Individuals consuming low levels of cholesterol, such as vegetarians, have a reduced incidence of heart disease. Certain food additive (e.g., sodium nitrite) have been implicated as carcinogenic; ironically, many of these same additives are designed to prevent illnesses and diseases caused by spoiled food. Food additives must receive both scientific scrutiny and regulatory control to ensure their safety.

Individual dietary requirements vary and make it difficult to establish exact dietary standards. Nevertheless, based on what is already known or is strongly suspected about the relationship between diet and disease, several recommendations can be made for Americans, which are, presumably, also valid suggestions for people in many other developed countries. Most individuals would be healthier, as a whole, if they consumed (a) only sufficient calories to meet body needs and maintain desirable weight (reduce calories if overweight), (b) less saturated fat and cholesterol, (c) less salt, (d) less sugar, (e) relatively more complex carbohydrates such as whole grains, cereals, fruits, and vegetables, and (f) relatedly more fish, poultry, legumes, and less red meat (U.S. Department of Agriculture, 1980).

Improved nutritional education is also essential for health promotion. Parents, teachers, physicians, and other health professionals should be knowledgeable about nutritional information and take advantage of the opportunity to impart knowledge to children, students, and the population in general. The media can also be a powerful influence as evidenced by the Stanford Heart Disease Prevention Program (Meyer, Nash, McAlister, MacCoby, & Farquhar, 1980). In this study a mass media campaign led to a reduction in the consumption of salt and cholesterol.

Weight loss in the obese and overweight individual is another important health promotion factor. Many nutritionally sound diets are available, but fad diets are ubiquitous. Overnight diet plans requiring no personal effort are, at best, dubious. Losing body weight gradually and systematically offers the greatest prognosis for maintaining the new weight. Wilson and Brownell (1980) completed a comprehensive review of controlled and uncontrolled clinical studies of weight loss programs. Behavioral techniques were reported to be superior to traditional medical and psychotherapeutic treatments in helping clients lose weight. The results of all programs are mixed, however, at what are generally regarded as the long-term follow-up points (one year or more). The basic principles of most behavioral weight loss programs (e.g., Stuart & Davis, 1972) involve self-monitoring of food intake, setting goals to alter eating behavior by changing external food-related cues, changing eating behaviors, altering patterns of exercise, and providing social reinforcement for the changed behaviors. Fundamental cognitive restructuring to influence the image of oneself as a trim-framed individual, while potentially extremely important, has received less attention.

The combination of a reduced diet with vigorous exercise is a very effective means of shedding excess poundage. The accepted figure for melting off a pound of fat involves the expenditure of 3500 calories (Getchell, 1979). Thirty minutes of vigorous exercise will burn approximately 300 calories in an average individual. The frequent weight-loss prescription of losing one pound per week commonly can be achieved by decreasing calorie intake by 400 calories per day and exercising for 30 minutes 4 times weekly.

Improved Safety Habits

Passive and active approaches can and are being taken to reduce accidental death and injury. In occupational settings, the work environment as well as job performance standards can be modified. Passive measures, such as the use of insulated tools, are the most efficient changes that can be made. The successful implementation of safety measures in the work place requires cooperation and effort from employers, employees, unions, and governmental agencies. Unfortunately, the development of hazard control technology has lagged behind the development of hazardous industrial chemicals and sources of energy such as microwaves, nuclear energy, lasers, and ultrasound.

Preventive action also can be taken to reduce accidents involving firearms, falls, burns, poisonings, and recreational activities. Comparative evidence from countries such as Australia, England, and Japan clearly shows that death and injury from handguns can be profoundly reduced by prohibiting or restricting their possession. Given the agenda in the United States to possess firearms, however, other measures such as using security and locks alarm systems, locating ammunition separately from the weapon, and ensuring the inaccessibility of firearms to children can also reduce accidents. Death and injury from burns can be substantially reduced through passive measures such as (a) the installation of smoke detectors and fire alarms, (b) the use of nonflammable materials in clothing and in the construction of furniture and other building structures that cater to large numbers of people (e.g., restaurants, commercial airlines, etc.), and (c) building designs which provide easy escape routes. The development of poison control centers to provide immediate information on poison antidotes has reduced morbidity and mortality rates from accidental poisoning. Individuals can also take steps to ensure that harmful substances are stored in proper containers and are out of the reach of children.

Passive and active measures also can reduce injuries and deaths from motor vehicle accidents. At least theoretically, one active measure, namely changing operator safety behaviors, could massively reduce motor vehicle accidents. The term "accident" is a misnomer in that it implies that the event is not due to any fault or misconduct on the part of the individual. Virtually all motor vehicle "accidents" are caused by driver carelessness, inattention, fatigue, and so on all of which are conditions or behaviors which can be modified. Motor vehicle accidents due to mechanical failure are exceedingly rare. Unfortunately, changing driver safety behavior requires a concerted effort from the operator. Although driver education and safety classes are certainly helpful, changing driver safety behavior requires constant vigilance while on the road. Unfortunately, this goal appears impossible to achieve on a large-scale basis.

The greatest risk factor in motor vehicle accidents that we have a potential to change involves the behavior of driving while intoxicated. Stiff penalties, including mandatory license suspension, driver education, combined with mandatory safety belts usage have all been helpful in reducing alcohol-related accident injury and death and should certainly be further developed.

Other actions taken to reduce morbidity and mortality from motor vehicle accidents are measures to protect those individuals who have accidents. Active measures have been ineffective for the most part. Although the use of lap and shoulder belts can almost halve the chances of serious injury or death, fewer than 20 percent of drivers use such restraints voluntarily in the United States. In other countries—Australia, for example—mandatory safety belt legislation has resulted in very high rates of compliance and lesser resistance than appears in the countries without such laws. Mandatory seat belt legislation in the United States has increased the use rate but has been faced with much adversity.

The greatest success in reducing motor vehicle injuries and death have resulted from passive measures. In 1966–1970 the U.S. government instituted federally mandated standards for improving the crashworthiness of vehicles. These changes reportedly saved an estimated 28,000 lives between 1966 and 1974 (Comptroller of the U.S., 1976; Robertson, 1977) and 37,000 lives between 1975 and 1978 (Robertson, 1981). Reducing the speed limits in the United States in 1974 to 55 miles per hour is estimated to have saved 4,000–5,000 lives each year. Other passive measures have yet to be implemented on a large-scale basis. Air bags have been demonstrated to be very effective in both laboratory and real-world settings and require no active effort from the drivers. Another safety measure only just now being tapped is the installation of a high center-mounted rear brake light, which has been shown to reduce rear-end collisions by about 50 percent (Malone, Kirkpatrick, Kohl, & Baker, 1978; Reilly, Kurke, & Buckenmaier, 1980; Rausch, Wong, & Kirkpatrick, 1982).

Physical Fitness Training

Exercise and physical fitness training can significantly improve one's physical and psychological health. A long-term program of vigorous exercise has been shown to be related to significant decreases in the risk for cardiovascular disease, coronary heart disease, high blood pressure, osteoporosis, arthritis, obesity, asthma, and diabetes (Haskell, 1984). Exercise may even slow down the aging process (Spirduso, 1983). Psychological benefits related to exercise include decreased depression and anxiety, increased self-esteem, self-reliance, and energy, and improved mood state and cognitive functioning (Folkins & Sime, 1981). Physical fitness training improves the efficiency of the heart, increases oxygen consumption throughout the body, and increases the strength of the striated muscles. Several large-scale studies have supported a relationship between exercise and improved health (Hammond & Garfinkel, 1969; Kannel & Sorkie, 1979; Paffenbarger, Wing, & Hyde, 1978).

Aerobic exercises such as brisk walking, jogging, swimming, cross-country skiing, and bicycling are the physical activities most frequently prescribed by health professionals to help prevent cardiovascular disease. Nonaerobic exercises, such as weight training, increase muscle tone and strength, but have no apparent reduction in risk for cardiovascular disease. When aerobic exercise is performed with sufficient intensity, duration, and frequency, improvements in cardiovascular, metabolic, and muscular fitness occur. This vigorous overload is referred to as the "training effect." This effect is achieved by aerobic exercise of at least 20–30 minutes 3–4 times weekly, sustained at an intensity sufficient to keep an individual's pulse rate at 70–80 percent of maximal heart rate (Getchell, 1979; Rigotti, Thomas, & Leaf, 1983).

Although there is a large amount of evidence to support the benefits of exercise to physical and mental health, most research indicates that the majority of people who begin an exercise program stop within the first few months. Compliance with exercise regimes is now the primary stumbling block in improving health through exercise. Some research indicates that social support, feedback, and praise during exercise, flexibility in exercise goal setting, and distraction-based cognitive strategies may enhance adherence in exercise programs (Martin et al., 1984). Continued research in this area is warranted.

Stress Reduction

There are three primary methods frequently used for reducing stress: (a) stress avoidance, (b) stress resistance, and (c) reduced arousal effects. Stress avoidance is the most effective stress management tool and involves avoiding stressful situations and changing one's exposure to potential stressors. Stress also can be avoided to a large extent by only establishing goals that can reasonably be achieved. Increasing the body's resistance to the negative effects of stress can lessen the impact of stressors. Individuals engaging in health promotion behaviors such as vigorous exercise, proper nutrition, smoking cessation, minimal alcohol consumption, and proper rest appear to be less affected by the impact of stress. Stress reduction also can be achieved by reducing arousal effects by planning for "fun time" or rest and relaxation. Active methods of controlling stress such as progressive relaxation (Jacobson, 1938), meditation, autogenic training (Schultz & Luthe, 1959), or biofeedback also can reduce arousal effects. Pelletier (1977) provides an excellent review of methods for controlling stress (see also Brown, 1978).

ARENAS FOR HEALTH PROMOTION & DISEASE PREVENTION

The last decade alone has seen recruitment of schools, employers, labor unions, and others from virtually every aspect of society into disease prevention efforts (McGinnis, 1985). There are numerous arenas in which preventive behavioral medicine practices can be implemented (see Andreoli & Guillory, 1983). The home provides the opportunity for the greatest influence on health promotion. Many health-related practices of parents (e.g., amount of cholesterol in foods prepared, use of child safety restraint devices in automobiles, etc.), directly influence the health of their children. Parents serve as role models for other health-related behaviors such as smoking, drinking of alcohol, and safety practices.

Schools are an ideal setting for imparting health promotion knowledge through specific classes such as health, physical education, biology, nutrition, and diverse education. Health-related practices such as physical fitness, nutritious school lunches, and immunization procedures also can be incorporated into school settings. Williams, Arnold, and Wynder (1977) demonstrated that children in school settings can be motivated to assume responsibility for their own future health and modify their lifestyles in a direction of reduced risk for disease. These researchers combined screening for disease risk factors, giving children their results in a Health Passport, and providing innovative learning activities in a health education curriculum. It has been shown that as the level of education increases, so does the likelihood of engaging in health-related practices (Johnson, 1981).

The work site is one setting that has just recently been tapped as an arena for health promotion. Cohen (1985) delineated several work site features particularly helpful to persons wishing to change their health habits. These features included (a) facilitation of regular program participation, (b) reinforcing social support from co-workers, (c) opportunities for environmental supports (e.g., healthy foods in the cafeteria, office smoking policies, etc.), (d) opportunities for positive reinforcement for participation, (e) decreased personal costs for health promotion activities, and (f) convenient location. The most advanced employee fitness programs to date are conducted in Japan. Japanese workers are also first in life expectancy and productivity (Cohen, 1985). Although there is clear evidence that employees participating in worksite exercise classes improve their physical fitness (Cox, Shepard & Corey, 1981; Pauly, Palmer, Wright, & Pfeiffer, 1982), much less evidence exists that these programs lead to increased productivity (Haskell, & Blair, 1980) or reduced absenteeism and turnover (Bjurstrom & Alexion, 1978). Clearly, more research is needed in this area.

Health care institutions, given that they are designed to provide health care, may have an easier task than other institutions in promoting health (Andreoli & Guillory, 1983). Hospitals usually have credibility in the eyes of the general public and have at least a mandate to provide preventive health services. The goal in this area should be to upgrade significantly the services provided, especially regarding the primary care physician. Califano (1979) reported that 80 percent of the patients surveyed had never been encouraged by a physician to engage in regular exercise. Primary care physicians should take a principal role to assess risk factors based on a patient's personal lifestyle and advise about appropriate prevention and intervention strategies.

Government, public, and private nonprofit organizations all have a responsibility to impart information and knowledge regarding health promotion via national health information programs. One of the biggest problems regarding information transfer involves getting research results to the public promptly and in terms that are understandable. The media provide one method of reaching the public. The Stanford Heart Disease Prevention Program (Meyers, Nash, McAlister, MacCoby, & Farquhar, 1980) demonstrated that the media can be a viable means to effect public changes in health habits.

PROBLEMS IN THE IMPLEMENTATION OF HEALTH PROMOTION PRACTICES

Our health promotion goals are clear; the obstacles to these goals are many. Impoverished social factors such as inadequate income, housing, diet, education, and healthful work places are all problems that must be resolved before further progress in disease prevention and health promotion can occur. Industries threatened with economic loss (e.g., tobacco industry) from health promotion programs may also create obstacles. The present knowledge base in disease prevention and health promotion has grown tremendously and many specific risk factors have been identified. Nevertheless, many more questions remain unanswered and continued research on prevention activities is essential.

Probably the major obstacle to the development of a healthier society is that modifying health-related behaviors is no easy task. Simply educating individuals on risk factors is usually less than adequate to motivate them to change their maladaptive behaviors. Brady (1983) provides an excellent example of this problem in his review of cigarette smoking. Cigarette smoking—a major risk factor for many serious diseases—continues to be a habit of millions. Seat belt use requires only seconds from an individual and can reduce injuries and fatalities dramatically. Nevertheless, only 1 in 5 individuals in the United States voluntarily employ these devices. If we are unable to convince people to spend several seconds daily to buckle a seat belt, how are we to convince them to engage in other health promotion behaviors requiring considerably greater effort? This is the challenge for behavioral scientists. We know what needs to be done—reduce clearly identified risk factors—but we do not appear to be clear about how to do it best!

Much of the research on compliance in health care is and should continue to provide us with methods for motivating individuals to reduce risk factors (e.g., Martin et al., 1984). Simultaneously, specific procedures to aid in the acquisition of health-related attitudes and behaviors (e.g., various goal-setting strategies, reinforcement strategies, relapse prevention training, etc.) need to be better established.

SUMMARY

After a sustained period of increasing death rates due to chronic illness, the trend has begun to change. While perhaps slowly, apparently, we have been "doing the right things" during the past 20 to 25 years, especially in regard to decreases in cardiovascular diseases (Stamler, 1985). Individuals have made significant lifestyle changes in eating, smoking, safety, and exercise habits. A long-term study by Pell and Fayerweather (1985) indicated that the incidence of myocardial infarction has decreased by 28 percent overall among 75,000 to 94,000 employees in a large company over the years 1957 to 1983. Nevertheless, mortality and morbidity rates due to lifestyle practices remain very high. Our efforts in research, education, and clinical practice must be continued and intensified. Health promotion and preventive behavioral medicine is a practice that works—it must be perpetuated and it must be refined to meet changes in the society which provide its context.

REFERENCES

Anderson, G. D., Blidner, I. N., & McClemont, S. (1984). Determinants of size at birth in a Canadian population. *American Journal of Obstetrics and Gynecology, 150*, 236–244.

Andreoli, K. G., & Guillory, M. M. (1983). Arenas for practicing health promotion. *Family and Community Health, 5*, 28–40.

Armor, D. J., Polich, J. M., & Stambul, H. B. (1976). *Alcoholism and treatment*, Santa Monica, CA: The Rand Corporation.

Aronow, W. S. (1978). Effect of passive smoking on angina pectoris. *New England Journal of Medicine, 299*, 21–24.

Belloc, N. B. (1973). Relationship of health practices and mortality. *Preventive Medicine, 2*, 67–81.

Belloc, N. B., & Breslow, L. (1972). Relation of physical health status and health practices. *Preventive Medicine, 1*, 409–421.

Belloc, N. B., Breslow, L., & Hochstim, J. (1971). Measurement of physical health in a general population survey. *American Journal of Epidemiology, 93*, 328–336.

Bjurstrom, L. A., & Alexion, N. G. (1978). A program of heart disease prevention for public employees. *Journal of Occupational Medicine, 20*, 521–531.

Bland, J. S. (1982). The improvement of health status by risk factor intervention: A tool of preventive medicine. *Journal of Holistic Medicine, 4*, 34–38.

Brady, J. P. (1983). Behavior, the environment, and health of the individual. *Preventive Medicine, 12*, 600–609.

Brandsma, J. M., Maultsby, M. C., & Welsh, R. J. (1980). *The out-patient treatment of alcoholism: A review and comparative study*. Baltimore, MD: University Park Press.

Bray, G. A. (1984). The role of weight control in health promotion and disease prevention in National Cancer Institute. *Smoking, tobacco, and cancer program: Annual report 1983*. Washington, DC: U.S. Department of Health and Human Services.

Caddy, G. R., & Gottheil, E. (1982). The role of programmed access to alcohol in alcoholism research and treatment. In M. Galanter, M.A. Rothschild, & J. Mason (Eds.), *Recent Advances in Alcoholism, I*. New York: Plenum Press.

Califano, J. A. (1979). *Healthy people: The Surgeon General's report on health promotion and disease prevention*. Washington, DC: U.S. Government Printing Office.

Cohen, W. S. (1985). Health promotion in the workplace: A prescription for good health. *American Psychologist, 40*, 213–216.

Comptroller of the United States. (1976). *Effectiveness, benefits, and costs of federal safety standards for protection of passenger car occupants*. Washington, DC: U.S. National Highway Traffic Safety Administration, Department of Transportation.

Correa, P., Pickle, L. W., Fontham, E., Lin, Y., & Haenszel, W. (1983). Passive smoking and lung cancer. *Lancet, 2,* 595–597.

Cox, M., Shephard, R. J., & Corey, P. (1981). Influence of an employee fitness programme upon fitness, productivity, and absenteeism. *Ergonomics, 24,* 795–806.

Davies, D. F. (1975). Progress toward the assessment of health status. *Preventive Medicine, 4,* 282–295.

DeLuca, J. R. (Ed.). (1981). *Fourth special report to the U.S. Congress on alcohol and health.* Rockville, MD: National Institute on Alcohol Abuse and Alcoholism.

Deutscher, S., Rockette, H. E., & Krishnaswami. (1984). Evaluation of habitual excessive alcohol consumption on myocardial infarction risk in coronary disease patients. *American Heart Journal, 108,* 988–995.

Ditman, K. S., Crawford, G. G., Forgy, E. W., Moskowitz, H., & MacAndrew, C. (1967). A controlled experiment on the use of court probation for drunk arrests. *American Journal of Psychiatry, 124,* 160–163.

Dwyer, J. (1984). Impact of maternal nutrition on infant health. *Resident and Staff Physician, 30,* 19–23.

Emrick, C. D. (1975). A review of psychologically-oriented treatment of alcoholism: II. The relative effectiveness of different treatment approaches and the effectiveness of treatment versus no treatment. *Quarterly Journal of Studies on Alcohol, 36,* 88–108.

Folkins, C. H., & Sime, W. E. (1981). Physical fitness training and mental health. *American Psychologist, 36,* 373–389.

Garcia-Palmieri, M. R., Costas, R., Cruz-Vidal, M., Sortie, P. D., & Havlik, R. J. (1982). Increased physical activity: A protective factor against heart attacks in Puerto Rico. *American Journal of Cardiology, 50,* 749–755.

Getchell, B. (1979). *Physical fitness: A way of life.* New York: John Wiley & Sons.

Hammond, E. C., & Garfinkel, L. (1969). Coronary heart disease, stroke, and aortic aneurysms: factors in the etiology. *Archives of Environmental Health, 19,* 167–182.

Haskell, W. L. (1984). Overview: Health benefits of exercise. In J.D. Matarazzo, A.M. Weiss, J.A. Herd, N.E. Miller, & S.M. Weiss (Eds.), *Behavioral health: A handbook of health enhancement and disease prevention* (pp. 409–423). New York: John Wiley & Sons.

Haskell, W. L., & Blair, S. N. (1980). The physical activity component of health promotion in occupational settings. *Public Health Reports, 95,* 109–118.

Haynes, S. G., Levine, S., Scotch, N., Feinleib, M., & Kannell, W. B. (1978). The relationship of psychosocial factors to coronary heart disease in the Framingham study. I. Methods and risk factors. *American Journal of Epidemiology, 107,* 362–383.

Jackson, R. T., Beaglehole, R., & Sharpe, N. (1983). Sudden death in runners. *New Zealand Medical Journal, 96,* 289–292.

Jacobson, E. (1938). *Progressive relaxation.* Chicago: University of Chicago Press.

Johnson, J. J. (1981). Urban black Americans. In A. Harwood (Ed.), *Ethnicity and medical care*. Cambridge, MA: Harvard University Press.

Jones, J. S., & Smith, D. W. (1973). Recognition of the fetal alcohol syndrome in early infancy. *Lancet, 2,* 999–1001.

Kamarck, T. W., & Lichtenstein, E. (1985). Current trends in clinic-based smoking control. *Annals of Behavioral Medicine, 7,* 19–23.

Kannel, W. B., & Lerner, D. J. (1984). Present status of risk factors for atherosclerosis. *Medical Times, 112,* 33–45.

Kannel, W. B., & Sorlie, P. (1979). Some health benefits of physical activity: The Framingham study. *Archives of Internal Medicine, 139,* 857–861.

Lichtenstein, E., & Brown, R. A. (1982). Current trends in the modification of cigarette dependence. In A.S. Bellack, M. Hersen, & A.E. Kazdin (Eds.), *International handbook of behavior modification and therapy*. New York: Plenum Press.

Malone, T. B., Kirkpatrick, M., Kohl, J. S., & Baker, C. (1978). *Field test evaluation of rear lighting systems*. Springfield, VA: National Technical Information Service.

Martin, J. E., Dubbert, P. M., Katell, A. D., Thompson, J. K., Raczynski, J. R., Lake, M., Smith, P. O., & Webster, J. S. (1984). Behavioral control of exercise in sedentary adults: Studies 1 through 6. *Journal of Consulting and Clinical Psychology, 52,* 795–811.

Massey, J. D., Moore, G. F., & Yonkers, A. J. (1984). Smokeless tobacco: A risk factor in oral cancer. *Ear, Nose, and Throat Journal, 63,* 453–458.

McGinnis, J. M. (1985). Recent history of federal initiatives in prevention policy. *American Psychologist, 40,* 205–212.

Metzner, H. L., Carman, W. J., & House, J. (1983). Health practices, risk factors and chronic disease in Tecumseh. *Preventive Medicine, 12,* 491–507.

Meyer, A. J., Nash, J. D., McAlister, A. L., MacCoby, N., & Farquhar, J. W. (1980). Skills training in a cardiovascular health education campaign. *Journal of Consulting and Clinical Psychology, 48,* 129–142.

Miller, W. R., & Caddy, G. R. (1977). Abstinence and controlled drinking in the treatment of problem drinkers. *Journal of Studies on Alcohol, 38,* 986–1003.

Miller, W. R., & Hester, R. K. (1986). The effectiveness of alcohol treatment: What research reveals. In W.R. Miller & N. Heather (Eds.), *Treating addictive behaviors: Processes of change* (pp. 121–174). New York: Plenum.

Mills, J. L., Braubard, B. I., Harley, E. E., Rhodes, G. G., & Berendes, H. W. (1984). Maternal alcohol consumption and birth weight: How much drinking during pregnancy is safe? *Journal of the American Medical Association, 252,* 1875–1879.

Morris, J. N., Everitt, M. G., Pollard, R., & Chave, S. P. W. (1980). Vigorous exercise in leisure-time: Protection against coronary heart disease. *Lancet,* pp. 1207–1210.

National Cancer Institute. (1984). *Smoking, tobacco, and cancer program: Annual report 1983*. Washington, DC.

National Cancer Institute. (1985). *Cancer rates and risks* (NIH Publication No. 85-69). Washington, DC: Department of Health and Human Services.

Ockene, J. K., & Camic, P. M. (1985). Public health approaches to cigarette cessation. *Annals of Behavioral Medicine, 7,* 14–18.

Paffenbarger, R. S., & Hale, W. E. (1975). Work activity and coronary heart mortality. *New England Journal of Medicine, 292,* 545–550.

Paffenbarger, R. S., Wing, A. L., & Hyde, R. T. (1978). Physical activity as an index of heart attack risk in college alumni. *American Journal of Epidemiology, 108,* 161–175.

Pauly, J. T., Palmer, J. A., Wright, C. C., & Pfeiffer, G. J. (1982). The effect of a 14-week employee fitness program on selected physiological and psychological parameters. *Journal of Occupational Medicine, 24,* 457–463.

Pell, S., & Fayerweather, W. E. (1985). Trends in the incidence of myocardial infarction and in associated mortality and morbidity in a large employed population, 1957-1983. *New England Journal of Medicine, 312,* 1005–1011.

Pelletier, K. R. (1977). *Mind as healer, mind as slayer: A holistic approach to preventing stress disorders.* New York: Dell.

Public Health Service. (1985). *Health United States: 1985.* Hyattsville, MD: Department of Health and Human Services.

Rausch, A., Wong, J., & Kirkpatrick, M. (1982). A field test of two single center, high mounted brake light systems. *Accident Analysis and Prevention, 14,* 39–45.

Ray, O. S. (1983). *Drugs, society, and human behavior.* St. Louis, MO: C.V. Mosby.

Reilly, R. E., Kurke, D. S., & Buckenmaier, C. C. (1980). *Validation of the reduction of rear-end collisions by a high-mounted auxiliary stop lamp.* Springfield, VA: National Technical Information System.

Rigotti, N. A., Thomas, G. S., & Leaf, A. (1983). Exercise and coronary heart disease. *Annual Review of Medicine, 34,* 391–412.

Robertson, L. S. (1977). State and federal new-car safety regulations: Effects on fatality rates. *Accident Analysis and Prevention, 9,* 151–156.

Robertson, L. S. (1981). Automobile safety regulations and death reductions in the United States. *American Journal of Public Health, 8,* 818–822.

Sackett, D. L., & Haynes, R. B. (1976). *Compliance with therapeutic regimens.* Baltimore: Johns Hopkins University Press.

Said, G., Patois, E., & Lellouch, J. (1984). Infantile colic and parental smoking. *British Medical Journal, 289,* 660.

Saunders, W. B. (Ed.). (1974). *Dorland's illustrated medical dictionary.* Philadelphia: W.B. Saunders Company.

Sausa, D. G. F., & Azevedo, E. S. (1984). Multivariate study of birthweight and maternal heterozygosity for sickle cells anemia in Bahia Brazil. *Human Heredity, 34,* 40–45.

Schultz, J., & Luthe, W. (1959). *Autogenic training: A psychophysiologic approach in psychotherapy.* New York: Grune & Stratton.

Sintonen, H. (1981). An approach to measuring and valuing health states. *Social Science and Medicine, 15,* 55–65.

Siscovick, D. S., & Weiss, N. S. (1984). The incidence of primary cardiac arrest during vigorous exercise. *The New England Journal of Medicine, 311,* 874–877.

Siscovick, D. S., Weiss, N. S., Hallstrom, A. P., Inui, T. S., & Peterson, D. R. (1982). Physical activity and primary cardiac arrest. *Journal of the American Medical Association, 248,* 3113–3117.

Sobell, M. B., & Sobell, L. C. (1975). The need for realism, relevance, and operational assumptions in the study of substance dependence. In H.D. Cappell & A. E. LeBlanc (Eds.), *Biological and behavioral approaches to drug dependence.* Ontario, Canada: Addiction Research Foundation.

Spirduso, W. W. (1983). Exercise and the aging brain. *Research Quarterly for Exercise and Sport, 54,* 208–218.

Stamler, J. (1985). Coronary heart disease: Doing the "right things." *The New England Journal of Medicine, 312,* 1053–1055.

Stuart, R. B., & Davis, B. (1972). *Slim chance in a fat world.* Illinois: Research.

Tager, I. B., Weiss, S. T., Rosner, B., & Speizer, F. E. (1979). Effect of parental cigarette smoking on the pulmonary function of children. *American Journal of Epidemiology, 110,* 15–26.

Tapp, J. T., & Goldenthal, P. A. (1982). A factor analytic study of health habits. *Preventive Medicine, 11,* 724–728.

Thompson, P. D. (1982). Cardiovascular hazards of physical activity. *Exercise Sports Science Review, 10,* 208–235.

Thompson, P. D., Funk, E. J., Carleton, R. A., & Sturner, W. Q. (1982). Incidence of death during jogging in Rhode Island from 1975 through 1980. *Journal of the American Medical Association, 247,* 2535–2538.

Trichopoulos, D., Kalandidi, A., Sparros, L., & MacMahon, B. (1981). Lung cancer and passive smoking. *International Journal of Cancer, 27,* 1–4.

United Nations. (1986). *Demographic yearbook 1984.* New York: Department of International Economics and Social Affairs.

United States Bureau of the Census. (1985). *Statistical abstract of the United States: 1985.* Washington, DC: United States Department of Commerce.

United States Department of Agriculture. (1980). *Nutrition and your health—Dietary Guidelines for Americans* (Home and Garden Bulletin No. 232). Washington, DC: United States Government Printing Office.

United States Public Health Service. (1964). *Smoking and health* (PHS Pub. No. 1103). Washington, DC: United States Government Printing Office.

Victor, M., Adams, R. O., & Collins, G. H. (1971). *The Wernicke-Korsakoff Syndrome.* Philadelphia: F.A. Davis.

Waller, B. F., & Roberts, W. C. (1980). Sudden death while running in conditioned runners aged 40 years or over. *American Journal of Cardiology, 45,* 1292–1300.

Weiss, S. H., Goedert, J. J., Sarngadharan, M. G., Bodner, A. J., The Aids Seroepidemiology Collaborative Working Group, Gallo, R. C., & Blattner, W. A. (1985). Screening test for HTLV-III (AIDS Agent) Antibodies. *The Journal of the American Medical Association, 253,* 221–125.

White, J. R., & Froeb, H. F. (1980). Small-airway dysfunction in nonsmokers chronically exposed to tobacco smoke. *New England Journal of Medicine, 302,* 720–723.

Williams, A. F. (1982). Passive and active measures for controlling disease and injury: The role of health psychologists. *Health Psychology, 1,* 399–409.

Williams, C. L., Arnold, C. B., & Wynder, E. L. (1977). Primary prevention of chronic disease beginning in childhood. *Preventive Medicine, 6,* 344–357.

Wilson, G. T., & Brownell, K. D. (1980). Behavior therapy for obesity: An evaluation of treatment outcome. *Advances in Behavior Research and Therapy, 3,* 49–86.

Wilson, J. (1981). The fetal alcohol syndrome. *Public Health, London, 85,* 129–132.

Wingard, D. L., Berkman, L. F., & Brand, R. J. (1982). A multivariate analysis of health related practices. A nine-year mortality follow-up of the Alameda County study. *American Journal of Epidemiology, 116,* 765–775.

2

Program Development Research For Public Health: The Example of Smoking*

J. Allan Best

Department of Health Studies
and
Director, Waterloo Smoking Projects
University of Waterloo, Ontario

Edward A. Smith

Department of Public Health,
University of North Carolina at Greensboro

Deborah J. Ossip-Klein

Department of Psychology
and Director, Smoking Research Program
The University of Rochester

* Preparation of this chapter was facilitated by a Canadian National Health Research and Development Program scholar award to Dr. Best, and a grant from the Ontario Ministry of Health (#01422). The authors wish to thank Russell Glasgow for helpful comments on previous drafts.

INTRODUCTION

The past 20 years have witnessed a remarkable shift in public health priorities and perspectives on primary prevention. Marc Lalonde's (1974) *A New Perspective on the Health of Canadians* proved a landmark document in a growing awareness of health policy makers and researchers that "diseases of lifestyle" are the predominant causes of morbidity and mortality in contemporary society. The historical antecedents and cross-cultural uniformity of this phenomenon have been well documented in Omran's "epidemiological transition" (1971) and supported by a wide range of other epidemiological data (cf. Belloc, 1973; Breslow & Enstrom, 1980; Califano, 1979; Matarazzo, 1984). In the wake of this evidence, there has been increased attention to the identification of behavioral risk factors and the development of guidelines for interventions. Biopsychosocial models of health behavior have matured rapidly, and applications of behavioral science principles and findings to health promotion/disease prevention look promising in many areas (see Hamburg, Elliott, & Parron, 1982; Matarazzo, Weiss, Herd, Miller, & Weiss, 1984; Weiner, 1981, for reviews). In this process, specific national objectives for health behavior change have been agreed upon (Richmond, 1980).

Amidst all of this concern, research, and policy development, however, there is an accompanying lag in the widespread efficacious diffusion of these behavioral principles. Certainly, there is a growing will on the part of health policy makers to act, as we face escalating health care costs and a health care delivery system ill-suited to "diseases of lifestyle" (Weiss, 1984). However, while convergence of interests is clear, and vigorous collaboration among the various health disciplines and professions is exciting, true integration of theory, research, and practice lags behind. Health promotion represents a "second revolution in public health" (Michael, 1982). The U.S. Institute of Medicine calls for a marriage between relevant science and health systems:

> In the foreseeable future, it should be possible to construct a reasonably unified biobehavioral science pertinent to health and disease, with major applications in all the health professions and by the public at large. (Hamburg, Elliot, & Parron, 1982, p. 320)

It is the process of moving forward—from the great *promises* of behavioral science principles to their *application* in diverse settings—which is the challenge of behavioral health science researchers.

To understand this challenge, it may be helpful to consider a very pragmatic scenario. Imagine yourself moving to a new job as medical officer of health for a city, or director of health promotion for the state health department. Suppose you have been given a clear mandate to be concerned with, and take responsibility for, the health and risk status of a defined population. Your job is to develop, implement, and manage a comprehensive network of services, programs, and policies which address priority needs. You recognize that a large potential influence on the health of your population may be achieved through lifestyle changes. What would you do? Are there well developed, robust strategies for defining the health promotion needs of a population? Do effective intervention programs exist, and are they in a form ready to be implemented? Is it the "art" or the "science" of disease prevention you have been asked to apply?

It is these sets of questions which the health scientist must keep in focus as she conducts research. The bridge linking biobehavioral science to health practice we might term a science of intervention research, or program development research. This fledgling discipline or methodology is the prime concern of this chapter. The chapter represents a beginning to develop a conceptual framework for integration. It is intended to have heuristic value—to stimulate thought and activity of prevention research producers and consumers.

The framework proposed here will rely on the basic model used by the U.S. National Cancer Institute to guide its research. This model depicts an organized progression from basic intervention research to widespread application of effective programs (Greenwald & Cullen, 1984). While subphases of the model have been elaborated on by Flay (1986), the five basic phases are: (a) hypothesis development, (b) method development, (c) controlled intervention trials, (d) defined population studies, and (e) demonstration and dissemination. The implications raised by this framework (as we interpret and apply it), as well as important issues to be considered in planning research programs within this progressive format, are discussed following a presentation of the framework.

Examples from literature on cigarette smoking prevention and cessation interventions are chosen to permit development of ideas and issues in some depth. Specifically, three areas relative to behavioral interventions in smoking research are investigated: self-help, physician intervention, and worksite promotion. The framework, however, is generalizable and should be useful to other areas involving potential social intervention mechanisms in prevention, early detection, and behavior change.

PHASE 1: HYPOTHESIS DEVELOPMENT

Hypothesis Development research addresses the question "What is the problem?" The goal of this first phase is to identify factors which may need to be considered when designing interventions. Determinants of health behavior are studied and epidemiological parameters of the problem are specified. Both theoretical models and empirical findings may be used to develop hypotheses to be tested in subsequent research.

For cigarette smoking, the health "problem" is well defined. Numerous studies have documented direct linkages between cigarette smoking and lung cancer, pulmonary disease, myocardial infarctions, fetal morbidity, and other health problems. However, given the complex relationship between the behavioral aspects of smoking, the individual's physiological status, and the biological dependence produced by nicotine, many questions remain (Best, Wainwright, Mills, & Kirkland, 1988).

The workplace, as a potential intervention channel, has generated many hypotheses regarding the development of efficient smoking cessation programs. Attempts to reduce smoking through interventions in the workplace, with or without the aid of a physician, and/or through the use of self-help materials, have tried to capitalize on both existing knowledge and the potential for change with this channel. Some of the hypothesized advantages of the worksite, for example, include long-term access of programs and the existence of captive populations. In addition, prevalence data suggest that employers can normally anticipate that approximately one third of employees are smokers. Of these, a substantial proportion are probably interested in quitting (Fielding, 1984). While worker acceptance of and participation in group programs is variable, with some surveys suggesting low demand (United States Department of Health and Human Services, 1983; Schneider, Benya, & Singer, 1984) and some surveys documenting low participation rates (Glasgow & Klesges, 1985), many researchers continue to find high levels of apparent interest in group programs.

The development of self-help mechanisms has also been guided by some basic hypotheses and knowledge regarding the cessation process. For example, cross-sectional studies have shown that up to 95 percent of ex-smokers have quit on their own (United States Department of Health, Education, and Welfare (USDHEW), 1979); approximately 60 percent of smokers have at least a desire to quit (National Center for Health Statistics (NCHS), 1982). In addition, most ex-smokers have not participated in formal smoking programs (Fisher, 1982; Lichtenstein, 1982). This had led many researchers to hypothesize that study of the "natural process" of smoking cessation would be productive in understanding both the motivational aspects of quitting and the techniques and rewards used by these ex-smokers (e.g., Perry & Richards, 1977; Perry, Richards, & Schulthies, 1977). By studying this natural process, conceptual models of smoking cessation have been aided in their development (Prochaska & DiClemente, 1983; Schlegel, d'Avernas, & Best, 1982). Prochaska, for example, suggests a five-stage process: (a) immotives, (b) contemplators, (c) recent quitters, (d) long-term quitters, and (e) relapsers.

The potential effects of physician intervention in altering smoking behavior are also based on Phase I information. As one example, a review of the biological, psychological, and social determinants of smoking highlights the barriers to change resulting from nicotine dependency (Best et al., 1988), and suggests promise for intervention incorporating physician prescription of nicotine replacements (Hughes & Miller, 1984). As a second example, surveys indicate that up to 70 percent of North Americans see a physician at least once a year (Kohn & White, 1976; National Center for Health Services Research (NCHSR), 1983; NCHS, 1982). These data suggest that even a nominal quit rate associated with physician intervention would have a tremendous population impact. The potential magnitude of this channel on smoking cessation, combined with the respected role of physicians, has generated many intervention models. Of special note are those studies dealing with high-risk target groups (e.g., survivors of myocardial infarction, pregnant women, and individuals with pulmonary disease) for whom the potential health impact of cessation is great.

Phase I research includes the development of basic principles determining health behavior and behavior change. These principles may include, for example, the (a) role of stimulus control and habit in determining chronic cigarette smoking, (b) interplay of biological and behavioral factors in a model of addiction, (c) mechanisms and processes of social support in facilitating behavior, or (d) stress factors in smoking relapse.

PHASE II: METHOD DEVELOPMENT

Phase II research is concerned with the development of potentially effective intervention and research methods. This *Method Development* phase involves pilot work to develop behavior change techniques, research protocols, and validation of measurement tools. Phase II research may employ uncontrolled evaluations of intervention techniques. On the other hand, Phase II could include highly controlled (but small and still preliminary) experiments to compare alternative intervention methods to appropriate control groups, and to assess the relative contribution of intervention components to outcomes. Correlational techniques may be used to study individual differences or environmental factors which either predict treatment impact or interact with intervention methods. The use of formative evaluations is appropriate at this stage, in helping to understand the perspective of both the program providers and the recipients. In sum, Phase II research involves the pilot development of intervention and research methods.

The majority of research in the three illustrative areas of smoking cessation is concentrated in this Method Development phase. Worksite intervention researchers have incorporated social support, physician involvement, and self-help mechanisms into their designs. Some of these designs involve controls, but many involve only the treatment group with either posttest only or a pre- and posttest design. Unfortunately there remains a lack of uniformity in reporting procedures (both regarding sampling and analysis) and an inconsistent use of biological measures (e.g., cotinine or CO) for verification of behavioral responses (Glasgow & Klesges, 1985).

These problems also exist in much of the physician intervention research (USDHHS, 1984) and in research involving self-help mechanisms (Glasgow & Klesges, 1985). There has been, however, some promising research using these three channels which are exemplary of Phase II method development research.

While the majority of smoking cessation studies at the worksite involve small samples, they do provide the required basis for further exploration. The use of monetary incentives, for example, appears to increase abstinence rates, in the short term at least (Sorman, 1979; Stitzer & Bigelow, 1982, 1983; Rand, Stitzer, Bigelow, & Mead, 1984; Stachnik & Stoffelmayr, 1983). Questions remain, however, as to the specific role attributable to incentives, as distinct from other program elements. In addition, the size of the award, its schedule, and nonmonetary alternatives (e.g., lottery tickets, tee-shirts, time off) have not been weighed. There remains the lingering question of what happens when the rewards are terminated; research in other areas suggests that this may lead to relapses.

Competition between worksites also appears promising (Klesges & Glasgow, 1986). Borrowing the concept from weight reduction programs, competition across worksites has a potential side benefit of developing a sense of group support and of making the quit attempt more fun. Management reactions which may interfere with or counteract such programs have not been researched but can be hypothesized and may include, for example, negative reactions toward individuals who don't contribute to the "team" effort. Other factors that need to be considered include the effect of competition on internal productivity (i.e., intercompany competition may or may not be preferable to intracompany competition) and the effect of employee loyalty to the company (e.g., employees with a sense of commitment may be more amenable to competition and a desire to "win" for the company).

The use of physician consults, either at the worksite or through worksite referral to the doctor's office, has reported successful outcomes. However, the lack of adequate control groups and biochemical validation suggests the need for confirmatory studies (Kornitzer, Dramaix, Kittel, & De Backer, 1980; Rose, Heller, Pedoe, & Christie, 1980; Rose, Hamilton, Colwell, & Shipley, 1982). The effect thus far also appears limited primarily to high-risk individuals (e.g., those at high risk of cardiovascular disease). Many Phase II questions regarding the use of physicians in conjunction with worksite-based programs still remain, however, and need further exploration. For example: What effect would alternative providers have (e.g., Would company nurses be as successful and thus more cost-efficient?)? Would similar effects be achieved without supplemental services (e.g., self-help manuals)?

Phase II research utilizing physician intervention with general patient populations has attempted to develop effective interventions based on protocols that are cost-efficient and pragmatic. The majority of this research has concentrated on the assessment of different techniques of direct physician advice to patients to quit smoking. Most of these studies indicate a reduction in smoking, both in noncontrolled designs (Handel, 1973; Pincherle & Wright, 1970; Rosser, 1979) and relative to control groups (cf. Mausner, Mausner, & Rial, 1968; Page, Walters, Schlegel, & Best, 1986). In addition, research by Wilson and his colleagues (Wilson, Wood, Johnston, & Sicurella, 1982) suggests that physician follow-up in the months following the quit attempt may be important in maintaining cessation. A review of physician intervention research can be found in a 1984 U.S. Surgeon General Report (USDHHS, 1984).

Nicotine gum, a fairly recent addition to the pharmacological armamentarium of physicians has generated a number of Phase II–method development studies. In controlled clinic-support studies, there is evidence that the gum alleviates withdrawal symptoms, and reduces smoking (Fagerstrom, 1982; Jarvis, Raw, Russell, & Feyerabend, 1982; Schneider et al., 1983; Killen, Maccoby & Taylor, 1984). Results in physician office studies are mixed (cf. Page et al., 1986; Russell, Merriman, & Edwards, 1983), but use of the gum as an adjunct continues to be seen as promising (Hughes & Miller, 1984). Intriguing results from the University of Waterloo (Schlegel, Manske, & Shannon, 1985) suggest an interaction effect: Gum may improve outcomes in relatively low-intensity interventions but actually interfere with more intensive treatments.

The special problems presented by high-risk populations who smoke have served as a natural catalyst for many physician-based intervention research programs at both this level and Phase III. For example, method development research has concentrated on the use of physicians to inform pregnant women of the known deleterious effects of smoking during pregnancy. This information, which links smoking to decreased birth weight, increased mortality, developmental retardation, hyperkinesis, and the inhibition of lactation (Landesmann, Dwyer, & Emmuel, 1979; USPHS, 1973; Denson, Nanson, & McWatters, 1975) has been passed on by doctors to pregnant women in the form of direct advice, leaflets, and posters (Baric, MacArthur, & Sherwood, 1976; Dalton, Hughes, & Cogswell, 1981). Results indicate greater reductions in cigarette smoking among those exposed, especially if the women were reached in their first trimester (Hughes, Epstein, Andrasik, et al., 1982). Research by Bauman, Ryan, Dent, and Koch (1983) added individualized feedback by having the women in the experimental group observe their CO levels while in a group setting. The addition of this condition, however, did not lead to increased cessation.

A number of studies of smoking cessation with high-risk populations have been conducted involving patients with pulmonary disease and cardiac disease (USDHHS, 1984). The majority involve prospective longitudinal data with intervention including: increased advice (Burt et al., 1974); behavior modification (Meyer & Henderson, 1974); and exercise (Sivarajan, Newton, Almes, et al., 1983). The use of controls has not been consistent in these studies, but the majority do report a higher cessation rate than found in the general patient population, and an overall direct relationship between severity of illness and cessation.

In the area of self-help techniques there has been an abundance of intervention techniques developed, but few have received the systematic attention required to get them beyond the Phase II method development stage. Self-help approaches have generally involved use of manuals with varying degrees of therapist contact. Overall success rates for "pure" self-help approaches (i.e., no personal contact beyond follow-up) are lower than for clinics with results varying across type of manual used. Generally, as level of therapist contact increases, abstinence rates increase as well, approaching clinic levels. However, as contact increases, the "self-help" nature of the intervention is questioned. (See Windsor & Bartlett, 1984, for a review of self-help programs for employees.)

The use of mailing self-help manuals (or chapters) to participants as another intervention method is encouraging (Brengelmann, 1978; Brengelmann & Sedlmayer, 1977). Research by Jeffrey and colleagues (Jeffrey, Danaher, Killen, Farquhar, & Kinnier, 1982), showed that reduction in smoking through this technique alone may be as productive as combining the same manual with other support, including individual consultations.

Smoking "relapse" prevention hotlines have also been used to reach self-quitters and show results similar to those of smoking clinics. Methods development research has identified means of obtaining and sustaining high utilization rates among subpopulations most likely to achieve long-term abstinence (Ossip-Klein, Shapiro, & Stiggins, 1984; Shapiro, Ossip-Klein, & Gerrity, 1985–1986).

Despite some flaws, methods development research in the area of self-help techniques has identified a number of potentially efficacious techniques for smoking reduction. Helpful manuals, for example, the American Lung Association's manual (Davis, Faust, & Ordentlich, 1984), and procedures (e.g., target dates) have been developed and modified. What remains, however, as in the case with much of the research in physician and worksite interventions, is the further organized development and refinement of these procedures in order to maximize their potential. The next step thus involves a transition in the research evolvement—a movement from method development to controlled intervention trials.

Phase II method development for worksite, physician, and self-help can be summarized as follows. Promising methods have been identified, including increased social support, prescription of nicotine-bearing chewing gum, use of incentives and competitions to increase and sustain motivation, and provisions of self-help guides or telephone hotlines to develop skills and to provide support. None of the methods can be seen as fully developed or "proven." Methodological problems remain, efficacy still is modest, and results are inconsistent. The challenge of applying biobehavioral science principles to changing smoking behavior in populations remains a humbling task.

PHASE III: CONTROLLED INTERVENTION TRIALS

In contrast to Phase II research which involves the pilot development of intervention and research methods, Phase III involves *evaluation* of promising interventions, primarily by means of controlled randomized trials. The samples involved need not be representative but the protocols should be carefully monitored and the research designs well conceived. Given that apparently useful intervention methods have been developed in Phase II studies, the question addressed in Phase III research is: Can these methods be efficacious when studied with adequate samples under controlled conditions? (An alternative to randomized trials may be the development of case control studies.)

It must be acknowledged that the boundaries between phases in this model are not always clear (Flay, 1986). One Phase II/III distinction relates to size: Many of the studies assigned to Phase II were methodologically well designed and controlled—they lacked only the large sample size required to ensure enough statistical power to detect intervention effects which might be relatively small in an absolute sense but still potentially very meaningful from a public health perspective.

There has been little Phase III worksite or self-help research. Multiple coronary risk trials have focused on high-risk men and shown modest but significant long-term effects on smoking cessation rates (e.g., Kornitzer, Dramaix, Kittel, & DeBacker, 1980; Rose et al., 1980). However, these results may not generalize to others not at high risk, nor to the circumstance where only a smoking, not a multiple-risk intervention, is applied. The one large self-help study in the literature (Davis et al., 1984) did report again a modest but significant intervention effect at 12 months for the American Lung Association's Freedom From Smoking manuals).

Likewise, Phase III physician intervention trials have largely been confined to high-risk groups. An exception, however, involves a design conceived by Russell and colleagues using a general patient population (Russell, Wilson, Taylor, & Baker, 1979). This study involved 28 physicians in a controlled design focusing on health education (but not involving specific skills for stopping smoking). The group with the maximum intervention had the highest quit rate (19%), while the control had the lowest (10%). An attempt to repeat this basic design, however, showed no difference between groups (Stewart & Rosser, 1982). A later study (Russell et al., 1983), involving a balanced design with 34 physicians (subject $N = 1938$), concluded that while there was no difference between the control group and those receiving physician advice, a pamphlet, and a warning of follow-up, there was a significant smoking reduction among those who got advice, the pamphlet, and nicotine gum.

Studies by Donovan and colleagues (Donovan, 1977; Donovan, Burgess, Hossack, & Yudkin, 1975) and Sexton and Hebel (1984) qualify as Phase III intervention trials oriented toward smoking reduction among pregnant women. Both studies basically confirm the success of intensified levels of information and contact. While Donovan does not report cessation rates, Sexton and Hebel indicate a 43 percent quit rate among those receiving a home visit, telephone, and mail contact, compared to a 20 percent reduction in the control group (confirmed via saliva thiocyanate).

Similar findings regarding intensity of contact and cessation are also suggested by Rose and Hamilton (1978), involving a study of pulmonary patients ($N = 1445$). At all follow-ups, those patients receiving a 15-minute appointment combined with a booklet were more than twice as likely to have stopped smoking than patients who were only using their normal physician.

These Phase III physician counseling and pregnant women trials again illustrate the difficulty in drawing clear distinctions between phases. As large, controlled trials they qualify for Phase III. But the *content* of the interventions did not rest on foundational Phase II methods development research. In general, larger intervention effects should be achievable when an adequate Phase II base is ensured.

PHASE IV: DEFINED POPULATION STUDIES

Phase IV research consists of *Defined Population Studies*. The concern is with (a) *effectiveness* (how well an intervention works under less controlled, more typical "real world" conditions), and (b) *external validity*, in contrast to the Phase III emphasis on efficacy (the impact of an intervention under highly controlled and relatively ideal research conditions) and internal validity. Key issues in the efficacy-effectiveness distinction are further discussed elsewhere (Flay, 1986; Meinhart, 1986; Wortman, 1983). Studies are designed to address the question "Will these methods be effective if disseminated, and what variables affect their effectiveness?"

Studies at this level thus require data collection at two levels: individual and organizational. It is not enough to know whether or not a mechanism works for individuals; we also need to understand any organizational or systems barriers that might impede the diffusion process. The populations being studied at this level (both individual and organizational) need to be representative of the target populations. To illustrate, a Phase III worksite smoking cessation clinic study would focus on abstinence among those who attend the clinic; Phase IV asks if abstinence among *all* company smokers increases as the result of the clinic. Similarly, the appropriate denominator for physician studies are all eligible smokers in the practice; for the American Lung Association self-help manuals mentioned earlier, all adult smokers in a community.

Few instances of Phase IV cessation studies exist. There are, however, some studies which yield insight into the direction such studies may take.

For example, preliminary data from worksite interventions suggest an inverse relationship between company size and both program efficiency and dissemination (Glasgow & Klesges, 1985). These tentative findings suggest a need for verification at multiple sites with company size and structure as variables of concern. This also suggests, however, a potential need for new Phase II type projects in which interventions are tried at a level which is less than company-wide (e.g., departments).

Given that some pilot (Phase II) studies suggest worksite-connected physician interventions achieve success, Phase IV studies might address questions on physician compliance. Li et al. (1984), for example, found few physicians were actually performing the prescribed regimen; other data, however, suggest higher compliance by physicians may be achieved through regular performance feedback (Ewart, Li, & Coates, 1983).

Also required at this level are studies which address the role of management and labor organizations in program acceptance and efficacy. The development of management support and the formation of committees with representation from groups with vested interest have been advocated as two mechanisms to improve program success (Klesges & Glasgow, 1986; Grove, Reed, & Miller, 1979; Bishop & Fisher, 1984; Stachnik & Stoffelmayr, 1983).

Because of their emphasis on diffusion variables, some research involving physicians may be considered as borderline—Phase IV research. These studies suggest disagreement between physicians' reports of advice to patients to quit smoking and the patients' reports of receiving this advice. Surveys of smoking patients indicate 22 percent (Stewart, Brook, & Kane, 1979) to 40 percent received advice from their physicians to quit smoking; over 85 percent of physicians indicate giving advice (Green & Horn, 1968; American Cancer Society, 1981; Battista, 1983). This pattern is also evident among pregnant patients (Danaher & Lichtenstein, 1978; Harris, 1979). These and other studies suggest that physician motivation and effort (Ewart et al., 1983) in addition to a physician's own smoking status (Danaher & Lichtenstein, 1978) may affect the dissemination process.

It should be pointed out that data at both the individual and organizational level may be addressed within a single study design. The trick is to organize the data collection process and measures to ensure that the needed information at these different levels is amassed. Two specific comments are germaine. First, during Phase IV, the worksite, practice, or community typically are (or should be) the unit of randomization, integration, and analysis; there remain, however, methodological problems which need to be worked out with these units of analysis (cf. Brown & Peterson, 1989). Second, within these large, controlled designs, there typically are opportunities to "piggyback" more basic research. For example, our recent Waterloo-McMaster Family Practice Smoking Cessation Project (Wilson, Taylor, Gilbert, Best, Lindsay, Willms, & Singer, 1988) is a Phase III/IV randomized controlled trial of the efficacy of physician training in smoking cessation counseling on a representative sample of patients. We have "piggybacked" a Phase I side study to work with a small separate group of patients to characterize in great detail the smoking cessation process with or without the prescription of nicotine-bearing chewing gum. These Phase I descriptive data will generate hypotheses about supplemental interventions which might be developed to complement physician counseling.

In sum, note that program *content* (e.g., prescription of Nicorette, use of incentives) and *participant characteristics* (e.g., level of social support, health status) are factors which tend to be investigated at Phases II and III. In contrast, *program setting* (e.g., worksite size) and *provider factors* (e.g., level of implementation or regiment compliance) tend to be studied at the Phase IV stage.

PHASE V: DEMONSTRATION AND DISSEMINATION

Phase V involves demonstration programs in the target populations. These address the question: "Are the intervention methods developed (from Phases III and IV) *in fact* effective when implemented as ongoing services in the community?" Evaluative research components must be incorporated in the demonstration project and procedures should ensure that the intervention follows the methodology previously validated. The ultimate goal of Phase V is the demonstration and further diffusion of the intervention mechanism; the impact of the intervention on a defined population's smoking status, morbidity, or mortality needs to be monitored. In the area of smoking cessation research, for example, the incidence of smoking-related diseases should be monitored in the target populations. Other measures, reflective of shorter term effects (e.g., lung expiration, days missed at work) should also be collected.

The five phases, possible conceptual models, and methodologies, are shown in Table 2.1. The entries to the table are illustrative only; the lists could be expanded and refined. Specific models and methodologies

Table 2.1.
Research Methodologies in Program Development Research

	Appropriate Conceptual Models	Typical Methodologies
I Hypothesis Generation	• Systems theory • Multiple determinant models	• Epidemiological surveys • Ethnographic interviews • Case histories
II Methods Development	• Causal modeling • Interactional models of behavior change • Determinants of behavior and change	• Tight experiments • Formative/process evaluation • Needs assessment/market research • Factor analysis
III Controlled Intervention Research	• Multifactorial influences on behavior, and behavior change	• Large randomized trials or cohort studies • Summative/efficacy impact evaluation • Economic analysis
IV Defined Population Studies	• Population health • Dissemination/diffusion/social marketing • Community organization	• Community trials • True and quasi experiments • Effectiveness/outcome evaluation
V Demonstration and Dissemination	• Health planning • Sociopolitical approaches to health policy	• Program evaluation

will vary with existing knowledge and data, the nature of the research question(s), the target behavior and population, research design, and the intended purpose or consumer of the research.

In conclusion, and to anticipate the following discussion of issues, let us sketch one example of a good Phase II and III research *without* Phase IV and V follow-up. As noted, the use of nicotine-bearing chewing gum as an adjunct in smoking cessation was reasonably established by the use of double-blinded placebo-controlled Phase II studies (Brantmark, Ohlin, & Westling, 1973; Russell, Wilson, Feyerabend, & Cole, 1976; Jarvis, Raw, Russell, & Feyerabend, 1982; Russell, Raw, & Jarvis, 1980), although its effects may be short-term only (Fagerstrom, 1982; Page, Walters, Schlegel, & Best, 1986; Schneider et al., 1983), and there have been negative reports (e.g., Malcolm, Sillet, Turner, & Ball, 1980; Puska, Bjorqvist, & Koskela, 1979). At the Phase III stage, Russell and his colleagues (1983) demonstrated a significant effect when the gum was added to physician advice; however, a warning signal sounded in that 50 percent of the patients did not even accept the offer of free gum. In a subsequent study in which patients had to pay for the gum, fully 70 percent did not have the prescription filled (Page et al., 1986). It seems clear that problems were to be expected at the diffusion stage. But no Phase IV or V research ensued! The product has been distributed internationally to the general public, without ensurance that physicians give clear instructions for its use, and without any monitoring of its effectiveness and follow-up. Note that the concern is not with the intervention per se—nicotine-bearing chewing gum seems to be efficacious. The concern is that provider and setting factors have not been assessed, and that the transition from efficacy to effectiveness occurred without adequate evaluation, perhaps in large part because researchers tend not to consider Phase IV and V as our responsibility.

IMPLICATIONS OF THE FRAMEWORK

The application of this framework to intervention research generates a number of issues which need to be addressed. We have organized these items around five specific areas.

Distinctions Between Phases

First, it should be recognized that the phases do not necessarily proceed in a tightly organized, linear fashion, and it often is difficult to clearly separate phases. There is reciprocity between the levels; for example, during Phase IV the complexity of the "real world" is such that unexpected influences on program effectiveness often will be identified, and researchers then may initiate a series of Phase II studies to better understand how these influences operate, and how they might be harnessed: A cyclic or "looping" perspective on the framework is needed. If, for example, it is found that physician intervention at the worksite has differential effects depending on client and/or physician characteristics (e.g., blue collar vs. white collar; male vs. female), more targeted pilot studies may be needed to understand these processes and potentially modify the intervention methods to accommodate these differences.

Needs for Integration

Diverse methodologies and disciplinary perspectives need to be integrated. A lot of synthesis already is occurring. For example, the synergism of the biological and behavioral sciences is a thread running through this entire volume. The methodologies of psychology and epidemiology are beginning to come together in behavioral epidemiology (Kaplan & Criqui, 1985). Matarazzo (1984) discusses the needs for disciplinary cooperation in a "science of behavioral health" between behavioral scientists. Especially as research moves into Phases IV and V, other perspectives may become important: community organization, demography, health planning, communications, political science, health policy, and so forth.

A second type of integration is the need to bridge scientific and practitioner perspectives. Effective consultation and collaboration between research providers (the scientists) and research consumers (those responsible for delivering services) should be required *throughout* the program development and implementation process. The key is to find ways in which the two groups can work together effectively and avoid adversarial positions. In fact, each can meaningfully contribute to the others' objectives. For example, researchers set specific goals which can potentiate the change practitioners want to produce. Conversely, research consumers have much to contribute with respect to the development of guidelines and standards for practical, attractive, and cost-effective methods.

An example of collaboration between research producers and consumers is the Freedom Line project, a smoking relapse prevention hotline, directed jointly by the University of Rochester Smoking Research Program and the American Lung Association-Finger Lakes Region, Inc. Interventions are provided to callers; initial interviews and follow-up information are collected systematically and used for ongoing research trials (Ossip-Klein et al., 1986).

To further illustrate, the opportunities and constraints presented by the worksite need to be understood from the manager's perspective. Likewise, if an intervention is to utilize a physician's office we must understand how that intervention would affect all roles in that structure—not just that of the physician. This process can result in a more effective and smooth intervention, thus aiding the consumer, and a more refined conceptual and theoretical base from which the researcher can identify important therapeutic processes and mediating variables (Glasgow & Klesges, 1985).

The Role of Substantive Models

Complementary substantive models must be selected to guide development of interventions and measures. The smoking cessation literature suggests, for example, that not only do people want to quit smoking, but also that many have tried (NCHS, 1982). Studies of self-quitters and those who have gone through organized programs, however, indicate a sequential series of readiness to quit; not all of those who want to quit are ready for the same intervention approach (cf. DiClemente & Prochaska, 1985). What is required then is the integration of needs assessment models (e.g., Who? How Many? Where?); intervention models (e.g., What will work with these people in this setting with this level of motivation?), and organizational models (What resources are available and how can they best be mobilized to provide the intervention?). Taken together, these complementary perspectives suggest a "network" of important considerations in comprehensive intervention development and delivery.

A key theoretical base that we have found productive in helping to tie together the strategies used in various intervention channels (e.g., worksite, primary care, schools, media, and community), is social learning theory, as developed by Bandura (1977, 1986). This theory, which identifies key determinants of behaviors and critical processes in behavior change, is appealing because it is comprehensive and empirically based. The theory emphasizes the importance of activities such as goal setting, performance feedback, and exposure to appropriate models in the change process. Bandura's theory provides the major conceptual framework for interventions used in a number of other major community intervention projects, including those conducted by the Stanford Heart Disease Prevention Program (Farquhar et al., 1984) and the Pawtucket Heart Health Project (Abrams et al., 1985; Lasater et al., 1984).

Taking Stock

As a means to promote the progression across phases, the field of health program development research needs to take stock on a regular basis. Questions need to be raised such as: Where do we stand with respect to the intervention research framework? What do we know about what works and what doesn't? Is it time yet to move to the next research phase? Various smoking prevention and cessation interventions, for example, are anywhere from Phase II to Phase IV in their current development; worksite cessation programs probably are mid-Phase II while certain aspects of physician intervention trials are Phase III, bordering on Phase IV. Self-help programs are Phase II, even though a multitude of such programs exist; apparently there is need to organize research in this area in order to mobilize a push toward Phase III-type research.

The question remains as to how researchers should assess the stage of development of their knowledge. Thorough literature reviews certainly are helpful, but other mechanisms such as consensus conferences and meta-analysis (Louis, Fineberg, & Mosteller, 1985) probably are needed to crystallize current status and catalyze a systematic approach to program development research.

We also need to think seriously about what we mean by a "science" of program development, and the diversity of paradigms that may be relevant to intervention research. Packer (1985) recently provided an overview of major paradigms, which has been useful in some of our smoking cessation process research. Thoreson (1984) has offered a thoughtful and eloquent discussion of the need to match scientific methods with the phenomena of concern and the conceptual models guiding the research. Both our theories and our methods must be sufficiently comprehensive to capture the full range of influences on health behavior and change. The concern is that developing models will be inadequately studied because popular scientific methods do not lend themselves well to complex health behavior program development and diffusion issues.

There also is a need to recognize different kinds of outcomes. Intervention researchers need to ask themselves "Are we engaged in research and development primarily to contribute to a scientific body of knowledge and understanding, or are our research studies intended primarily to promote social change?" Research certainly can serve both masters, but in practice it is very difficult indeed to achieve a good balance between these quite different outcomes. Similarly, we need to balance effectiveness and application. For example, while from a scientific perspective self-help manuals may not achieve impressive, nor consistent, effects (e.g., Davis et al., 1984; Owen & Ewins, 1982; Schlegel, Manske, & Shannon, 1985), the practical benefits of their low cost and high acceptability to a large population may far outweigh scientific concerns. Essentially, this is a question of cost-effectiveness: What is the "bang for the buck"? Given limited resources, should our concern be a specific program's effectiveness (i.e., the *percentage* of smokers who quit) or should it be the total *number* of people who quit smoking?

There is a conundrum for the scientist in that our understanding of the determinants of health behavior and change still is far from complete, and there is a sense that if we understood the problems better, we could develop more effective interventions. However, this must be balanced against pressing population health needs for effective services; the reality currently is that while our programs are less than perfect, in many arenas they can have a population impact if carefully disseminated. On a day-to-day basis, the problem is that researchers typically move too slowly, while programmers often move too quickly. Thus, to strain an old metaphor, the train is in the station and will be leaving shortly, with or without us—researchers can catch the train if they have the will, but they may have to leave some of their luggage behind.

The popularity of books, articles, audiotapes, and, most recently, videotapes are strong indicators that self-help mechanisms are being marketed—whether or not they are effective and regardless of their scientific basis. Rosen (1987) provides an overview of related issues. Between 10 and 15 percent of U.S. businesses currently provide smoking programs (Fielding, 1985; Walsh, 1984). Certainly research has not kept in stride with the demand for these services. The question raised is do we compromise the scientific process in order to serve the health needs of the community by developing (and modifying) programs given the limitations of our knowledge?

Research Funding

A final implication concerns research funding. If one considers the list of concerns raised thus far, it suggests the importance of *focused* research initiatives for at least two reasons. First, intervention research often requires large, sustained operating grants which tax the resources and flexibility of general contribution programs. Second, the need for diverse, evolving methodologies from quite different disciplines challenges the sophistication, good will, and trust of many a review panel. Thus, mechanisms such as those which focus on intervention research themes and center and program grants are more consistent with the needs of intervention research. Furthermore, Matarazzo (1984) argues that major development of scientist programs providing training and salary support will be needed to achieve necessary disciplinary integration. Funding for resource and coordination centers might also be a priority (Ontario Council of Health Task Force on Smoking, 1982).

ISSUES IN PROGRAM DEVELOPMENT RESEARCH

The five implications just presented, of the five-phase framework, are general, cutting across the phases. In addition, there are important specific issues to be considered at points, as the framework is applied to substantive public health problems. Some of these derive from the *intervention perspective* on the problems of change as we begin to wed substantive models and data (e.g., what we know about smoking prevention and cessation and what works) with the research design. Others relate more to the *research process itself,* and the need for continuing conceptual and methodological refinement of the model. The following two sections discuss these intervention and research perspectives; the chapter then ends with a summary and conclusion section.

The Intervention Perspective

For behaviors that we want to modify, we need models of the determinants of that behavior and the process of changing that behavior and, flowing from these models, effective intervention strategies. Smoking, like other health behaviors, is complex, determined by an interplay between constitutional, pharmacological, learning, and social/environmental factors (Best et al., 1988). Little is known about the processes and problems of change, but available evidence suggests relatively discrete stages of change (cf. DiClemente & Prochaska, 1985; Prochaska & DiClemente, 1983). Most people do not suddenly alter health lifestyle. Rather, a more typical pattern would be an increasing awareness of the need for change, associated with increased motivation, followed by a series of change attempts, before ultimate success. This suggests that programs for a population can have various objectives. For example, the aim of a mass media program may be limited to increasing awareness of a problem; while a special clinic may assume adequate motivation, and focus on the development of necessary skills for change. An associated concept focuses on readiness for change. Different proportions of the population may be ready for different services. A relatively large segment of the population may be open to comparatively low-investment media programs, but a much smaller percentage will be ready for intensive change programs. This concept suggests the need for "market research" to identify the characteristics of each target group, and to develop an integrated series of interventions designed to reach individuals at different stages in readiness for change. These concepts have become cornerstones for planning community-based smoking interventions, as illustrated by cardiovascular multiple-risk community studies (cf. Farquhar et al., 1984; Lasater et al., 1984; Blackburn et al., 1984). Despite the relative lack of data on the process of smoking cessation, increasingly effective interventions are becoming available, perhaps in part because of a growing appreciation of the need to address the diverse determinants of smoking (Lichtenstein & Mermelstein, 1984), and in part because population-level impacts seem possible (Flay, 1986).

A related concept, neglected thus far in the smoking prevention and cessation literature, follows from a realization that a given individual may require a series of interventions, to help her move through the various stages of change. It is useful to think of a sequenced or "step care" approach, to ensure continuing individual effort and change (Best, 1978). A person may begin with minimal-help approach such as a mass media program, physician counseling, or self-help print materials. If he is unsuccessful, he may move on to a group program. Finally, the more recalcitrant person may require intensive, individual counseling. A key question is how we help the struggling smoker "recycle," to try again with more intensive interventions (Prochaska, 1985).

High-risk populations, for example, may be an easily targeted group. Motivation to quit smoking appears to be tied to severity of illness—concurrently, cessation is highest among those most ill (USDHEW, 1979; Pederson, 1982; Pederson & Baskerville, 1983). Patients with pulmonary disease, for example, have had quite favorable cessation rates following brief physician advice (e.g., Davison & Duffy, 1982; Cooperstock & Thom, 1982; Daughton, Fix, Kass, & Patil, 1980), as have survivors of myocardial infarction (e.g., Baile, Bigelow, Gottlieb, Stitzer, & Sacktor, 1982; Cooperstock & Thom, 1982; Kirk, Lund, Woolcock, & Greenhalgh, 1980). Likewise, pregnant women represent a target population whose peak motivation may be high but temporary, suggesting they need to be reached early.

Groups not at high risk, on the other hand, may be experiencing different levels of readiness. For example, while historically the tie between readiness and smoking cessation self-help manuals has not been addressed (Lichenstein, 1982) it doesn't imply that those who fail did not receive the appropriate treatment; experience with these manuals may perhaps be viewed as one of the first steps taken by those attempting to quit (Glasgow & Klesges, 1985). Similarly, the immediate effects of mass media campaigns may not be forthcoming. Rather, there may be a "sleeper" effect with the media representing an early influence on motivation or helping to develop a perceived supportive environment (Best, 1980).

A third intervention concept weds individual change process to social and organizational change. Given that an intervention program is in place, what are the most effective mechanisms to integrate the individual's stage of readiness within the intervention being offered? Promising approaches to prevention and cessation should be further developed and evaluated in defined population studies of local communities to examine the effectiveness of an integrated network of cessation services (Best & Ossip-Klein, 1985). Support for this recommendation comes from (a) encouraging signs of effectiveness for comprehensive community programs, (b) a consensus that a diversity of coordinated programs and services is required to be maximally effective, and (c) evidence that repeated efforts with individual smokers and services aimed at relapse prevention and maintenance of nonsmoking increase success. Networks may be most effective if they build on natural social support systems, such as the family and worksite units. Networks of smoking programs and services must rely on data-based planning and monitoring. For example, regular tracking in the community of smoking rates for different groups, readiness for change, and preference for alternative services should be developed. The concept of integrated networks is extraordinarily complex and still underdeveloped.

The Research Perspective

Issues from the research perspective revolve around the interface between the intervention per se and the context in which it is delivered. The outcome of any behavioral intervention is a function of interactions between intervention methods, client characteristics, provider variables, and the setting, using the language of the therapeutic change literature (Vanden Bos, 1985); the parallel concepts from information processing are message, audience, source, and channel (Flay, DiTecco, & Schlegel, 1980). Research and evaluation designs must reflect this complexity.

First, the research questions must be framed to reflect this complexity within each phase. For example, in Phase II, there is likely to be concern with client or audience variables, as they influence intervention efficacy. Client characteristics either are seen as organismic variables, taken as a given (e.g., level of nicotine dependence) and as a basis for tailoring interventions, or (b) mediating variables to be addressed by the intervention (e.g., self-efficacy). At this stage of knowledge, little is known about these individual level mediating variables and how they are affected by smoking programs. We do know that low-level smokers sometimes respond better than heavy smokers (Kornitzer et al., 1980; Li et al., 1984; Rand et al., 1984; Ockene, Hymowitz, Sexton, & Broste, 1982); undoubtedly there are other individual characteristics that may be more useful in achieving program success. There is some evidence, for example, that when subjects attribute success to their own actions they are more likely to quit smoking (Chambliss & Murray, 1979) but this may interact with other individual traits such as locus of control or self-efficacy (Colletti & Kopel,

1979; Hunt 1979; Nentwig, 1978). This attribution process is also reflected in a study by Schlegel, Manske, and Shannon (1985) in which the effects of nicotine gum as an aid to cigarette cessation was more effective when self-administered than when there was intense therapist involvement.

In contrast to the concern over client variables in Phase II, at Phase IV there will be greater concern with setting and provider variables, factors which influence intervention effectiveness as the intervention moves from a research to a service context. At the worksite, for example, smoking cessation programs must take into account not only adherence to the intervention strategies and characteristics of the workers to be served, but must also recognize, and control for, contextual variables. Such contextual variables may include company size, policies, degree of management support, the history of health promotion, sex ratio, job stability, union/management relations, percentage of smokers, growth orientation of the company, and the relative work and socioeconomic status of the contact person (Glasgow & Klesges, 1985; Terborg, 1986). This shift in research emphasis may be manifested in such questions as: What affects the motivation of management to accept programs? In this regard, data may be needed which underscores the nonhealth benefits accrued through programs (e.g., decreased turnover, improved morale, enhanced public relations).

This leads to a second issue: variables affecting the *diffusion* of interventions become a whole new, separate domain for empirical investigation. Program effectiveness varies as a function of efficacy, availability, and audience acceptance (Flay, 1986). In addition it is recognized that programs typically are *adapted* more than *adopted* (cf. Berman, 1980). Again, we can either accept the system as an "organismic given," or we can use implementation research as a tool for innovation and social change (cf. Basch, 1984; Best, Bass, & Owen, 1977; Fuchs, 1983; Kreuter, Christenson, & Davis, 1984). A key observation here is, that as a science progresses, there is a movement from correlational *description* of mediator variables to *manipulation* and *control.* There is a strong tendency currently in Phase IV and V intervention research to take the delivery system as a given, to model these uncontrolled sources of variance in our data analyses, but not to treat setting and provider variables as factors to be controlled. The promise of community intervention research suggests that delivery systems can be influenced. The next question is whether or not, given an understanding of dissemination variables affecting intervention outcomes, greater control will improve outcomes and efficiency of complex behavioral programs for which uniform delivery is not easily achieved.

A third, again related issue, concerns the transition from Phase III to IV. Often, a crisis arises around the transition from the randomized controlled trials of Phase III, to the demonstration projects in defined populations of Phase IV. The nature of the phenomena at issue, and of questions about them, change. Research methodology, project outcomes, and funding mechanisms often are all changed simultaneously. The U.S. National Heart, Lung, and Blood Institute's Demonstration and Evaluation program (NHLBI, 1983) illustrates this transition. The program emphasizes the importance, in addition to scientific data, of intervention packages ready for dissemination, training procedures, evaluation tools, and so on.

Further, as our focus shifts through the phases from individual to population impacts the issue of tailoring programs to individual and target audiences needs to be considered empirically. Our increasing conceptual sophistication may run away with us. For example, researchers talk about smoking cessation programs tailored to the needs of pregnant women, the worksite, teenagers, and heavy smokers. Even within the worksite there is a perceived need for separate programs for different status individuals (e.g., blue collar vs. managerial) (Glasgow & Klesges, 1985). Are these groups in fact so different that a good generic program cannot be as effective as a specially designed and evaluated intervention? Review of the smoking prevention literature certainly suggests remarkably consistent findings despite program variation (Flay, 1985), and the same is true of group smoking cessation clinics (Best & Bloch, 1979). Generalizability of interventions should be carefully assessed through Phases III and IV, and the incremental value of tailored interventions tested empirically.

Finally, note the tradeoff between intervention complexity and diffusion ease. As the intervention becomes more sophisticated, efficacy may increase (but not necessarily so: see Lichtenstein, 1982). However, ease and quality of dissemination and implementation may decrease, and it is not at all clear what the optimal level of intervention sophistication will be in a particular context. More is not always better; overly complex management or treatment procedures with self-help manuals, for example, may be less effective (e.g., Lando, Shirley, Gregory, & McCullough, 1979) and lead to decreased adherence (Best, 1980; Pomerleau & Pomerleau, 1977). Similarly, individualized tailoring of treatment (e.g., Owen & Ewins, 1982) or providing physiological feedback such as CO readings for smokers (Glasgow, Klesges, Godding, & Gegelman, 1983; Glasgow, Klesges, & Vasey, 1987; Bauman et al., 1983) may not add to a procedure's effectiveness. A balance between complexity and diffusion ease must be a priority consideration through the research phases.

SUMMARY AND CONCLUSIONS

A model for health intervention research has been outlined, and a host of illustrative implications and issues has been introduced. The status of smoking cessation research in three specific areas, the use of self-help manuals, physician, and worksite interventions has been used to exemplify the application of this framework to a substantive area. The purposes have been to develop a framework which may be useful in planning and organizing intervention research, and to suggest that there *is* sufficient conceptual and methodological complexity to indicate a need to think in terms of an interdisciplinary arena of intervention research. No one existing discipline or perspective can adequately encompass the breadth of the endeavor; the development of a coherent "science" would have considerable pragmatic advantage.

It is important to ask whether the framework really adds anything or if it simply relabels with new jargon the approach any thoughtful scientist would take in developing new interventions. We think one strength of the framework is that it *does* mesh well with usual approaches. The value of the framework is in organizing and highlighting research issues and methodologies. Distinctive contributions of diverse disciplines are suggested. The level of analysis gradually moves from the individual to groups to populations. An interest in factors influencing dissemination and implementation is stimulated; a new perspective is expected to emerge on methodological, conceptual, and sociopolitical challenges inherent in the transition from research to service settings. However, the discussion also highlights the importance of continuing to develop the framework. Modest beginnings are being made, and future opportunities for health intervention researchers are bright.

REFERENCES

Abrams, D. B., Pinto, R. P., Monti, P. M., Jacobus, S., Brown, R., & Elder, J. P. (1985). *Health education vs. social network support for relapse prevention in a worksite smoking cessation program.* Poster presented at the meeting of the Society of Behavior Medicine, New Orleans, LA.

American Cancer Society. (1981). The impact of providing physicians with quit-smoking materials for smoking patients. *CA-A Cancer Journal for Clinicians, 31,* 75–78.

Baile, W. F., Bigelow, G. E., Gottlieb, S. H., Stitzer, M. L., & Sacktor, J. D. (1982). Rapid resumption of cigarette smoking following myocardial infarction: Inverse relationship to myocardial infarction severity. *Addictive Behaviors, 7,* 373–380.

Bandura, A. (1977). *Social learning theory.* Englewood Cliffs, NJ: Prentice-Hall.

Bandura, A. (1986). *Social foundations of thought and action. A social cognitive theory.* Englewood Cliffs, NJ: Prentice-Hall.

Baric, L., MacArthur, C., & Sherwood, M. (1976). A study of health education aspects of smoking in pregnancy. *International Journal of Health Education, 19* (2/Supplement), 1–27.

Basch, C. E. (1984). Research on disseminating and implementing health education programs in schools. *Journal of School Health, 54,* 57–66.

Battista, R. N. (1983). Adult cancer prevention in primary care: Patterns of practice in Quebec. *American Journal of Public Health, 73,* 1036–1039.

Bauman, K. E., Ryan, E. S., Dent, C. W., & Koch, G. G. (1983). The influence of observing carbon monoxide level on cigarette smoking by public prenatal patients. *American Journal of Public Health, 73,* 1089–1091.

Belloc, N. B. (1973). Relationship of health practices and mortality. *Preventive Medicine, 1,* 409–421.

Berman, P. (1980). Thinking about programmed and adaptive implementation: Matching strategies to situations. In D. Mann & H. Ingram (Eds.), *Why policies succeed and fail.* Beverly Hills: Sage.

Best, J. A. (1978). Targeting and self-selection of smoking modification methods. In J. L. Schwartz (Ed.), *Progress in smoking cessation.* New York: American Cancer Society.

Best, J. A. (1980). Mass media, self-management and smoking modification. In P. O. Davidson (Ed.), *Changing health lifestyles* (pp. 346–370) New York: Brummer/Mazel.

Best, J. A., Bass, F., & Owen, L. E. (1977). Mode of service delivery in smoking cessation program for public health. *Canadian Journal of Public Health, 68,* 469–473.

Best, J. A., & Bloch, M. (1979). Compliance in the control of cigarette smoking. In R. B. Haynes, D. W. Taylor, & D. L. Sackett (Eds.), *Compliance in health care.* Baltimore: Johns Hopkins University Press.

Best, J. A., & Ossip-Klein, D. J., 1985. Smoking cessation: Rapporteur's report. In W. F. Forbes, R. C. Frecker, & D. Nostbakken (Eds.), *Proceedings of the 5th World Conference on Smoking and Health* (Vol. 2). Ottawa: Canadian Council on Smoking and Health.

Best, J. A., Wainwright, P. E., Mills, D. E., & Kirkland, S. A. (1988). Biobehavioral approaches to smoking control. In W. Linden (Ed.), *Biological barriers in behavioral medicine* (pp. 63–99). New York: Plenum.

Bishop, D. B., & Fisher, E. B. (1984). *Employer assisted smoking elimination: The second year* (9/83–10/84). Annual report to the American Lung Association of Eastern Missouri, St. Louis, MO.

Blackburn, H., Luepker, R. V., Kline, E. G., Bracht, N., Carlaw, R., Jacobs, D., Mittelmark, M., Stauffer, L., & Taylor, H. L. (1984). The Minnesota Heart Health Program. A research and demonstration project in cardiovascular disease prevention. In J. D. Matarazzo, S. M. Weiss, J. A. Herd, N. E. Miller, & S. M. Weiss (Eds.), *Behavioral health: A handbook of health enhancement and disease prevention* (pp. 1171–1178). New York: Wiley.

Brantmark, B., Ohlin, P., & Westling, H. (1973). Nicotine-containing chewing gum as an antismoking aid. *Psychopharmacologia, 31,* 191–200.

Brengelmann, J., & Sedlmayr, E. (1977). Experiments in the reduction of smoking behavior. In W. Steinfield et al. (Ed.), *Health consequences, education, cessation activities, and government action.* Washington, DC: DHEW Publication No. (NIH) 77-1413.

Brengelmann, J. (1978). The treatment of smoking through the mail. In J. Schwartz (Ed.), *Progress in smoking cessation.* New York: American Cancer Society.

Breslow, L., & Enstrom, J. E. (1980). Persistence of health habits and their relationship to mortality. *Preventive Medicine, 9,* 469–483.

Brown, K. S., & Peterson, A. V. (1989). Statistical methods for the analysis of longitudinal data from school based smoking prevention studies. *Preventive Medicine, 18,* 290–303.

Burt, A., Thornley, P., Illingworth, D., White, P., Shaw, T. R. D., & Turner, R. (1974). Stopping smoking after myocardial infarction. *Lancet, 1* (7852), 304–306.

Califano, J. A., Jr. (1979). *Healthy people: The Surgeon General's report on health promotion and disease prevention.* Washington, DC: U.S. Government Printing Office.

Chambliss, C., & Murray, E. J. (1979). Cognitive procedures for smoking reduction: Symptom attribution versus efficacy attribution. *Cognitive Therapy and Research, 3,* 91–95.

Colletti, G., & Kopel, S. A. (1979). Maintaining behavior change: An investigation of three maintenance strategies and the relationship of self-attribution to the long-term reduction of cigarette smoking. *Journal of Consulting and Clinical Psychology, 47,* 614–617.

Cooperstock, R., & Thom, B. (1982). Health, smoking and doctor's advice. *Journal of the Royal College of General Practitioners, 32,* 174–178.

Dalton, E. R., Hughes, C. A., & Cogswell, J. J. (1981). Cigarette smoking in pregnancy: A health education problem. *Public Health (London), 95,* 207–214.

Danaher, B. G., & Lichtenstein, E. (1978). *Become an ex-smoker.* Englewood Cliffs, NJ: Prentice-Hall.

Daughton, D. M., Fix, A. J., Kass, I., & Patil, K. D. (1980). Smoking cessation among patients with chronic obstructive pulmonary disease (COPD). *Addictive Behaviors, 5,* 125–128.

Davis, A. L., Faust, R., & Ordentlich, M. (1984). Self-help smoking cessation and maintenance programs: A comparative study with 12-month follow-up by the American Lung Association. *American Journal of Public Health, 74,* 1212–1217.

Davison, G., & Duffy, M. (1982). Smoking habits of long-term survivors of surgery for lung cancer. *Thorax, 37,* 331–333.

Denson, R., Nanson, J. L., & McWatters, M. D. (1975). Hypkerkinesis and maternal smoking. *Canadian Psychiatric Association Journal, 20,* 6–12.

DiClemente, C. O., & Prochaska, J. O. (1985). Processes and stages of self change: Coping and competence in smoking behavior change. In S. Schiffman & T. A. Wills (Eds.), *Coping and substance abuse* (pp. 319–343). New York: Academic Press.

Donovan, J. W. (1977). Randomized controlled trial of anti-smoking advice in pregnancy. *British Journal of Preventive and Social Medicine, 31,* 6–12.

Donovan, J. W., Burgess, P. L., Hossack, & Yudkin, G. D. (1975). Routine advice against smoking in pregnancy. *Journal of the Royal College of General Practitioners, 25,* 264–268.

Ewart, C. K., Li, V. C., & Coates, T. J. (1983). Increasing physicians' antismoking influence by applying an inexpensive feedback technique. *Journal of Medical Education, 58,* 468–473.

Fagerstrom, K. A. (1982). A comparison of psychological and pharmacological treatment in smoking cessation. *Journal of Behavioral Medicine, 5,* 343–351.

Farquhar, J. W., Fortmann, S. P., Maccoby, N. et al. (1984). The Stanford Five City Project: An overview. In J. D. Matarazzo, S. M. Weiss, J. A. Herd, N. E. Miller, & S. M. Weiss (Eds.), *Behavioral health: A handbook of health enhancement and disease prevention* (pp. 1154–1165). New York: Wiley.

Fielding, J. E. (1984). Health promotion and disease prevention at the worksite. *Annual Review of Public Health, 5,* 237–265.

Fielding, J. E. (1985). Smoking: Health effects and control. *New England Journal of Medicine, 313,* 555–561.

Fisher, E. B., Jr. (1982). Cessation of smoking: Self-motivated quitting. *The health consequences of smoking: Cancer. A report of the Surgeon General* (DHHS Publication No. PHS 82-50179). Washington, DC: U.S. Government Printing Office.

Flay, B. R. (1986). Efficacy and effectiveness trials in the development of health promotion programs. *Preventive Medicine, 15,* 451–474.

Flay, B. R. (1985). Psychosocial approaches to smoking prevention: A review of findings. *Health Psychology, 4,* 449–488.

Flay, B. R., DiTecco, D., & Schlegel, R. P. (1980). Mass media in health promotion: An analysis using an extended information-processing model. *Health Education Quarterly, 7,* 127–147.

Fuchs, V. R. (1983, August). *Setting priorities in health education and promotion.* Paper presented at the Sun Valley Health Forums, Glen Cove, NY.

Glasgow, R. E., & Bernstein, D. A. (1981). Behavioral treatment of smoking behavior. In L. A. Bradley & C. K. Prokop (Eds.), *Medical psychology: A new perspective.* New York: Academic Press.

Glasgow, R. E., Klesges, R. C., Godding, P. R., & Gegelman, R. (1983). Controlled smoking, with or without carbon monoxide feedback, as an alternative for chronic smokers. *Behavior Therapy, 14,* 386–397.

Glasgow, R. E., Klesges, R. C., & Vasey, M. (1983). Controlled smoking for chronic smokers: An extension and replication. *Addictive Behaviors, 8,* 143–150.

Glasgow, R. E., Klesges, R. C., Klesges, L. M., Vasey, M. W., & Gunnerson, D. F. (1985). Long-term effects of a controlled smoking program: A 2 ½ year follow-up. *Behavior Therapy, 16,* 303–307.

Glasgow, R. E., & Klesges, R. C. (1985). Smoking intervention programs in the workplace. In *The health consequences of smoking: Cancer and chronic disease in the workplace. A report of the Surgeon General.* Rockville, MD: Office of Smoking and Health.

Glasgow, R. E. (1986). Smoking. In K. Holroyd & T. Creer (Eds.), *Self-management of chronic disease: Handbook of clinical interventions and research*. New York: Academic Press.

Green, D. E., & Horn, D. (1968). Physician's attitude toward their involvement in smoking problems of patients. *Diseases of the Chest, 54,* 180–181.

Greenwald, P., & Cullen, J. W. (1984). The scientific approach to cancer control. *CA—A Cancer Journal for Physicians, 34,* 328–332.

Grove, D. A., Reed, R. W., & Miller, L. C. (1979). A health promotion program in a corporate setting. *Journal of Family Practice, 9,* 83–88.

Hamburg, D. A., Elliott, G. R., & Parron, D. L. (1982). *Health and behaviors: Frontiers of research in the biobehavioral sciences*. Washington, DC: National Academy Press.

Handel, S. (1973). Change in smoking habits in a general practice. *Post Graduate Medical Journal, 49,* 679–681.

Harris, J. E. (1979). Cigarette smoking in the United States, 1950–1978. In *Smoking and Health: A report of the Surgeon General* (DHEW Publication No. PHS 79-50066). Washington, DC: U.S. Government Printing Office.

Hughes, J. R., Epstein, L. F., & Andrasik, F., et al. (1982). Smoking and carbon monoxide levels during pregnancy. *Addictive Behaviors, 7,* 271–276.

Hughes, J. R., & Miller, S. A. (1984) Nicotine gum as an aid to smoking cessation. *Journal of the American Medical Association, 252,* 2855–2858.

Hunt, P. T. (1979). A study of three cognitive-behavioral indices of self control in smoking cessation. *Dissertation Abstracts International, 40,* 2368.

Jarvis, M. J., Raw, M., Russell, M. A. H., & Feyerabend, C. (1982). Randomized controlled trial of nicotine chewing gum. *British Medical Journal, 285,* 537–540.

Jeffery, R. W., Danaher, B. G., Killen, J., Farquhar, J. D., & Kinnier, R. (1982). Self administered programs for health behavior change: Smoking cessation and weight reduction by mail. *Addictive Behaviors, 7,* 57–63.

Kaplan, R. M., & Criqui, M. H. (Eds.). (1985). *Behavioral epidemiology and disease prevention*. New York: Plenum.

Killen, J. D., Maccoby, N., & Taylor, C. B. (1984). Nicotine gum and self regulation training in smoking relapse prevention (SHDPP). *Behaviour Therapy, 15,* 234–248.

Kirk, C. J. C., Lund, V. J., Woolcock, N. E., & Greenhalgh, R. M. (1980). The effect of advice to stop smoking on arterial disease patients, assessed by serum thiocyanate levels. *Journal of Cardiovascular Surgery, 21,* 568–569.

Klesges, R. C., & Glasgow, R. E. (1986). Smoking modification in the worksite. In M. F. Cataldo & T. J. Coates (Eds.), *Health and industry: A behavioral medicine perspective* (pp. 231–254). New York: Wiley Interscience.

Kohn, R., & White, K. L. (Eds.). (1976). *Health care: An international study* (Report of the World Health Organization/International Collaboration Study of Medical Care Utilization). London: Oxford University Press.

Kornitzer, M., Dramaix, M., Kittel, F., & De Backer, G. (1980). The Belgian Heart Disease Prevention Project: Changes in smoking habits after two years of intervention. *Preventive Medicine, 9,* 496–503.

Kreuter, M. W., Christenson, G. J., & Davis, R. (1984). School health education research: Future issues and challenges. *Journal of School Health, 54,* 27–32.

Lalonde, M. (1974). *A new perspective on the health of Canadians: A working document.* Ottawa: National Health and Welfare.

Landesman-Dwyer, S., & Emanuel, I. (1979). Smoking during pregnancy. *Teratology, 19,* 119–125.

Lando, H. A., Shirley, R. J., Gregory, V. R., & McCullough, J. A. (1979). *A broad-spectrum treatment in eliminating smoking: Preparation, aversion, and maintenance.* Paper presented at the annual meeting of the American Psychological Association. New York.

Lasater, T., Abrams, D., & Artz, L., et al. (1984). Lay volunteer delivery of a community based cardiovascular risk factor change program: The Pawtucket experiment. In J. D. Matarazzo, S. M. Weiss, J. A. Herd, N. E. Miller, & S. M. Weiss (Eds.), *Behavioral health: A handbook of health enhancement and disease prevention* (pp. 1166–1170). New York: Wiley.

Li, V. C., Coates, T. C., Spielberg, L. A., Ewart, C. K., Dorfman, S., & Huster, W. J. (1984). Smoking cessation with young women in public family planning clinics: The impact of physician messages and waiting room media. *Preventive Medicine, 13,* 447–489.

Lichtenstein, E. (1982). The smoking problem: A behavioral perspective. *Journal of Consulting and Clinical Psychology, 50,* 804–819.

Lichtenstein, E., & Mermelstein, R. J. (1984). Review of approaches to smoking treatment: Behavior modification strategies. In J. D. Matarazzo, S. M. Weiss, J. A. Herd, N. E. Miller, & S. M. Weiss (Eds.), *Behavioral health: A handbook of health enhancement and disease prevention.* New York: Wiley.

Louis, T. A., Fineberg, H. V., & Mosteller, F. (1985). Findings for public health from meta-analysis. *Annual Review of Public Health, 6,* 1–20.

Malcolm, R. E., Sillett, R. W., Turner, J. A. M., & Ball, K. P. (1980). The use of nicotine chewing gum as an aid to stopping smoking. *Psychopharmacology, 70,* 295–296.

Matarazzo, J. D. (1984). A 1990 challenge for the health service professions. In J. D. Matarazzo, S. M. Weiss, J. A. Herd, N. E. Miller, & S. M. Weiss (Eds.), *Behavioral health. A handbook of health enhancement and disease prevention* (p. 1292). New York: Wiley.

Matarazzo, J. D., Weiss, S. M., Herd, J. A., Miller, N. E., Weiss, S. M. (Eds.). (1984). *Behavioral health: A handbook of health enhancement and disease prevention.* New York: Wiley.

Mausner, J. S., Mausner, R., & Rial, W. Y. (1968). The influence of a physician on the smoking behavior of his patients. *American Journal of Public Health, 58,* 46–53.

Meinert, C. L. (1986). *Clinical trials. Design, conduct and analysis* (Vol. 8). New York: Oxford University Press.

Meyer, A. J., & Henderson, J. B. (1974). Multiple risk factor reduction in the prevention of cardiovascular disease. *Preventive Medicine, 3,* 225–236.

Michael, J. M. (1982). The second revolution in health: Health promotion and its environmental base. *American Psychologist, 37,* 936–941.

National Center for Health Services Research (NCHSR). (1983). *National health care expenditures study-data preview* (DHHS Publication No. (PHS)83-3361). Washington, DC: U.S. Government Printing Office.

National Center for Health Statistics (NCHS). (1982). *Current estimates from the National Health Interview Survey: United States* (Vital and Health Statistics, Series 10, No. 141. DHHS Publication No. (PHS)82-1569, 106 pp.). Washington, DC: U.S. Government Printing Office.

Nentwig, C. G. (1978). Attribution of cause and long-term effects of the modification of smoking behavior. *Behavioral Analysis and Modification, 2,* 285–295.

National Heart, Lung, and Blood Institute (NHLBI). (1983). *Guidelines for demonstration and education research grants*. Washington, DC: National Heart, Lung, and Blood Institute.

Ockene, J. K., Hymowitz, N., Sexton, M., & Broste, S. K. (1982). Comparison of patterns of smoking behavior change among smokers in the Multiple Risk Factor Intervention Trial (MRFIT). *Preventive Medicine, 11,* 621–638.

Omran, A. R. (1971). The epidemiological transition: A theory of the epidemiology of population change. *Milbank Memorial Fund Quarterly, 29,* 509–538.

Ontario Council of Health Task Force on Smoking. (1982). *Smoking and health in Ontario: A need for balance*. Toronto: Ontario Council of Health.

Ossip-Klein, D. J., Shapiro, R. M., & Stiggins, J. (1984). Freedom Line: Increasing utilization of a telephone support service for ex-smokers. *Addictive Behaviors, 9,* 227–230.

Owen, N., & Ewins, A. (1982, November). *Correspondence courses for quitting smoking*. Paper presented at annual meeting of the Association for the Advancement of Behavior Therapy, Los Angeles, CA.

Packer, M. J. (1985). Hermeneutic inquiry in the study of human conduct. *American Psychologist, 40,* 1081–1093.

Page, A. R., Walters, D., Schlegel, R. P., & Best, J. A. (1986). Smoking cessation in family practice: The effects of advice and nicotine chewing gum prescription. *Addictive Behaviors, 11,* 443–446.

Pederson, L. L. (1982). Compliance with physician advice to quit smoking: A review of the literature. *Preventive Medicine, 11,* 71–84.

Pederson, L. L., & Baskerville, J. C. (1983). Multivariate prediction of smoking cessation following physician advice to quit smoking: A validation study. *Preventive Medicine, 12,* 430–436.

Perry, M. G., & Richards, C. S. (1977). An investigation of naturally occurring episodes of self-controlled behaviors. *Journal of Consulting Psychology, 24,* 178–183.

Perry, M. G., Richards, C. S., & Schulthies, K. R. (1977). Behavioral self-control and smoking reduction: A study of self-initiated attempts to reduce smoking. *Behavior Therapy, 8,* 360–365.

Pincherle, G., & Wright, H. B. (1970). Smoking habits of business executives: Doctor variation in reducing cigarette consumption. *Practitioner, 205,* 209–121.

Pomerleau, O. F., & Pomerleau, C. S. (1977). *Break the smoking habit: A behavioral program for giving up cigarettes*. Champaign, IL: Research Press.

Prochaska, J. O. (1985). *Patterns of changes in smoking behavior*. Paper presented at the NHLBI Smoking Relapse Workshop, Bethesda, ME.

Prochaska, J. O., & DiClemente, C. C. (1983). Stages and processes of self-change of smoking: Toward an integrative model of change. *Journal of Consulting and Clinical Psychology, 51,* 390–395.

Puska, P., Bjorkqvist, S., & Koskela, K. (1979). Nicotine-containing chewing gum in smoking cessation: A double blind trial with half year follow-up. *Addictive Behaviors, 4,* 141–146.

Rand, C., Stitzer, M., Bigelow, G., & Mead, A. (1984). *Contingent reinforcement for smoking abstinence*. Poster presented at American Psychological Association, Toronto, Canada.

Richmond, J. B. (1980). *Promoting health-preventing disease: Objectives for the nation*. Washington, DC: National Academy Press.

Rose, G., Heller, R. F., Pedoe, H. T., & Christie, D. G. S. (1980). Heart disease prevention: A randomized controlled trial in industry. *British Medical Journal, 280,* 747–751.

Rose, G., & Hamilton, P. J. S. (1978). A randomized controlled trial of the effect on middle-aged men of advice to stop smoking. *Journal of Epidemiology and Clinical Health, 32,* 275–281.

Rose, G., Hamilton, P. J. S., Colwell, L., & Shipley, M. J. (1982). A randomized controlled trial of anti-smoking advice: 10-year results. *Journal of Epidemiology and Community Health, 36,* 102–108.

Rosen, G. M. (1987). Self-help treatment books and the commercialization of psychotherapy. *American Psychologist, 42,* 46–51.

Rosser, W. W. (1979). Ways of helping patients to stop smoking. *Canadian Family Physician, 25,* 923–926.

Russell, M. A. H., Wilson, C., Feyerabend, C., & Cole, P. V. (1976). Effect of nicotine chewing gum on smoking behavior and as an aid to cigarette withdrawal. *British Medical Journal, 272,* 391–393.

Russell, M. A. H., Wilson, C., Taylor, C., & Baker, C. D. (1979). Effect of general practitioners' advice against smoking. *British Medical Journal, 278,* 231–235.

Russell, M. A. H., Raw, M., & Jarvis, M. J. (1980). Clinical use of nicotine chewing-gum. *British Medical Journal, 280,* 1599–1602.

Russell, M. A. J., Merriman, R., & Edwards, A. R. (1983). Effect of nicotine chewing gum as an adjunct to general practitioners' advice against smoking. *British Medical Journal, 287,* 1782–1785.

Schlegel, R. P., d'Avernas, J., & Best, J. A. (1982). *Self-management and smoking cessation: A critical analysis and integrative model*. Unpublished manuscript, University of Waterloo, Waterloo, Ontario, Canada.

Schlegel, R. P., Manske, S. R., & Shannon, M. E. (1985). BUTT OUT! Evaluation of the Canadian Armed Forces smoking cessation programme. *Proceeding of the 5th World Conference on Smoking and Health*. Winnipeg, Canada.

Schneider, N. G., Jarvik, M. E., Forsythe, A. B., Read, L. L., Elliot, M. L., & Schweiger, A. (1983). Nicotine gum in smoking cessation: A placebo-controlled, double-blind trial. *Addictive Behaviors, 8,* 253–261.

Schneider, S. J., Benya, A., & Singer, H. (1984). Computerized direct mail to treat smokers who avoid treatment. *Computers and Biomedical Research, 17,* 409–418.

Sexton, M., & Hebel, R. (1984). A clinical trial of change in maternal smoking and its effect on birth weight. *Journal of the American Medical Association, 251* (7), 911–915.

Shapiro, R. M., Ossip-Klein, D. J., & Gerrity, E. T. (1985–86). Perceived helpfulness of messages on a community-based telephone support service for ex-smokers. *International Journal of the Addictions, 20* (11&12), 1837–1847.

Sivarajan, E. S., Newton, K. M., & Almes, M. J., et al. (1983). The patient after myocardial infarction. Limited effects of outpatient teaching and counseling after myocardial infarction: A controlled study. *Heart and Lung, 12,* 63–75.

Sorman, K. (1979). This quit-smoking program works. *American Lung Association Bulletin, 65,* 2–6.

Stachnik, T., & Stoffelmayr, B. (1983). Worksite smoking cessation programs: A potential for national impact. *American Journal of Public Health, 73,* 1395–1396.

Stewart, A. L., Brook, R. H., & Kane, R. L. (1979). *Smoking. Conceptualization and measurement of health habits for adults in the Health Insurance Study* (Vol. 1, Rand Publication Series R-2374/ 1-HEW). Santa Monica: Rand Corporation.

Stewart, P. J., & Rosser, W. W. (1982). The impact of routine advice on smoking cessation from family physicians. *Canadian Medical Association Journal, 126,* 1051–1054.

Stitzer, M. L., & Bigelow, G. E. (1982). Contingent reinforcement for reduce carbon monoxide levels in cigarette smokers. *Addictive Behaviors, 7,* 403–412.

Stitzer, M. L., & Bigelow, G. E. (1983). Contingent payment for carbon monoxide reduction: Effects of pay amount. *Behavior Therapy, 14,* 647–656.

Terborg, J. R. (1986). Health promotion at the worksite: A research challenge for personnel and human resources management. In K. H. Rowland & G. Ferus (Eds.), *Research in personnel and human resource management* (Vol. 4). Greenwich, CT: JAI Press.

Thoresen, C. E. (1984). Overview. In J. D. Matarazzo, S. M. Weiss, J. A. Herd, N. E. Miller, & S. M. Weiss (Eds.), *Behavioral health: A handbook of health enhancement and disease prevention* (pp. 297–307). New York: Wiley.

U. S. Department of Health and Human Services (USDHHS). (1984). *The health consequences of smoking: Chronic obstructive lung disease.* Washington, DC: U.S. Government Printing Office.

U.S. Department of Health and Human Services (USDHHS). (1983). *The health consequences of smoking: Cardiovascular disease.* Washington, DC: U.S. Government Printing Office.

U.S. Department of Health, Education, and Welfare (USDHHS). (1979). *Smoking and health: A report of the Surgeon General.* Washington, DC: U.S. Government Printing Office.

U.S. Public Health Service (USPHS). (1973). *The health consequences of smoking. Smoking and pregnancy* (A Report of the Surgeon General). Washington, DC: U.S. Government Printing Office.

Vanden Bos, G. R. (Ed.). (1985). Psychotherapy research. *American Psychologist, 41,* 111–214.

Walsh, D. C. (1984). Corporate smoking policies: A review and analysis. *Journal of Occupational Medicine, 76,* 17–22.

Weiner, H. (1981). Brain, behavior and bodily disease: A summary. In H. Weiner, M. A. Hofer, & A. J. Stunkard (Eds.), *Brain, behavior, and bodily disease* (Vol. 59). New York: Rowen Press.

Weiss, S. M. (1984). Community health promotion demonstration programs: Introduction. In J. D. Matarazzo, S. M. Weiss, J. A. Herd, N. E. Miller, & S. M. Weiss (Eds.), *Behavioral health: A handbook of health enhancement and disease prevention* (pp. 1137–1139). New York: Wiley.

Wilson, D., Wood, G., Johnston, N., & Sicurella, J. (1982). Randomized clinical trial of supportive follow-up for cigarette smokers in a family practice. *Canadian Medical Association Journal, 126,* 127–129.

Windsor, R. A., & Bartlett, E. E. (1984). Employee self-help smoking cessation programs: A review of the literature. *Health Education Quarterly, 11,* 349–359.

Wortman, P. M. (1983). Evaluation research: A methodological perspective. *Annual Review of Psychology, 34,* 223–260.

3

Policy Issues Influencing Behavioral Medicine: An International Analysis

Jonathan S. Raymond

Gordon College
Wenham, MA

Patrick H. DeLeon

United States Senate Staff

Gary R. VandenBos

University of Bergen
Bergen, Norway

Jerrold M. Michael

University of Hawaii
Honolulu, HI

Behavioral medicine research and practice are influenced by health policy and can influence health policy as well. There is a continually occurring, multifaceted, multidirectional flow of "influence" among behavioral medicine research, policy, and practice.

By "health policy," we mean the priorities, goals, guidelines, regulations, and laws which directly or indirectly affect the delivery of health care services, the regulation of the environment for health, the conduct of health-relevant research, and the training of professionals for local, state, national, and international government agencies, legislative bodies, university faculties, foundations, associations, and other public and private groups (DeLeon & VandenBos, 1984).

A number of definitions have dominated the thinking about "behavioral medicine" since the term was first publicly used by Birk (1973) to describe the merits of biofeedback to treat medical disorders such as asthma, tension and migraine headaches, and epilepsy. In general terms, Birk saw behavioral medicine as the application of behaviorism to medicine.

Expanding beyond the parameters of biofeedback, Pomerleau and Brady (1979) define "behavioral medicine" as:

> (a) the clinical use of techniques derived from the experimental analysis of behavior—behavior therapy and behavior modification—for the evaluation, prevention, management, or treatment of physical disease or physiological dysfunction; and (b) the conduct of research contributing to the functional analysis and understanding of behavior associated with medical disorders and problems in health care. (p. xii)

A second widely employed definition arose out of the 1977 Yale Conference on Behavioral Medicine; that definition states:

> Behavioral medicine is the field concerned with the development of behavioral science knowledge and techniques relevant to the understanding of physical health and illness and the application of this knowledge and these techniques to prevention, diagnosis, treatment, and rehabilitation. Psychosis, neurosis, and substance abuse are included only insofar as they contribute to physical disorders as an end point. (Schwartz & Weiss, 1978a, p. 3)

Later the Yale group redefined "behavioral medicine" thus:

> The interdisciplinary field concerned with the development and integration of behavioral and biomedical science knowledge and techniques relevant to health and illness and the application of this knowledge and

> these techniques to prevention, diagnosis, treatment, and rehabilitation. (Schwartz & Weiss, 1978b, p. 249)

By "behavioral medicine," we mean the emerging field of inquiry and practice that is occasioned by the synergistic merging of the behavioral and medical sciences and professions. This is a broad working definition that encompasses much more than just clinical practice issues. It includes research, public information, community action, education, training, policy formation, and policy implementation. In this sense, we are in accord with the Yale redefinition which acknowledges the importance of prevention, diagnosis, treatment, and rehabilitation. We, however, choose to place the greatest emphasis on prevention as we believe that simple behavioral preventive interventions are the most relevant to improvement in the world's health.

This chapter focuses on policy issues that can influence the international development and utility of behavioral medicine. It is critical that international health policy discussions maintain the broad perspective encompassed in the above definition, as all too often such discussions become restricted to a limited clinical definition of behavioral medicine (with a resulting provincialism reflecting Western—and at times singularly American—points of view that emanate from a preoccupation with Western-style, curative medicine). In our opinion, a restrictive posture precludes comprehensive, globally relevant consideration of the full range of world health needs (and options for the application of behavioral medicine interventions).

By an international analysis, we mean the identification and examination of those issues that reflect the pressing realities of health and disease throughout the developing and developed world. An international perspective is critical because the vast majority of the world's health problems differ from those found in the developed nations. In addition, 80 percent of the world's population (primarily those in developing countries) require health care delivery systems less costly than those found in the United States, Australia, England, Sweden, and other developed countries. The majority of the world's population receives (and will continue to receive) "health care" that integrates modern medical practices with indigenous practices.

For researchers and practitioners in behavioral medicine, we are in an unprecedented era of behavioral-medical synergism. For many years, the behavioral and medical sciences have moved forward in parallel in both research and practice. Until recently, there have been only occasional moments in the history of major collaborative contributions between the behavioral and medical fields (and these have been restricted primarily to psychology and psychiatry within the speciality of mental health, and, perhaps, psychology and optometry in the area of vision care).

Recently, however, interdisciplinary collaborative initiatives of behavioral and medical scientists have produced significant gains in understanding and practical applications in the health field (Hamburg, Elliott, & Parron, 1982). Indicators of progress include new journals and state-of-the-art texts, new professional associations (for example, the Society for Behavioral Medicine, and the health psychology division of the American Psychological Association), new organizational entities within government research institutes and centers, and new departments (and doctoral programs) within schools of medicine and public health, as well as joint psychology-nursing training programs (Keller & Baumann, 1986; Mitchell, Barnard, Booth, Magyary, & Spieker, 1986). This behavioral-medical synergism is a very recent phenomenon. Consequently, its products, as contributions to the health field, suggest that behavioral medicine is in a stage of infancy.

EXISTING REALITIES

Several existing international realities first should be acknowledged. These are unavoidable. They serve as a context for discussing the broad policy issues facing the field.

First, behavioral medicine, as a hybrid field, presently exists in the service of curative medicine. A quick perusal of the refereed journals and texts published in the field reveals that nearly all topics relate to tertiary care and service delivery.

Yet, in our judgment, the most pressing health policy issues, which affect the bulk of the world's population, are directly related to the realities of health economics (and, for example, the fact that national health budgets are being significantly curtailed by governments in developing nations struggling to pay off their foreign debts). The cost of curative medical systems continue to escalate, and these costs are viewed by public officials as "squeezing all available resources" from meager national treasuries (while at the same time morbidity and mortality rates are on the rise due to the health conditions that we feel are in reality preventable). Inequities and disparities exist in health status between developed and developing countries. In Japan, the risk of dying within one year after birth is one out of 142 and in the Scandinavian countries, it is one out of 125. In Bangladesh, however, it is one out of eight. Persons living in developing countries have an average life span of about 50 years, while individuals living in Western Europe and North America have an average life span that is 50 percent longer (WHO, 1986).

Second, it is clear that prevention, preventive health strategies, and preventive medicine are not the major themes around which behavioral medicine research and practice are organized. Although not insubstantial, resources in support of behavioral medicine research are devoted almost exclusively to curative, tertiary themes and foci (DeLeon, Kjervik, Kraut, & VandenBos, 1985).

Preventive-oriented research remains a very small portion of the health and behavior research programs supported in the United States. For example, the United States as a nation spends less than $0.50 per capita on preventive care, while at the same time spending approximately $1440 per capita on curative measures (Inouye, 1984). This is at a time when the Surgeon General of the United States has reported that seven of the top ten causes of death in the nation could be significantly reduced if those at risk would modify their daily life styles (DHEW, 1979; DHHS, 1980). There are a few potential exemptions to this situation, however. Initiatives developed by the U.S. State Department's Agency for International Development (AID) can be viewed as natural mechanisms for proponents of behavioral medicine to contribute to preventive health outcomes on a very large scale. Broad-scale immunization, oral rehydration therapy, birth spacing, breastfeeding, growth monitoring, and nutrition programs could all benefit from the synergism of behavioral medicine, in both research and practice. However, it would appear that little contribution from behavioral medicine is happening in this area. Precious few of the AID resources (for example, under its Child Survival Initiative) are actually either being influenced by the field of behavioral medicine or serving to shape the field's destiny. Similarly, behavioral medicine would appear to be contributing little to the health care initiatives of UNICEF and the World Health Organization (WHO).

Third, there exists a compelling and significant opportunity to apply behavioral medicine to global health needs in a preventive fashion. The fundamental challenge that confronts behavioral medicine from an international perspective is not one of achieving new medical breakthroughs, but rather of applying behavioral science methods to improving the worldwide utilization of techniques and technology which are already available to modern medicine.

In the developing world, 40,000 children under the age of five die each day from disease and conditions which are preventable (USAID, 1985). If all the world's children were to benefit from basic immunizations, clean water supplies, adequate sanitation, nutritious diets, and the application of appropriate technology to treat diarrheal diseases when necessary (for example, through oral rehydration therapy), the tragic deaths of 15 million children each year could be avoided (McPherson, 1986). By our collective daily failure to act in accordance with existing knowledge and technology, millions of children, parents, and their communities experience suffering, death, and needless disability each year.

Another graphic example may be found in a disease which many individuals in the Western world rarely think about—malaria. Today nearly 2,400 million people—just over half of the world's population—live in areas where malaria is an active health risk. In much of the developing world, malaria is one of the top five causes of infant and child mortality (Fox & Brent, 1984; Rodgers, 1980). It has been estimated that there are now about 200 million cases of malaria (Nossal, 1984). At especially high-risk are pregnant women (who apparently lose their antimalarial immunity during pregnancy) who contract acute falciparum malaria at rates four to twelve times higher than their nonpregnant peers (Wyler, 1982). The frequency of this disease can be greatly reduced, if existing behavioral medicine knowledge is appropriately applied.

Vitamin A deficiency is prevalent in most developing nations. Informed estimates suggest that in Asia alone, as many as five million children may develop xerophthalmia (nutritional blindness) every year (Sommer, Tarwotjo, Hussaini, & Susanto, 1983). In one study in Indonesia, 16 percent of all deaths in children, from ages one to six, was directly associated with mild vitamin A deficiency (Sommer, 1983). Vitamin A deficiency is also known to increase the risk of mortality from other infections (diarrhea, respiratory ailments)—in some age groups eight to twelve times the rates among children without the deficiency.

Acute respiratory infections, malaria, and vitamin A deficiency are but three of a long list of existing realities directly implicated in the deaths of millions of children in the world each year who are under the age of six. The list of other modifiable, but pressing health problems includes malnutrition in general (with its accompanying infections—diarrhea, in particular), iron deficiency anemia, low birth-weight neonates, poor family spacing, foul water supplies, poor breastfeeding and weaning practices, and deaths due to six particular vaccine preventable diseases—diptheria, pertusis (whooping cough), tetanus (including neonatal tetanus), measles, polio, and tuberculosis (Grant, 1986a).

The barriers to radically improving the health of the world's children are essentially attitudinal, dispositional, and behavioral. The task can be viewed as being twofold: (a) the rapid social mobilization of existing resources and technologies directed toward children's health through intensive national mobilization campaigns in all areas of Child Survival initiatives (Grant, 1986b) including immunizations, nutrition/growth monitoring, breastfeeding, oral rehydration therapy, and clean drinking water, and (b) the worldwide development of national primary health care systems which extend down to the rural, village level and provide lasting continuity of care and assurance of health for all. We cite this as but one area of concern in which a broader conceptualization of behavioral medicine is essential to adequately addressing the pressing realities of the global challenge facing the field.

Fourth, the successful application of behavioral medicine to global preventive health will require more than applications arising solely out of an American (or Western) scientific enterprise. Indigenous contributions to the field are critical and essential.

This presents us with a major challenge. Today's understanding of the potential interface of the behavioral sciences and medicine has been developed primarily by Western scientists, using Western methods, and studying Western young adults (readily available and accessible to university researchers). This results in major problems of generalizability of findings and methods. Even the basic operating assumptions are problematic. For example, individualism, which is a perspective more readily accepted in the West, permeates the philosophy and theoretical frameworks of modern (Western) behavioral science. Individualism, with its dominant focus on the individual as the center of inquiry, influences the choice of topics and problems studied and the hypotheses generated (Gergen, 1973). Yet, in most of the world, individualism has a less dominant conceptual role than the notion of collectivism—with its focus on the group, family, or community. From a global perspective, collectivism is the dominant world view—it influences much of the world's health behavior.

Laypersons, philosophers, politicians, concerned clinicians, and scientists from the developing world are keenly aware of the need for more indigenous theoretical frameworks and constructs that acknowledge the collective nature of human behavior, including health-related behavior. Unfortunately, however, there is a relative dearth of clinicians or scientists in parts of the world with expertise and a focused interest in behavioral medicine. For example, a recent international meeting on social science and tropical medicine which was held in Kuala Lumpur, Malaysia drew only 50 scholars. Most of those were from Western, more developed countries and only a few otherwise were from the developing world.

Some progress is being made, however. It is the formal policy of the World Health Organization (WHO) to address this paucity of trained indigenous manpower and to build up the reserve of scientists in behavioral medicine through their doctoral fellowship program in social psychology and tropical medicine (UNDP/World Bank/WHO,

1985). In our judgment, increasing the worldwide population of scientific expertise in behavioral medicine and creating interfaces between the international behavioral medicine community and national and international policy makers is absolutely essential to the ultimate potential contribution of behavioral medicine to any global or national strategy for health. More resources will especially be needed to even begin to reach the projected requirements for indigenous scientific and scholarly leadership in behavioral medicine.

SUMMARY OF EXISTING REALITIES

Acknowledging existing realities permits the clearer presentation of possibilities in the development of policy. We have highlighted what, in our judgment, is the current state of affairs in the world's health. What has been presented should serve as the context for an international analysis of what ought to be in the way of policy influencing behavioral medicine. This context has been presented so that the field of behavioral medicine might move forward by becoming more responsive to the needs and opportunities that will undoubtedly continue to present themselves internationally. However, before moving on to discuss the various possibilities for policy to influence behavioral medicine, and vice versa, we feel that several of the points which emerged from the previous discussion merit summarization.

1. The field of behavioral medicine, while still in its infancy, is nevertheless experiencing rapid, substantive development and scholarly advancement as the relationship of health and behavior is acknowledged increasingly in policy and practice.
2. But behavioral medicine has yet to embrace and contribute to the field of preventive medicine in any substantive way and therefore has made little unique contribution to those issues which impact the health of most of the world's populations.
3. The field of behavioral medicine is experiencing increasing formal support from the research enterprise. This support comes from both government and private sectors. However, it is primarily concentrated in contributions to curative medicine.
4. There is a significant opportunity for behavioral medicine to contribute to the improvement of the world's health. This will be accomplished by moving beyond curative medicine and focusing on contributions to preventive strategies, especially at the community and village level.

5. The pervasive "Western" bias within the theories, practices, research, and problem selection within behavioral medicine must be overcome. Significant theoretical frameworks and constructs will need to be developed that go beyond existing and emerging Western contributions.
6. Contributions of behavioral medicine to the improvement of world health will be in direct proportion to the increase in the world's population of indigenous scientists and clinicians in the field and to their contact with and influence among key decision makers (i.e., health policy leadership) at both an international and national level.

OPPORTUNITIES FOR PSYCHOLOGY

As we have indicated, many of the pressing health problems facing the Third World today could be significantly addressed by adopting a rationally based, prevention-oriented health delivery system. Such a system, at a minimum, must ensure that the personnel and economic resources that are available are systematically targeted towards areas of greatest need. To implement this approach and to ensure that the most current state-of-the-art clinical knowledge is effectively utilized, these nations need a cadre of health policy leadership that is not emotionally tied to the status quo or to outdated models of health delivery. Expertise in systems theory and management, rather than specific clinical skills per se, must be given a premium (and, above all else, students must be recruited from the indigenous populations).

Of all the health care disciplines that should be interested in aggressively pursuing an international behavioral medicine agenda, psychology may very well, in our opinion, have the most to offer the field. Psychology's true uniqueness as a profession (whether one is considering its health care specialists, or its research specialists, or its educational specialists) is that its practitioners and scientists are fundamentally empirically oriented. Psychology is above all else a *behavioral science*. Its expertise is not in having developed complex theoretical models for explaining human behavior—although admittedly many psychologist have done this—but rather in its constantly insisting that there be an empirical basis for explaining observable behaviors. However, it is also an open question in our minds as to whether the field of psychology will ever accept its collective responsibility in this area.

Psychology is a relatively young profession, even in the United States. It was only with the passage of the Missouri State Practice Act in 1977 that psychology became licensed/certified in each of the U.S. jurisdictions (DeLeon, Donahue, & VandenBos, 1984). Similarly, it was only with the enactment of President Reagan's Comprehensive Criminal Code Reform Act, as a provision of the Fiscal Year 1985 Continuing Resolution (P.L. 98-473), that psychology was expressly recognized under the U.S. Federal Criminal Code (DeLeon, VandenBos, & Kraut, 1986). This recognition and utilization of psychologists in other developed and developing countries is not so advanced as in the United States.

Today, psychology is just beginning to explore seriously the outer limits of its potential scope of practice (DeLeon, 1986). Practitioners in the United States, for example, are just beginning to address the issue of whether behavioral scientists (i.e., psychologists) should seek psychotropic prescription privileges (Adams, 1986; Burns, DeLeon, Chemtob, & Welch, in press; Fox & Brent, 1987; Inouye, 1984; Samuels, 1985). Internationally, psychology should explore and expand its involvement in health psychology and behavioral medicine.

For more than a decade now, farsighted leaders within the professional psychology community (Cummings & VandenBos, 1979; Fox & Bent, 1984; Rodgers, 1980) have stressed the critical need for psychology to possess its own clinical treatment facilities in order to be able to systemically develop psychologically based comprehensive treatment programs. Such "homes for psychology" would also provide excellent training experiences for the next generation of psychology's leaders. Today, there are nearly a third more practicing psychologists in the United States than there are psychiatrists (Dorken, Stapp, & VandenBos, 1986), but to our knowledge no psychology training program possesses its own inpatient facility. A number of psychology departments and professional schools do, however, administer outpatient clinics. It makes little sense that psychology's students cannot (or should not) receive inpatient training under the direction of their mentors. We suggest that this state of affairs not only reflects the relative professional youth of psychology, but more significantly, the extent to which psychology's training programs have not yet accepted their fundamental responsibility to guide the development/evolution of the profession. Internationally, groups such as the European Federation of Professional Psychological Associations are working with WHO to enhance the recognition of roles and contributions of psychology and psychologists (and expand the range and location of professional training and practice).

If one steps back and looks at the administrative accomplishments of individual psychologists, these quickly become very impressive (DeLeon, Kjervik, Kraut, & VandenBos, 1985). In the United States, psychologists presently serve as the administrators of major treatment facilities and as clinical directors of comprehensive clinical programs. Psychologists serve at the highest levels of academia. Nearly one-third of the chief mental health officers in individual state mental health systems are psychologists. Within the U.S. federal government psychologists currently serve as the acting director of the National Institute of Mental Health, director of the National Institute on Drug Abuse, director of the National Institute on Disability and Rehabilitation Research, and the Assistant Secretary for Human Development Services. A psychologist even once served as Secretary of the then-Department of Health, Education and Welfare. Few of these psychologists (or other behavioral scientists) have concentrated in international health or behavioral medicine. Although individual psychologists have achieved considerable administrative success, there is very little recognition (or appreciation) of their accomplishments within the collective awareness of psychology. Psychology training programs, both internationally and in the United States do not seem to hold these individuals out as role models. If our universities do not highlight and appreciate the accomplishments of these individuals (and the career options implied for current graduate students), the behavioral science contribution to international behavioral medicine will be limited.

When individual psychologist have decided to become involved, they have met with considerable success and acceptance (Averasturi, 1983). But again, this has been on an individual (and not institutional) basis. Within the American Psychological Association (APA), dedicated psychologists have worked to raise APA's collective consciousness regarding international issues (Brengelmann & Wittchen, 1986; David, 1986; Derksen, 1986; Kennedy & David, 1986; McPherson, 1986; Wagner, 1986). Where, we would rhetorically ask, has been the follow-up by either psychology's educational institutions or psychology's national association (i.e., the APA)? Given the youth of the profession, however, one might first ask whether it is even reasonable to expect either to have acted.

Historically, it has been exclusively medicine (i.e., physicians) that has reached out and offered themselves to serve as the health leadership of the Third World. In our judgment, the fact that physicians have traditionally been accepted reflects the absence of any systematic competition from the other health disciplines, rather than their specific clinical expertise per se. Simply stated, there is nothing in a medical school curriculum, as contrasted to what a psychologist or optometrist might experience, that uniquely qualifies the physician per se to be "captain of the international health ship." In fact, it could be argued that physicians' "love affair" with curative medicine is part of the problem in adequately meeting the most pressing world health problems with behavioral and prevention-oriented interventions. In the United States, some policy makers are arguing for consideration of an expanded array of intervention models within international health circles. For example, during the (United States) Senate Appropriation Committee's deliberations on the Fiscal Year 1986 Appropriation bill for the Department of Health and Human Services (HHS), at the request of Senator Inouye, language was included in the relevant Senate report stating:

> The Committee feels that it is very much in our national interest for HHS to actively engage in international health activities. The Committee is aware that most recently the Public Health Service spent $69,500,00 for international health activities. The Committee encourages HHS to continue to provide support for such activities and to develop a comprehensive report for the Congress on its international activities during this fiscal year. (Senate Report #99-151, pp. 125–126)

The following year, during its deliberations on the Fiscal Year 1987 Appropriations bill for the Department of Health and Human Services, the Senate Appropriation Committee included two related directives:

> The Committee continues to be supportive of efforts by the Department in the area of international health and urges the U.S. Public Health Service to work collaboratively with the Agency for International Development in this regard. The Committee would be interested in learning of possible projects which could be jointly funded by the two Departments during the hearings on the fiscal year 1988 budget. (Senate Report #99-408, p. 131)

And,

> The Committee strongly urges the NIA (National Institute on Aging) to pursue appropriate cross-cultural and cross-national studies with such countries as Japan, the United Kingdom, Italy, Sweden, Finland, the Peoples Republic of China, and Nigeria. The Committee understands that promising activities have already been undertaken by the NIA and that a number of these nations have expressed considerable interest in furthering cooperative efforts with the NIA. Examples of the types of research that could be addressed include Alzheimer's disease, cancer, heart disease, osteoporosis, and broad-based comparisons of overall health and functioning characteristics of older people in their communities. The availability of an international data base on aging would remove a significant barrier to cross-national demographic research on the elderly especially those of 85 years and older. The Committee further requests a report from the NIA on its international activities prior to the budget hearings on next year's bill. (Senate Report #99-408, p. 102)

That same year the Senate Appropriations Committee, during its deliberations on the Foreign Assistance and Related Programs Appropriation bill for Fiscal Year 1987, also included a part under the health account of the Agency for International Development (AID) that stated:

> Aging—The Committee is aware of the projected rapid increases of older people around the world in developing and developed nations. Accordingly, it is timely that AID begin to allocate a proportion of its health resources into international research on problems affecting older persons. The Committee recommends that at least $5,000,000 be set aside for this purpose. AID is directed to collaborate with the Department of Health and Human Services for this purpose. AID is directed to collaborate with the National Institute on Aging for the Department of Health and Human Services in such activities as comparative international epidemiological studies on Alzheimer's disease and related dementias, osteoporosis, and other health problems affecting older people. The Committee understands that preliminary observations by the NIA have suggested significant differences in the prevalence of such chronic conditions in different cultures and environments, and that systematic studies of these differences may provide important insight into causes, prevention, and treatment of these maladies. The Committee further directs that a detailed report be developed describing those projects funded under this new initiative. (Senate Report #99-443, p. 59)

We cite this development of the growing U.S. Congressional interest in international gerentology as a concrete area within which psychology could make a major contribution to behavioral medicine. Given the projected magnitude of the future needs within the United States with the ever-aging American population similar to the rest of the world—including developing countries, the Appropriations Committees (with their jurisdiction over the Department of Health and Human Services), included a total of $15 million for new domestic geriatric health manpower training initiatives during their deliberations on the Fiscal Years 1986 and 1987 Appropriations bills. Yet, even with this growing Congressional interest (and with the documented potential contribution that psychology could make to the quality of life of the American senior citizen population), problems of statutory recognition continue to exist for U.S. psychology. During the closing hours of the 99th Congress (after the training funds had been made available by the Appropriations Committees), the Congressional Authorization Committees enacted legislation formally establishing a new *medical and dental school* geriatric training initiative which, unfortunately, made no legislative reference to behavioral science or psychology.

As noted earlier, there is a clear and pressing need, both internationally and in the United States related to geriatric health needs and psychology has much to offer. In fact, much of what is needed can be viewed as constituting efforts to improve the overall quality of life during one's twilight years (i.e., instituting modifications in lifestyle and expectations), which is clearly the province of behavioral scientists. Yet, psychology was not active enough during the political process (i.e., during the health policy formulation process) to ensure that its unique expertise was formally recognized. The funding for the international geriatric programs is not limited to medical or dental schools; however, psychology's training programs must once again play "catch up ball" in order to eventually have an opportunity to make appropriate contributions to training, research, policy, and practice.

Yet, in our judgment, even with the setback described above, steady progress is being made. The senior author has been actively involved in the health policy formulating process as the director of the International Center for Health Promotion and Disease Prevention at the University of Hawaii's School of Public Health. As indicated earlier, it is incumbent upon those at the public policy level, who are interested in behavioral medicine, to ensure that a high priority is given to various prevention activities. Further, as DeLeon and Pallak (1982) have pointed out, perhaps the best vehicle for psychology to accomplish this objective is through collaborative efforts with our nation's schools of public health.

As a provision of the Health Promotion and Disease Prevention Amendments of 1984 (P.L. 98-551), our nation's schools of public health were successful in having a network of health promotion and disease prevention centers authorized. The original legislative authority provided that up to thirteen such centers could be established, over a three-year period of time. Further, during the Congressional deliberations on the Consolidated Omnibus Budget Reconciliation Act of 1985 (COBRA) (P.L. 99-272), similar authority was also provided under the Medicare provisions of the Social Security Act. As conceptualized, these centers were to be truly interdisciplinary in nature (and psychology was expressly included, as a coequal partner with medicine and nursing).

The health promotion and disease prevention movement is still only in its infancy (DeLeon & VandenBos, 1983). Very few realize that it was only back in 1974 that Marc Lalonde, the then-minister of national health and welfare for Canada, brought prevention centrally into the public policy arena for the first time when he released his far-reaching report entitled *A New Perspective on the Health of Canadians*. Five years later the U.S. government released *Healthy People: The Surgeon General's Report on Health Promotion and Disease Prevention*

(DHEW, 1979). And in 1982, the prestigious Institute of Medicine released its report *Health and Behavior: Frontiers of Research in the Biobehavioral Sciences* (Hamburg, Elliot, & Parron, 1982). For psychology, however, the most significant development in its evolution as a true health profession has been the recent establishment of a joint nursing-psychology degree program at the University of Wisconsin (Keller & Baumann, 1986; Mitchell et al., 1986). Nevertheless, the underlying question still remains: Will psychology's training institutions eventually mature enough to seriously address the national and international ramifications of the "behavioral medicine" movement?

POLICY POSSIBILITIES

What possible policy developments would move forward the field of behavioral medicine, thereby permitting its contributions to have a more substantive impact on world health?

By definition, a statement of policy is inherently prescriptive. It is a statement of what ought to be. We shall now offer some comments and suggestions related to policy issues which influence behavioral medicine. The potential impact of behavioral medicine will be stated in the language of prescription. Policy implications implicit in what follows should be adopted broadly, by international, regional, and national entities—both public and private—and applied liberally in the future.

International agencies charged with responsibilities relevant to world health stand to gain much by embracing behavioral medicine. Although upon occasion the U.S. Congress takes the lead (as evidenced in the Senate Appropriation Committee's interest in international gerontology noted earlier), international agencies, with their control of day-to-day priorities, are in unique positions to occasion incentives for the field to move in the direction of serving preventive strategies and initiatives. WHO and UNICEF are especially capable of influencing the field's participation in and contributions to the "Health For All/Primary Health Care" movement and the "Child Survival and Development Revolution." As a matter of policy, they should target their messages more effectively to the behavioral medicine audience (using behavioral health concepts and terminology), so as to receive the attention and support of the multidisciplinary field of behavioral medicine (and achieve the maximum improvement in world health).

Yet, it is also important to emphasize that, given the relative youthfulness of the behavioral medicine movement, researchers and practitioners in the field must be willing to familiarize the relevant agencies with their expertise, as well as familiarizing themselves with the missions, initiatives, policies, and perspectives of international health-related agencies (such as World Health Organization, United Nations Children's Fund, Canadian International Development Agency, Japanese Agency for International Assistance, and the U.S. Agency for International Development). And, as we have noted with the field of psychology, the various training institutions have a special obligation (and opportunity) to demonstrate creative leadership.

Academics must actively listen to the messages being delivered by the leadership of agencies dedicated to international health, and they must actively seek out (and participate in formulating) opportunities for the field of behavioral medicine to contribute to the major global health agendas. This can, admittedly, be done more easily by universities which have specific regional and international missions (DHHS, 1980).

We would suggest, in particular, that for the foreseeable future, policies and actions which favor immediate support of the Child Survival and Primary Health Care initiatives of WHO and UNICEF by proponents of behavioral medicine will yield tangible opportunities for scholarly contributions. In terms of a longer, more strategic approach to fundamentally shifting internal support to international health objectives, universities should look inwardly to the possibility of internationalizing their curricula, especially in the schools of medicine, nursing, public health, and health psychology. Curricula should include the development of new course work which both supports behavioral medicine and is international in scope and perspective. New academic courses are especially needed in behavioral epidemiology with an emphasis on infectious diseases, which currently have priority in much of the developing world. Courses are also critically needed in operations research and specifically in community health care financing and economics for the developing world (Derkson, 1986; Dorken & Stapp, & VandenBos, 1986). However, as our world's population grows steadily older, there will also be an increasing need for more Western-like chronic disease curricula.

As a matter of fundamental policy, visiting scholar programs should be immediately instituted and strengthened within univerisities. Support should be sought from international agencies, governmental agencies, and private charitable institutions. As we indicated earlier, there can be a major "blow out" process without such a component. Preventive medicine training likewise should be supported and strengthened with strong international field experiences promoted in developing country settings. Such programs, as a matter of policy, should be interdisciplinary in nature and should engage participants and residents in national primary health care strategies and/or child survival campaigns, for example. Likewise, short, intensive leadership training in Child Survival and Development and Primary Health Care programming should be viewed as an area of behavioral medicine and should receive immediate support and active attention by all institutions concerned with the world's health.

Basic communication presents a major challenge to the internationally relevant development of the field of behavioral medicine. Not only are new international journals needed, but also priority should be given to international health issues and behavioral medicine by the current journals of all disciplines. Policies that promote enhanced professional communications, and especially contributions by scholars indigenous to the developing world, are critical and essential.

Western scholars and clinicians who choose to internationalize their contributions must be careful to go beyond academic tourism, to reach beyond their cultural biases, and to push past their potential provincialism. Language skills are crucial to overcoming many of these constraints. Researchers and clinicians working in the international arena of behavioral medicine should be conversant in the native tongue to collaborate effectively with their international peers. Policies promulgated by universities and donor agencies in support of language acquisition and skill building are called for, especially for visiting scholars and internationally collaborating researchers.

We feel that it is imperative that the social and behavioral sciences in the developing world themselves be supported and nurtured so that they will flourish and begin to contribute in major ways to the behavioral-medical interface and creative synergism which is at the very heart of behavioral medicine. Policies targeted toward the Third World (which build basic faculties) that promote and strengthen scholarship in the social-behavioral science sciences, and that link scholars in the social-behavioral science to the medical sciences, and that open ministries of health and the private sector to the skills and activities and applications of sociobehavioral scientists, are critical and essential.

International collaboration by individuals, between faculties and agencies, and among universities and institutions, is critical and essential to the advancing contribution of behavioral medicine to world health. Policies which foster a diversity of linkages and collaboration are very important. Presently, in the United States, various universities and the Centers for Disease Control (CDC) of the U.S. Department of Health and Human Services are linked together through cooperative agreements between CDC and the Association of Schools of Public Health as well as the Association of Schools of Medicine. This arrangement has resulted in several million dollars of preventive health research being conducted each year by universities in accordance with CDC's agenda. Under this approach research protocols are mutually shaped and agreed upon with all collaborating entities benefitting. Such action-oriented linkage should be expanded and emulated in the world health arena.

Under the leadership of the International Center for Health Promotion and Disease Prevention at the University of Hawaii, 10 schools of public health and departments of community medicine throughout Asia and the Pacific region have joined together to form the Asia-Pacific Academic Consortium for Public Health (Michael & Grossman, 1985). With funding from WHO and AID this Consortium, since its chartering meeting in January 1984, has initiated several joint research projects, sharing faculty in each project. The Consortium has also exchanged scholars and students between member universities, jointly sponsored major international conferences, and started a new journal for the Asia-Pacific region. In all of its endeavors to date, the activities of the Consortium have included themes, topics, projects, and ideas in the mainstream of what we would call international behavioral medicine as discussed above. Policy in support of such international academic consortia is critical if the field of behavioral medicine is to develop and become truly responsive to the challenges of world health. Policies that support the abiding participation of donor agencies, key national and international agencies, professional associations, governments, and private individuals in the activities of such consortia bode well for the future international relevance of behavioral medicine and for the eventual erradication of major health-related global problems (WHO, 1986).

SUMMARY OF POSSIBILITIES IN POLICY

We have identified 10 possible areas of policy development that if acted upon would undoubtedly result in significantly influencing the contributions of behavioral medicine on world health and also serve to further develop the field. These policy areas are diverse in their potential for action by a wide range of agencies and constituencies. Some areas are natural for guiding action by international agencies and others by professional associations, ministries of health, or universities, for example. The 10 possible areas of policy evolution include the following:

1. International agencies should seek to benefit from embracing behavioral medicine to further their own goals and missions. They should actively apply incentives to engage practitioners and

researchers in behavioral medicine and target their messages more deliberately to behavioral medicine audiences.

2. Professionals and academics in behavioral medicine should become familiar with the mission, policies, and goals and objectives of international agencies and understand the potential opportunities for professional expressions and contributions to the field of world health made possible through the action agendas of international agencies.
3. Universities, as a matter of policy, should internationalize their curricula in support of world health foci and priorities on informed leadership development and action. They should also strengthen their visiting scholars program, especially with indigenous peers from developing and least developed countries who are drawn from the ranks of behavioral medicine.
4. Universities should also strengthen their preventive medicine residency programs to provide field experience in child survival and primary health care initiatives in developing and least developed countries, with an emphasis on behavioral medicine and the priority diseases of the designated country; these residency programs should be open to interested parties of all clinical disciplines, including nursing and psychology.
5. International agencies, ministries of health, universities, and others should support the conduct of short, intensive leadership training opportunities in child survival and primary health care strategies as a broad approach or complement to behavioral medicine.
6. All entities concerned with the contribution of behavioral medicine to world health should support and promote enhanced communication for health through the establishment of international journals, special foci conferences, and other mechanisms of professional exchange including providing increased exposure to international issues through the current scholarly journals of the various disciplines.
7. Indigenous scholarship in the social-behavioral sciences should be actively nurtured and supported by universities and donor agencies to build a foundation of theory and research for behavioral medicine which is practical, relevant, and indigenous.
8. Western scholars in behavioral medicine should be supported and urged to acquire skill in indigenous languages by international health agencies and donors whose policy it is to promote language acquisition as an integral component of receiving support for collaborative research and/or training with indigenous peers.
9. International collaboration should be actively encouraged and promoted by universities, governments, international agencies,

international donors, and others concerned with the merits of behavioral medicine.

10. International academic consortia need to be established and supported to address the world's major health-related challenges through behavioral medicine. Such consortia should link several universities together and promote international collaboration across countries and among faculty of several schools or universities.

CONCLUSION

Existing realities regarding world health present a compelling case for a broad definition of behavioral medicine, one broad enough to encompass (and in fact, emphasize) preventive approaches to global health problems. A number of possibilities exist for the participation of a diverse array of entities, including international health-related agencies, universities, governments, professional associations, donor agencies, foundations, and individuals.

The global initiatives of the "Child Survival and Development Revolution" and the "Health For All/Primary Health Care Movement" provide immediate opportunities for researchers and practitioners to address the major health issues confronting much of the world's population. The challenges facing behavioral medicine, regarding its international contribution to world health, are not primarily a matter of achieving new scientific discoveries or technological breakthroughs. Rather, they have to do with the perceptions, dispositions, and behaviors which exert profound influence on health policies and the priority to be given to preventive actions such as immunizations, breastfeeding, focused nutrition programs, and oral rehydration therapy as well as the commitment of resources to the development and financing of extensive national primary health care systems at the village or community level.

Behavioral medicine has a great deal to contribute to the goals of world health if policies are adopted in several quarters and sectors which liberate behavioral medicine to be internationally relevant and responsive. It is an article of faith that under the right conditions, consistent with the discussion above of existing realities and policy potentials, behavioral medicine will thrive. It will become a highly relevant field making a major impact on the health and well-being of much of the world's population, both in the immediate and in the distant future.

We particularly discussed the problems confronting psychology in some depth, because in our judgment this provides an excellent illustration of the dilemma facing all of behavioral medicine. Those who choose a health career are surprisingly hesitant to become personally involved in the political/health policy process. This is especially true for those with responsibility for our health professions' training institutions. As a result, those who establish health policy are often not aware of the evolving trends within the various professions, nor are those who are shaping the destiny of the various health professions aware of the goals and aspirations of the health policy leadership. The unfortunate result is that society is not as well served as those involved would wish.

Behavioral medicine, in a supportive policy context, can do much to reduce and eliminate the inequities which exist today in the world's health. The extent to which it succeeds depends upon the degree to which it is permitted by policy (or insists upon the right) to focus on the existing realities, and to address the inequities of living conditions and quality of life which perpetuate the ongoing preventable loss of human life.

REFERENCES

Adams, D. (1986, January). A prescription for psychologists. *Georgia Psychologist, 39*(1), 13–15.

Averasturi, L. G. (1983). Presentation at the APA Public Policy forum. American Psychological Association. Washington, DC.

Birk, L. (1973). *Biofeedback: Behavioral Medicine.* New York: Grune & Stratton.

Brengelmann, J. C., & Wittchen, H. U. (1986). Professional psychology and private health services: Developing trends in the Federal Republic of Germany. *American Psychologist, 41,* 306–308.

Burns, S. M., DeLeon, P. H., Chembtob, C. M., & Welch, B. L. (in press). Psychotropic medication: A new technique for psychology? *Psychotherapy.*

Cummings, N. A., & VandenBos, G. R. (1979). The general practice of psychology. *Professional Psychology, 10,* 430–440.

David, H. P. (1986). Population, development, and reproductive behavior: Perspectives for population and health psychology. *American Psychologist, 41,* 309–312.

DeLeon, P. H. (1986). Increasing the societal contribution of organized psychology. *American Psychologist, 41,* 466–474.

DeLeon, P. H., Donahue, J., & VandenBos, G. R. (1984). The interface of psychology and the law. In J. R. McNamara (Ed.), *Critical issues, devel-*

opments, and trends in professional psychology: Vol 2 (pp. 235–256). New York: Praeger.

DeLeon, P. H., Kjervik, D. K., Kraut, A. G., & VandenBos, G. R. (1985). Psychology and nursing: A natural alliance. *American Psychologist, 40,* 1153–1164.

DeLeon, P. H., & Pallak, M. S. (1982). Public health an psychology: An important, expanding interaction. *American Psychologist, 37,* 934–935.

DeLeon, P. H., & VandenBos, G. R. (1983). The new federal health care frontiers—Cost containment and "Wellness." *Psychotherapy in Private Practice, 1,* 17–32.

DeLeon, P. H., & VandenBos, G. R. (1984). Public health policy and behavioral health. In J. D. Matarazzo, S. M. Weiss, J. A. Herd, & N. E. Miller (Eds.), *Behavioral health: A handbook of health enhancement and disease prevention* (pp. 150–163). New York: Wiley.

DeLeon, P. H., VandenBos, G. R., & Kraut, A. G. (1986). Federal recognition of psychology as a profession. In H. Dorken & Associates (Eds.), *Professional psychology in transition: Meeting today's challenges* (pp. 99–117). San Francisco: Jossey-Bass.

Department of Health, Education, and Welfare (HEW). (1979). *Healthy people: The surgeon general's report on health promotion and disease prevention* (DHEW Pub. No. (PHS) 79-55071). Washington, DC: U.S. Government Printing Office.

Department of Health and Human Services (HHS). (1980). *Promoting health, preventing disease: Objectives for the nation* (Stock No. 017-001-00435-9). Washington, DC: U.S. Government Printing Office.

Derksen, J. J. (1986). Clinical psychologists in the primary health care system in the Netherlands. *American Psychologist, 41,* 313–314.

Dorken, H., Stapp, J., & VandenBos, G. R. (1986). Licensed psychologists: A decade of major growth. In H. Dorken and Associates (Eds.), *Professional psychology in transition: Meeting today's challenges* (pp. 3–19). San Francisco: Jossey-Bass.

Fox, R. E. (1987). *Prescription privileges: Their implications for the practice of psychology.* Invited address at the Division 29 Midwinter Meeting. New Orleans, LA.

Fox, R. E., & Brent, R. J. (1984). Current status and future directions of professional psychology. In J. R. McNamara (Ed.), *Critical issues, development, and trends in professional psychology: Vol. 2* (pp. 257–293). New York: Praegar.

Gergen, K. J. (1973). Social psychology as history. *Journal of Personality and Social Psychology, 26* (2), 131–138.

Grant, J. P. (1986a, July). *To reach the unreached: A world commitment to child health and well-being.* A paper presented to the annual meeting of the International Pediatrics Congress. Honolulu, HI.

Grant, J. P. (1986b). *The state of the world's children 1986.* Oxford: UNICEF and Oxford University Press.

Hamburg, D. A., Elliott, G. R., & Parron, D. L. (Eds.). (1982). *Health and behavior: Frontiers of research in the biobehavioral sciences.* Washington, DC: Institute of Medicine, National Academy Press.

Inouye, D. K. (1984b). 1984 Ira Hiscock Public Lecture. University of Hawaii, School of Public Health, Honolulu, HI.

Keller, M. L. & Baumann, L. J. (1986). Comment: Further comments on psychology and nursing. *American psychologist, 41,* 1169–1170.

Kennedy, S., & David, H. P. (1986). Psychology and policy around the world: Widening psychology's sphere of influence. *American Psychologist, 41,* 296–297.

McPherson, M. P. (1986a). *The AID Child Survival Strategy* (mimeograph). Washington, DC: United States Agency for International Development.

McPherson, F. M. (1986b). The professional psychologist in Europe. *American Psychologist, 41,* 302–305.

Michael, J. M., & Grossman, J. (1985). The Asia-Pacific Academic Consortium for Public Health, *Mobius, 5*(3), 17–20.

Mitchell, S. K., Barnard, K. E., Booth, C. L., Magyary, D. L., & Spieker, S. J. (1986). Comment: The natural alliance of psychology and nursing: Substance as well as practice. *American Psychologist, 41,* 1170.

Nossal, G. J. V. (1984). *The biotechnology revolution and new vaccines, in protecting the world's children: Vaccines and immunization.*

Pomerleau, O. F. & Brady, J. P. (1979). *Behavioral medicine: Theory and practice.* Baltimore: Williams and Wilkins.

Rodgers, D. A. (1980). The status of psychologists in hospitals: Technicians or professionals. *Clinical psychologists, 33*(4), 5–7.

Samuels, R. M. (1985). From the President: A prescription for psychologists. *The Independent Practitioner, 5*(3), 2–3.

Schwartz, G. E., & Weiss, S. M. (1978a). Yale conference on behavioral medicine: a proposed definition and statement of goals. *Journal of Behavioral Medicine, 1,* 3–12.

Schwartz, G. E., & Weiss, S. M. (1978b). Behavioral medicine revisited: an amended definition. *Journal of Behavioral Medicine, 1,* 249–252.

Sommer, A., Tarwotjo, I., Hussaini, G., & Susanto, D. (1983). Increased mortality in children with mild vitamin A deficiency. *Lancet, 2.*

Stinson, W. (1982). Community Financing of Primary Health Care, American Public Health Association. *International Health Programs Monograph Series 1* (No. 4).

UNDP/World Bank/WHO Special Programme for Research and Training in Tropical Diseases. (1985). *1985 Seventh Programme Report; Chapter 12, Social and Economic Research.* Geneva, Switzerland.

United States Agency for International Development. (1985). *Child Survival: A Report to Congress on the AID Program.* Washington, DC: Author.

Vandiver, F. E. (1984). Universities: The next iteration? *Science, 225.*

Wagner, D. A. (1986). Child development research and the Third World: A future of mutual interest? *American Psychologist, 41,* 298–301.

WHO. (1986). *Intersectoral Action for Health: The role of intersectoral cooperation in national strategies for Health For All* (technical discussions). Geneva, Switzerland.

WHO. (1985a). Basic principles for control of acute respiratory infections in children in developing countries: A joint UNICEF/WHO statement.

WHO. (1985b). Basic principles for the control of malaria: A joint UNICEF/WHO statement.
WHO. (1984). *Roles of universities in health for all.* Geneva, Switzerland.
WHO. (1981). *Global strategy for health for all by the year 2000.* Geneva, Switzerland.
Wyler, D. J. (1982). Malaria: Resurgence, resistance, and research. *New England Journal of Medicine.*

II

THE MUSCULOSKELETAL SYSTEM

4

Pathophysiology of Musculoskeletal Pain and Dysfunction

Rene Cailliet

University of Southern California

Pain that originates from musculoskeletal tissue, be it from injury, abuse, inflammation, or mechanical abnormality, is a predominant symptom of everyday medical practices. Musculoskeletal tissues are the site of impulses that eventually will be interpreted as nociceptive pain which is, in turn, considered to be acute and extracentral in comparison to central or chronic pain. The neurological pathways of nociceptive pain from peripheral tissue sites are well documented. These peripheral stimuli are transmitted via somatic and sympathetic fibers.

Transmission of impulses from these musculoskeletal tissue sites are via the dorsal roots which enter the tracts of Lissauer, specifically Rexed Zone I and II, the substantia gelatinosum (S.G.), where they then synapse to cross over to be transmitted via the ascending tracts of the spinothalamic column to the thalamus, a region of the mid-brainstem. In this concept the initiation of these nociceptive impulses originate within the connective tissue of the musculoskeletal tissues. The end organs of the nerve fibers that transmit impulses, which ultimately will be "pain sensation," are located in these soft tissues.

The term "soft tissue" remains ambiguous in the context of neuromusculoskeletal tissue. The essential components of soft tissue are: (a) collagen fibers as the component of capsular tissue, (b) collagen tissues as a component of ligaments, (c) collagen fibers within tendons, (d) collagen fibers within cartilage that are subserved by synovial tissue, (e) muscular tissues, and lastly (f) fibrous tissue. These are the tissue components of "soft tissue" which function physiologically but are also pathologically the cause of pain and dysfunction. Each of these six tissues have mechanical efficiency to ensure normal pain-free movement. Trauma of these tissues may also, however, result in pain production and impaired function.

As most soft tissues are involved in the movement of joints, joints must perform their motions efficiently according to their alignment, contours, enclosing tissues, and their muscular action component.

In evaluating musculoskeletal function each aspect of musculoskeletal action and the tissues involved must be documented. Each joint has a precise movement both in its direction as well as its limitation (MacConaill, 1965; Paockop, Kovirokko, Toderman, & Gozman, 1979). When there is pain and malfunction it is mandatory that the specific motion and the tissues involved in the causation of pain and malfunction be fully appreciated. Only when this specific mechanism and tissue site of abnormality is elucidated can the cause of pain and malfunction be understood.

SOFT TISSUE COMPONENTS

Before fully understanding malfunction and pain, it is necessary that normal function be appreciated. Collagen is the predominant component of soft tissue. Histologically, a collagen fiber is a tri-helix band of aminoacid molecules. Each tri-helix collagen fiber is a spiral chain of aminoacids. These aminoacid chains interact within the fiber.

Numerous fibers of collagen intertwine specifically to form a precise connective tissue which in turn is so constructed as to serve a precise function. Connective tissue which requires elasticity (flexibility) is loosely organized and by virtue of this organization, as well as the percentage of collagen components, permits this flexibility. Flexibility is ensured by the fact that the intertwining collagen fibers glide upon each other at their intersection. They attach at various distances from their intersections, and it is the elasticity of the collagen fibers between these points of intersection contact that determine the extent of the elasticity. Each single collagen fiber has plasticity or elasticity inherent in its structural ability to uncoil. Once the collagen fiber is uncoiled it will resume its original coiled length upon release of the external force. If excessive force is applied, however, causing excessive lengthening, the aminoacid chains literally disconnect and the fiber cannot retract to its original structural length. If the collagen fibers at their intersections become adherent, which is not normal, these new points of contact become shorter. Hence, the connective tissue becomes less elastic.

Normal elasticity of connective tissue must exist in joint capsules and be maintained to ensure normal joint movement. That normal elasticity is also pain-free. If flexibility of connective tissues is markedly decreased, there is not only impairment in the total joint range of motion, but it is apparent that pain can then occur when this elasticity is exceeded by attempting to achieve full joint motion. Limited joint range of motion, disability, and pain result from this soft tissue inelasticity.

There are many aspects of connective tissue that still remain unknown and conjectural. How the aminoacids that form the collagen fibers remain bound to each other is not completely clear. Neuroanatomists, soft tissue physiologists, and physiological chemists differ as to whether the bindings of aminoacids are chemical or electrical. How these bonds are disrupted or possibly reunited after injury is also not fully understood. What is accepted, however, is: (a) the macromicroscopic structure of connective tissue has been clarified; (b) repeated elongation, that is passive stretching, is mandatory for maintenance of tissue normalcy; (c) excessive elongation of the aminoacid chains can be pathological from disruption of the collagen fibers; (d) failure to repeatedly and adequately elongate connective tissue within their physiological limits results ultimately in inelasticity—this is termed contracture; and (e) joints require elasticity of these connective tissues and will remain normal unless the connective tissue is excessively stretched. Excessive flexibility creates an unstable joint. If the connective tissue becomes constricted, the joint becomes constricted. Either of these conditions result in dysfunction and, conceivably, pain.

Another component of soft tissue is fibrous tissue. Fibrous tissue fibers structurally differ from collagen. Fibrous fibers are essentially elongated unicellular tissues with tapered ends. Fibrous tissue, although it has a slight elasticity, functions essentially to limit movement. It has, therefore, a limited amount of elasticity. Fibrous tissue is preset in larger proportion within the soft tissue of joints where limited movement is intended. Its presence in the connective tissue of joints prevents excessive movement to protect the other connective tissues within that joint capsule.

Even tough fibrous tissue has limited elasticity, it must be stretched frequently to its physiological elongation to maintain its normal function. Failure to repeatedly elongate fibrous tissue allows the fibrous fiber to shorten.

In contradiction to collagen fibers, fibrous tissue fibers have a tendency to proliferate. Under conditions of very limited oxygen supply, fibrous tissue thrives, whereas the more specialized collagen tends to deteriorate. Injury of the soft tissue with resultant inflammation and also resultant ischemia predisposes to proliferation of fibrous tissue. Fibrous tissue tends to proliferate and increase its percentage, causing the total connective tissue to be more fibrous and therefore less elastic. A truism of soft tissue injuries is that "crude fibrous tissue replaces the very specialized efficient tissues of the body in the presence of injury, inflammation and ischemia." Therefore the tissues around joints, the so-called periarticular tissues, will as a rule, from injury, misuse, or inflammation, tend to contain an excessive percentage of fibrous tissue and a decreasing percentage of the more specialized collagen tissues. Hence limitation of the joint results with dysfunction and resultant pain. It is apparent, therefore, that injury to soft tissue results in the deterioration or destruction of highly specialized tissues such as collagen and muscular tissues and has a tendency to be replaced by fibrous tissue. This propensity of fibrous tissue is the main component of what can be called "scar." Scar in essence is a replacement of soft tissue by fibrous fibers which tend to retract and render the tissue inelastic.

There is a third soft tissue component known as elastin. As its name denotes it is a tissue that is highly elastic and has slight resiliency. There are a few places in the body where connective tissue is formed exclusively of elastin. The physical capability of elastin is its ability to recoil immediately upon any external force being released. Thus elastin tissue has excessive flexibility before it can be damaged.

The ligamentum flavum of the vertebral column is an example of elastin tissue. When the spine flexes, the ligamentum flavum which lines the inner aspect of the spinal canal elongates proportionately. As the spine reextends, this ligamentum flavum immediately and simultaneously recoils. This rapid elongation and recoiling allegedly prevents the synovial tissues of the posterior facet joints from being entrapped as their articular surfaces approach.

Elastin tissue has no blood supply and no innervation. Deterioration of elastin appears to involve chemical structural changes resulting from aging and microtrauma in a manner not fully understood. Microscopically, elastic fibers fibrillate, fragment, and become invaded with fibrous tissue. Having no blood supply, elastin tissue maintains elasticity which must be maintained by repeated stretching and elongation.

Joints normally have a precise movement and a specific limitation. The tissue about these joints, therefore, must have a precise proportion of each of the three components of soft tissue. There must be a specific proportion of collagen to fibrous to elastin material, depending on the precise joint function normally expected. An example of this proportion is the capsule of the shoulder glenohumeral joint which has an excessive range of motion for normal function. This motion must also be pain-free. The glenuhumeral capsule has a connective tissue that has a high percentage of collagen, a moderate percentage of elastin, and a lower percentage of fibrous tissue fibers. The collagen fibers intersect at wide distances. Full pain-free range of motion for normal function therefore demands that the percentages of collagen, elastin and fiber remain identical and each component remain thoroughly elastic. Failure to maintain this normal percentage of the components of the connective tissue and to maintain the elasticity of each of these components leads to inflexibility. Restriction of the glenohumeral joint capsule results in the so-called "frozen shoulder" which is usually a limited painful shoulder movement.

The hip joint, the femoral acetabular articulation, has a higher percentage of fibrous tissue with much less elastin and collagen fibers that are more closely intersected. The front part of the capsule of the hip has connective tissue in that it is constructed to prevent the joint from excessive hyperextension. To prevent this motion, a ligament is formed within the capsule which prevents that portion of the joint from elongating excessively. This ligament, known as the "Y" ligament of Bigelow, the iliopectineal ligament, is essentially a thickened portion of the capsule which restricts that precise movement. This structural potion of the capsule is so constructed that the collagen fibers lay parallel to each other and thus have limited extensibility. With less criss-cross intersection of collagen fibers the capsular tissue has less flexibility.

A tissue that has parallel collagen fibers, each of limited elongation, is the tendon. The achilles tendon is a prime example of the function of parallel collagen fibers. Tension within the achilles tendon gives it it's functional capacity of conveying adequate strength to the gastrocsoleus muscle that permits full body weight, and weights can be added to be elevated against gravity.

Another excellent example of the structure and function of connective (soft) tissue is the ligamentum nuchae of the neck. This tissue is essentially wholy fibrous. By its limited elongation it maintains the head and neck erect, against gravity, with minimal muscular effort.

Both tendons and ligaments, by virtue of having limited intrinsic blood supply and minimal nociceptor nerve endings, are uncommon tissue sites for nociceptor impulses resulting in pain.

CARTILAGE

Cartilage is a "soft tissue" which contributes a precise function in joint movement. Cartilage primarily acts as a "shock absorber" and simultaneously functions to create lubrication of the joint. It performs these two functions by virtue of its structure. When this structure is damaged there is resultant impairment of joint range of motion. There is also a very definite potential for resultant pain from this cartilage change. Cartilage is essentially a "sponge cover" of the end of any two bones that oppose each other to form a joint.

The matrix of cartilage is a complex chemical mucopoly-saccharide, approximately 80 percent water throughout which collagen fibers are enmeshed. The matrix of cartilage is secreted via the cells known as chondrocytes which are located at the base of cartilage. These chondrocytes receive their nutrition from a filtration of blood.

The blood that supplies this filtrate comes from blood vessels that approach the cartilage within the bones of the joint, but no blood vessel penetrates and enters the cartilage. The blood filtrate internally filters through the thin layer of bone at the base of the cartilage, from the blood vessels of the bone ends.

Nutrition of the cartilage, therefore, requires imbibition of the fluid that has been brought to the very margin of the bone (MacConaill, 1950). This imbibition is performed by virtue of "a sponge action" of the cartilage. Imbibition or so-called sponge action is similar to the action of a sponge within fluid. When the sponge is squeezed, fluid leaves the sponge to enter its surrounding fluid, and simultaneously when the sponge is released, allowing it to expand, it imbibes the fluid from without to within the sponge. The sponge effect of compression and relaxation is the basis of nutrition of the cartilage (Cailliet, 1969). As well as being instrumental in the nutrition of the cartilage, imbibition also instigates the lubrication of the joint. When compressed the cartilage extrudes mucinoid material into the joint. This mucinoid coats the cartilage and decreases friction between the two opposing surfaces or the cartilages of the joint. Cartilage acts as a shock absorber, lubricates the joint, and maintains its own nutrition by imbibition: alternate compression and expansion. The matrix of the cartilage "secretes" these fluids. The mechanical structure of the cartilage that allows this compression expansion are collagen fibers enmeshed within the matrix. They are coiled within the cartilage and act like sponges. Upon sustaining compression, they literally flatten; upon the compression being removed, they expand. Cartilage thus performs its mandated function of weight bearing-shock absorption by alternate compression and relaxation imbibition. For a joint to have a normal pain-free function it must therefore have adequate normal cartilage.

The lubricating fluid expressed from cartilage compression must, in turn, be contained within a flexible capsule. In essence, normal joint function mandates significant normal cartilage lining, frequent compression and elaxation, adequate blood flow, and physiological flexibility of the enclosing capsule: all soft tissue qualities (Raden, Paul, & Rose, 1975).

MUSCLES

All joints move by virtue of muscular action. Muscles attach to and from bony appendages and the joints function by virtue of mechanical leverage. When a muscle contracts it shortens and therefore approximates the bony portions of the joint to which these muscles are attached.

Muscles that are prime movers are termed the agonists in that, as they shorten, they move the joint in a specific direction and do so with a specific force and for a specific duration and distance. Similarly, muscles whose site and attachment move the joint in the opposite direction must elongate to permit this movement. These "opposing" muscles are called antagonist. This process is termed "reciprocal relaxation of antagonist muscles," which means the opposing muscles must proportionately and simultaneously elongate as the moving muscles shorten. There is a reflex neurological mechanism within the spinal cord that ensures that when flexors contract, extensors reciprocally relax (Eldred, 1967). This reflex functions by virtue of sensory impulses in the contracting antagonistic muscles sending a message to the spinal cord terminal which instantaneously, automatically, and proportionately relaxes the opposing antagonistic muscle. The operation of this reciprocal relaxation neurological mechanism requires an intact nerve supply to the muscle. The "message" sent to the central nervous system is via the autonomic nervous system of Spindle cells and Golgi apparatus: The former, muscle proprioceptors, are located within the muscle fibers (intrafusal fibers) and the latter within the tendons of that muscle.

The Spindle system conveys rapidity of elongation and contraction, and the Golgi system correlates the force expended for the needed action. These are instantaneous actions coordinated at the cord level but adversely influenced, cortically, by faulty intention, unpreparedness, fatigue, sugar, impatience, and depression.

As stated, the proper neuromuscular activity depends on normalcy of the end organs: the joint cartilages, ligaments, joint capsules, and adequate extrafusal nerve supply precise action. Normal muscular function is neurologically programmed. The action is willed and thus initiated. Repeated action that leads to essentially automatic coordinated movement is facilitated chemically and electrically by the neurologically coordinated patterns. This implies that repetition facilitates and enhances the neurological patterns, making them more efficient, more precise, and operated with much less effort. Willed movement patterns become more automatic. Just as constant normal repetition enhances movement, there are many factors that can interrupt or interfere with normal smooth coordinated movements. Some of the factors that interefere with normal neuromuscular mechanisms include fatigue, anger, anxiety, depression, tension, or other psychophysiological neuromuscular factors. These "factors" interefere with normal neuromuscular mechanisms with resultant erratic uncoordinated movements. Too much force may be exerted to perform the desired act. Too little effort may be expended thus not accomplishing the desired act. The distance may be misjudged. The muscles involved in the intended action may exert excessive contraction: too abrupt a contraction or too excessive a distance. The movement is erratic, ineffectual, and potentially damaging to the tissues involved.

The interfering factors of neuromuscular function not only make the agonist muscles erratic but momentarily interfere with the reciprocal relaxation reflex. By not synchronously relaxing, the antagonistic muscle may be mechanically injured. In addition to the impairment of the neuromuscular coordination by emotional factors, there is a secondary involvement of the autonomic nervous system. Up to this point it has been the somatic nervous system that has controlled muscular action. This is the nervous system under "voluntary" control. In essence, the willed function of desired movement is transmitted from the brain to the spinal cord to the muscle through the somatic nervous system which is under voluntary control. This neurological mechanism is one in which acquired skill and efficient movement can be enhanced by training. It can, of course, be impaired with inadequate training, infrequent utilization, fatigue, and all of the other emotional components previously described.

The other system, the autonomic system, is not under voluntary control and is transmitted through an entirely different portion of the nervous system. This system is essentially one which goes to blood vessels, glands, and to organs that are automatic in their functions such as the heart, lungs, kidney, stomach, and so on. This autonomic nervous system also goes to the somatic muscles of the skeleton and has a precise function, mostly automatic, rather than being under voluntary control (Goldstein, Grinker, Heath, Oken, & Shipman, 1964). Muscle tone is considered to be a function of both the somatic and the autonomic nerve supply to the muscle. Muscle contraction that is initiated by the emotions occurs via the autonomic nervous system. The term "tension," from a muscular viewpoint, can be considered as a sustained muscle contraction initiated via the autonomic nervous system as a residual or sequelae of emotional tension (Cameron, 1944). This is mediated both electrically and chemically with a marked influence of hormonal secretions which are secondary to emotional arousal. Sustained muscle contraction may be termed "muscular tension," essentially a persistent contraction of the muscle which, when in the agonist muscle, make function inefficient and, in the antagonist muscle, causes failure of relaxation, thus disruption of normal movement.

There also is muscular "spasm." The spasm is a reflex muscular contraction of an isometric nature. This isometric label indicates sustained contraction or shortening with failure of relaxation or elongation. Muscular spasm may be protective in that it is purposeful. Purposeful, hence protective, spasm may be the result of pain or inflammation in which the spasm prevents joint movement. This protective spasm should be short-lived, in essence be sustained for the duration of inflammation or injury healing. In this context muscle spasm is essentially normal or at least desirable. Muscle spasm or sustained muscular contraction that is excessive or prolonged as a result of anxiety, apprehension, anger, of depression is not only purposeless, but also detrimental. Such sustained muscular contraction interferes with normal neuromuscular function. This sustained contraction, however, is also a common source of nociceptive stimuli which become the cause of pain as well as dysfunction. The mechanism of muscular pain is well documented (Sicuteri, Franchi, & Michelacci, 1974). A muscle that contracts normally releases metabolites of this muscular activity. These are the waste products that normally remain in the tissue rather briefly and are eliminated when the muscle relaxes and new blood flow to that muscle returns. These waste products, however, are potentially irritating to the muscle. They include lactic acid, substance P, histamine, and numerous other chemicals. As a rule these chemical "metabolic waste products" are not produced in excess nor allowed to remain too long within the muscular tissues. Normal muscle contraction also constricts the blood vessels within that muscle belly during the contraction phase. This causes a brief transient period of ischemia.

This period of ischemia is normally limited in duration and intensity. The limitation of the period of ischemia is controlled by a well-balanced delicate neurophysiological chemical mechanism. The metabolites of muscular contraction chemically effect the nerve endings within the muscle that reflexly transmit impulses to the spinal cord and initiate a reflex relaxation with corresponding resumption of blood flow. If a muscle contraction is held for too long a period of time there is an accumulation of irritating metabolites. The sustained muscular contraction further constricts the blood vessels and thus increases the ischemia. This ischemia, due to vasocontriction, sustains an increasing amount of accumulation of metabolites which in turn are irritants, causing the muscle to contract excessively and a vicious metabolic cycle results. The sustained muscular contraction now becomes a definite source of pain as the accumulated metabolites and the ischemic muscles initiate pain producing nocioceptive stimuli.

In addition to the component of muscular contraction in sustained isometric contraction termed "spasm" or "tension," there are also the side effects upon the connective tissues of the joints involved. The connective tissues that surround the muscles as well as the connective tissues that surround the joints in the capsule now cannot passively elongate to their normal elasticity. This now causes the capsule to constrict, which it does by virtue of the sustained contraction and the created ischemia. The ischemia enhances the invasion of fibrous tissues and the deterioration of collagen fibers. The ischemia also encourages the intersecting collagen fibers of the connective tissue to adhere with further limitation.

This vicious cycle is a pattern that is exhibited in the tense, anxious, angry patient in whom the emotional factors now become evident in the physical aspects of the musculoskeletal system. The tense, angry, anxious person now is "uptight" in that movement is restricted, limited, erratic, uncoordinated. Musculoskeletal pain, impairment, and disability now become self-apparent. The following algorithm is postulated to account for the mechanisms by which pain and dysfunction affects the neuromusculoskeletal system.

SUMMARY

Normal pain-free neuromusculoskeletal function demands normal structural joint alignment, normal joint capsular flexibility, normal muscle strength and endurance, and normal neuromuscular coordination. This normal pain-free motion also presumes no interference from autonomic emotional dysfunction. Failure to maintain physical flexibility and physiological strength and endurance by proper exercise may result in impairment. Excessive autonomic interference may also cause a transient type of malfunction and pain but also lays the groundwork for structural malfunction. Repeated persistent abnormal psychoneurological factors can lead to structural abnormalities. The connective tissue component of function and malfunction and its relationship to soft tissue musculoskeletal pain is thus evident. Normal musculoskeletal function is under voluntary control and can be maintained by proper activities, exercises, and proper application of the activities of daily living. The interfering emotional autonomic and somatic neurological component can be modified and influenced by training, medication, counseling, and other therapeutic modalities.

REFERENCES

Cailliet, R. (1969). Mechanics of joints. In S. Licht (Ed.), *Arthritis and physical medicine* (Vol. 2). Baltimore, MD: Waverly Press.

Cameron, D. E. (1944). Observation in the patterns of anxiety. *American Journal of Psychiatry, 101,* 36.

Eastoe, J. J. (1967). Composition of collagen and allied proteins. In G. N. Ramachandran (Ed.), *Treatise on collagen* (Vol. 1). London: Academic Press.

Eldred, E. (1967). Functional implication of dynamic and static components of the spindle response to stretch. *American Journal of Physical Medicine, 46,* 129–140.

Goldstein, I. B., Grinker, R. R., Heath, H. A., Oken, D., & Shipman, W. G. (1964). Study in psychophysiology of muscle tension: I. Response specificity. *Archives of General Psychiatry, 11,* 322.

MacConaill, M. A. (1965). Mechanical anatomy of motion and posture. In S. Licht (Ed.), *Therapeutic exercises.* Baltimore, MD: Waverly Press.

MacConaill, M. A. (1950). The movement of bones and joints: The synovial fluid and its assistants. *Journal of Bone and Joint Surgery* (B), *32*(2), 244–252.

Paockop, D. J., Kovirokko, K. J., Toderman, L., & Gozman, N. O. (1979). The biosynthesis of collagen and its disorders. *New England Journal of Medicine, 301*(1), 13–23; *31*(2), 77–85.

Radin, E. L., Paul, I. L., & Rose, R. M. (1975). Mechanical factors in the aetiology of osteoarthroses. *Annals of Rheumatic Diseases, 34* (Supp.), 132–133.

Sicuteri, F., Franchi, J., & Michelacci, S. (1974). Biochemical mechanisms of ischemic pain. In *Advances in neurology* (Vol. 4, pp. 39–44). New York: NY: Raven Press.

5

Functional Assessment of the Musculoskeletally Impaired Patient

Cynthia C. Smith

Private Practice
Bethesda, MD

Frances Oakley
Gloria Furst
Lynn Gerber

National Institutes of Health
Bethesda, MD

INTRODUCTION

Classical concepts of rehabilitation are characterized by a pathologically oriented view of the individual that is reflected in the assessment process. More recent trends in rehabilitation, however, focus on the concept of function and adaptation, thereby necessitating a change in the assessment process. Since the goal of rehabilitation is to restore and enhance adaptive function, functional assessment constitutes an essential component of the process. Input from a variety of disciplines including occupational therapy, physical therapy, physical medicine, and speech therapy provide a comprehensive approach to assessment and treatment. This chapter identifies the dimensions that comprise an individual's adaptive level of functioning and presents a model which can be used for assessing function in people with musculoskeletal impairment.

DIMENSIONS OF FUNCTION

In the broadest sense, function is described as the performance or action of a person. How and why people perform is a complex process. A person's actions are an attempt to satisfy the external demands of the environment while, at the same time, an attempt to satisfy internal demands for performance. Internal demands include needs, beliefs, values, interests, and personal desires for competence. In other words, a person's performance is in response to the complex process of maintaining a state of equilibrium between internal and environmental demands. The relationship between the person and the environment is a dynamic process in which not only the person, but also the environment, may support or constrain function. Furthermore, each person encounters a variety of environments such as work, school, or home in which he or she must perform with each environment dictating various expectations for performance.

Function can be characterized as either adaptive or maladaptive. The concept of adaptation acknowledges that daily living involves the process of adjusting to environmental conditions (Kielhofner, 1985). Adaptive functioning occurs when a harmonious relationship between the person and the environment has been achieved. For example, to judge a person as functioning adaptively in the role of worker, he or she should be able to derive a sense of satisfaction, meaning, and enjoyment in working while simultaneously performing work responsibilities in a satisfactory manner.

Maladaptive functioning, on the other hand, occurs when the relationship between the person and the environment is in disequilibrium—that is, the person's internal demands and/or the demands of the environment are not satisfied.

To assess a person's adaptive level of functioning, it is not enough to assess the internal status of the person. The process of interaction between the person and his or her environment as well as the environmental factors that influence this process must be assessed. The same person may function adaptively in some environments while functioning maladaptively in others (Kielhofner, 1985).

THE MODEL OF HUMAN OCCUPATION

The Model of Human Occupation (Kielhofner, 1980a, b; Kielhofner & Burke, 1980; Kielhofner, Burke, & Igi 1980) conceptualizes individuals as open systems in interaction with the environment via a cycle of intake, output, feedback, and throughput (see Figure 5.1). Intake is the incorporation of information into the system, output is the export of some action, feedback is the reception of information regarding the process and consequences of the system's output, and throughput is the internal rearrangement that occurs when information comes into the system through intake and feedback. The model of human occupation provides a framework to assess a person's level of functioning on a continuum from adaptive to maladaptive. In this model, adaptive functioning is described in part by the person's internal status or throughput. Function is measured by skills, habits, roles, interests, values, and feeling of competence, and in part by interactions with the environment. The internal status or throughput of an individual comprises three interrelated subsystems which are arranged hierarchically in the following descending order: volition, habituation, and performance (see Figure 5.2).

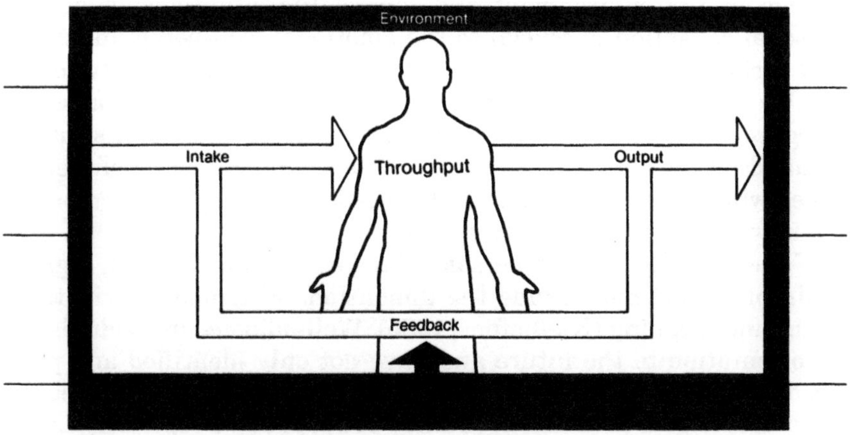

FIGURE 5.1. The Human System in Interaction with the Environment

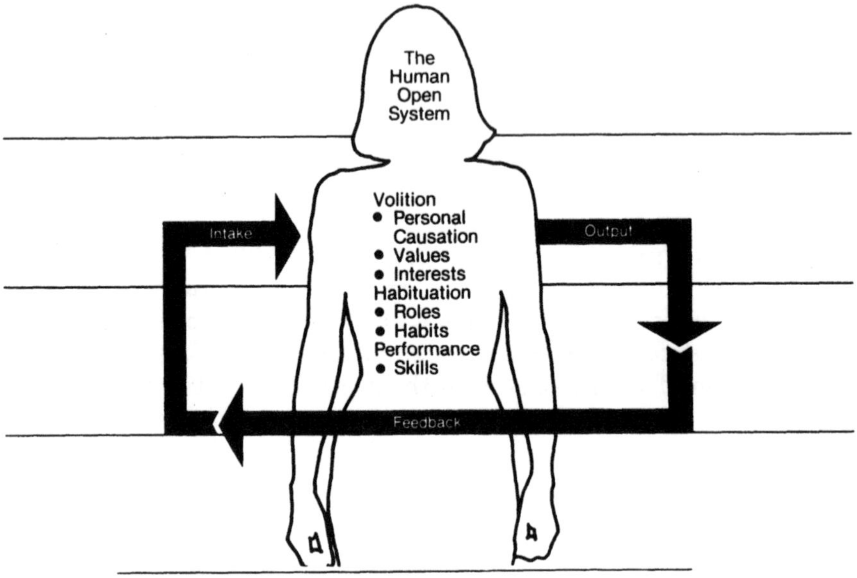

FIGURE 5.2. The Model of Human Occupation

Volition Subsystem

The volition subsystem is responsible for initiating or enacting behavior and contains three components that influence decisions for action: personal causation, values, and interests. Personal causation refers to an individual's feelings of efficacy regarding his or her ability to effect change in the environment and control life situations. A sense of personal causation is crucial to the emotional well-being and competent performance of an individual. People who are successfully adapted display socially adjusted behavior, are able to accurately process feedback from the environment, are able to assess their skills and the demands of the environment, and have encountered successful experiences which foster a positive self-concept and a sense of competency (Oakley, Kielhofner, & Barris, 1985).

Values are defined as personal images of what is good, right, or desirable to do and include the dimensions of temporal orientation, goals, and meaning (Kielhofner, 1985). Well-adjusted individuals have an orientation to the future and have not only identified and prioritized their goals, but also are capable of identifying and executing behavior for goal attainment (Oakley et al., 1985). People who have no goals or have difficulty establishing priorities for such are candidates for maladaptation because they cannot use existing skills effectively to organize daily life.

Meaning is also important for successful adaptation and is derived from interaction with one's environment. Meaning not only provides a framework for interpreting and ordering events that occur, but links the events in such a way as to create a sense of continuity or wholeness.

Interests are preferences for action. Well-adjusted individuals typically have identified areas of interest which they routinely pursue (Oakley et al., 1985).

The components of the volition subsystem—personal causation, values, and interests—work together as the motivating force to enact behavior.

Habituation Subsystem

The habituation subsystem is responsible for triggering and maintaining everyday behavior into patterns and routines. Habits and roles are the components of this subsystem. Habits are automatic routines of behavior that support role performance while roles provide opportunities for performance. People who are considered to be adaptive typically have incorporated into their lives a number of vocational and avocational roles that provide a sense of identity and satisfaction in maintaining a balance among these roles while allowing adequate time for rest and sleep (Oakley et al., 1985).

Performance Subsystem

The performance subsystem is responsible for producing action and its component is skills. Skills consist of motor, cognitive, and perceptual elements that allow a person to produce behavior.

Environment

The environment refers to the objects, tasks, social groups, and culture with which a person interacts. The components (personal causation, values, interests, goals, roles, habits, and skills) of the three subsystems, in interaction with the environment, provide a framework to identify and assess adaptive behavior. If the components are intact, in harmony, and congruent with environment demands, then the output is adaptive behavior. If, on the other hand, components are absent, in disharmony, or incongruent with environmental demands, then the output is maladaptive behavior.

PHYSICIANS CONSIDERATION IN MUSCULOSKELETAL DISORDERS

Patients with musculoskeletal disorders present with a wide variety of problems, which may initially seem to be confined to performance, but when the problem persists or intensifies, has impact on the normal routines and stereotype behaviors forcing reevaluation of values and goals.

Musculoskeletal disorders include those processes that affect bones, joints, ligaments, tendon, and muscle. Some of these disorders are systemic and inflammatory and involve more than a few joints and/or muscles. Systemic illness is characterized by abnormalities in the blood suggestive of an inflammatory process. These abnormalities are manifested by anemia, high sedimentation rate, and often the presence of abnormal circulating antibodies. Diseases that are systemic include rheumatoid arthritis, psoriatic arthritis, Reiter's syndrome, systemic lupus, polymyositis, and some forms of juvenile arthritis to name a few. Diseases or processes that are usually confined to a few joints or musculotendinous junctions may have local inflammation and lack the blood abnormalities described above. Examples include lower back pain, fibrositis, osteoarthritis, gout, and pseudogout. Discussion of the classification of musculoskeletal disorders and their natural history is available (Rodman, Shumacher, & Zvaifler, 1983; Kelly, Harris, Ruddy, & Sledge, 1985).

A number of musculoskeletal disorders are associated with problems in other organ systems of the body and need to be identified as part of a complete evaluation. Most notably, systemic lupus can involve heart, kidneys, and central nervous system; rheumatoid arthritis can involve lung and peripheral nervous system; polymyositis can involve the heart and lung; psoriatic arthritis and Reiter's involve the skin; and juvenile arthritis may involve the eyes.

PHYSICIAN EVALUATION

During the initial evaluation of a patient with musculoskeletal problems, determination of anatomical abnormalities by careful physical examination is done. This includes neurological evaluation, determination of joint alignment and deformity, muscle strength and range of motion of joints. Laboratory results are useful in determining whether the process is systemic and/or inflammatory. When these tests demonstrate a systemic, inflammatory process, medications are selected to try to control it. Whereas if the process is a local one and there is little evidence for inflammation, medication is less often used and treatments tend to be confined to the affected anatomical area. Radiographic abnormalities often support clinical impressions and confirm the need for pharmacological intervention in an attempt to control a destructive process.

The examination must extend past the static measurements of alignment, strength, and range of motion. More complex activity and dynamic measurements are necessary to evaluate a patient's performance level. Grip strength, the time it takes to walk 50 feet, and stride characteristics add important information. All of these are observed, quantifiable, "objective" measures.

Stamina—the ability to sustain a certain level of performance—is measurable, but is rarely done in patients with musculoskeletal disability. Information about sustained performance and stamina is usually obtained from history or self-report in the form of an activities of daily living questionnaire. A review of currently used assessments is available (Gerber, 1985).

The conclusion of a survey of rheumatologists performed to determine what they believed was important to know about patients with musculoskeletal disease concluded that mobility, pain, role activity and level of independence in self-care were the important measures to assess (Bombardier, Tugwell, Sinclair, Dok, Anderson, & Buchanan, 1982). With information in each of the above areas, referrals to orthopedics, physical therapy, occupational therapy, and social work could be made. These parameters could then be used as outcome measures as well.

Important to note is that often the outcome measures are self-reports about what the individual can do. It is often of interest to know what a patient is doing. Disability in part may be the disequilibrium between what one can do or states he can do and what is actually done. The health care professional needs to know if such disparity exists.

Patients with inflammatory disease of the musculoskeletal system frequently cannot predict a level of performance from day to day. Unlike persons who have an event that occurs at a moment in time, and that remains fixed, rheumatic diseases tend to be relapsing and remitting. It is not unusual for a patient to be immobile in the morning but functional in the evening or to have good and bad days, which may vary with the weather, moon, stars, and so on. This inability to predict what one's performance level may be can limit rehabilitation potential. The severity of the disease, the rapidity with which function declines, and the length of time it takes to induce a remission or stabilize the functional level are all parameters important to consider in determining whether the level of function is commensurate with the anatomical and physiological problems. When anatomy and function are not aligned, a review of the physical, laboratory, and psychosocial findings must be performed. A review of medications and referral to occupational therapy and social service should be made to further explore the dysfunctions.

CLINICAL JUDGMENT

Clinical judgment is based upon a collection of information that measures strength, range of motion, pain, laboratory indices of inflammation, and clinical measures of inflammation and swelling. It also includes a sense of how the patient is doing globally and compared with the previous visit and a much prior one if that information is available. Upon these objective, subjective, comparative, and global assessments, referral criteria and selection of medications are made and outcomes to treatment are assessed.

MUSCULOSKELETAL DISORDERS AND THE HUMAN OPEN SYSTEM

As noted earlier, the model of human occupation provides a framework for assessing the motivational and behavioral as well as physical, social, and environmental factors that influence the actions of an individual and together define function. Following is a brief discussion of how musculoskeletal disorders effect the components of the human open system and how these components can be evaluated.

Effect on the Performance and Habituation Subsystem

Most patients with musculoskeletal disabilities are primarily concerned with problems related to performance, therefore evaluation of this subsystem first facilitates cooperation with a more complete assessment of all subsystems. The performance subsystem, the ability to execute motor activities, is affected variably by muscle spasticity, weakness and/or atrophy, joint deformities, pain, and fatigue. Attempts to perform previously routine activities and daily habits following disability can result in feedback that performance is inadequate. Because the skills required to perform the routine daily activities necessary for performance of social roles have been altered, and new, disability-related routines and habits such as medication, exercise, and home therapy need to be included, the habituation subsystem is also affected.

Effect on the Volition Subsystem

Personal interests, values, and feelings of competency within the volition subsystem that influences decisions for action may all be affected by the feedback into the system that interaction with the environment(s) has been altered. Reduced belief in the ability to do routine activities effectively and the expectation that future attempts to act may also not meet performance expectations may result in loss of self-esteem. Personal goals and standards are both directly related to knowledge of present and future abilities to function. Persons with musculoskeletal disabilities may be severely hampered in their ability to predict present or future function and therefore have great difficulty with establishing goals and meeting their standards of performance that existed prior to disability.

Potential Maladaptations

Changes in the ability to conform to role behaviors such as attending classes, doing household activities, shopping, social encounters, working, child care, and so on may have several consequences. The disabled individuals, as well as those around them, may no longer expect participation in roles considered to be meaningful and valuable prior to disability. New roles, acquired because of disability, may be perceived as less valuable. For example, a working parent who cannot return to work and must assume the role of homemaker may derive little self-esteem if this new role is not valued by the individual as well as others. Alternatively, the disabled individual may continue to participate in role activities established prior to disability inadequately and/or ineffectively. The result, again, can be loss of self-esteem as well as a tendency to withdraw from any participation in role activities. The value and meaning of various role and leisure activities is often altered as changed physical abilities necessitate changing priorities for action. Activities which previously had developed into habits or routines requiring little thought or preparation may become more difficult and time consuming to do. These activities, therefore, may change in value because of the challenge required to deal with them. Self-care and household activities often become more important after disability as do preoccupation with activities related to the role of patient such as exercises, rest, and medication routines. A frequent occurrance in this process of changing habits and roles is reduced participation or lack of participation in recreation and leisure activities and roles of friend, spouse, and so on, in order to fulfill productive roles that have become more difficult. The result of these changes on volition can be an imbalance in the relationship of work, leisure, and rest which can lead to maladaptation.

Communication and interaction skills become increasingly important for those with chronic, progressively disabling diseases. As physical abilities decrease, and an increasing number of routine activities become more difficult or impossible to accomplish alone, adaptation depends on the ability to appropriately seek help and cooperation from others. For example, a disabled individual may be able to vacuum a room or work on a large stack of reports at the office only if another person is asked to take out the vacuum cleaner or move the reports from where they are stored.

Table 5.1 is a partial list of some of the evaluation tools which may be used for assessing the status of the open system of persons with musculoskeletal disabilities. A brief description and references for each assessment is included in an annotated reference at the end of

Table 5.1.
Evaluation Tools for Assessment of Musculoskeletal Disabilities

Performance Subsystem	Reference
Skills	
Passive range of motion	A
Active range of motion	A
Eye hand/fine-hand coordination	A
Rheumatoid Arthritis Hand Assessment	B
Physical capacities evaluation	A
Activities of Daily Living	A
Household Activities	A
Home Evaluation	A
Functional Status Index	C
Health Assessment Questionnaire	D
Habituation Subsystem	
Roles	
Occupational History	E
Occupational Therapy Functional Screening Tool	F
Activity Questionnaire	G
Role Checklist	H
Habits	
Occupational History	
Occupational Therapy Functional Screening Tool	
Activity Questionnaire	

this chapter. A more complete list of evaluations of volition, habituation, and the environment, including descriptions and sources for each evaluation can be found in Keilhofner (1985). Many evaluations for assessing the performance subsystem are available in occupational, physical, and/or speech therapy departments. Two case examples are presented to demonstrate application of some of the evaluation tools for assessing function of musculoskeletally disabled individuals.

CASE STUDY: SPASMODIC TORTICOLLIS

William

This 54-year-old white male, diagnosed with spasmodic torticollis, presented with symptom of abnormal head posture with chin elevated and turned to the right. He was referred to rehabilitation medicine for training in relaxation procedures to decrease neck musculature tension.

William had been followed for one year by the referring neurologist and had been placed on a drug regimen (Artane, Librium, Laprison). Previous evaluation by physical medicine at another hospital described abnormal posturing and treatment at that time was physical therapy to maintain neck mobility. Current evaluation by physical medicine substantiated these findings and referred William to Occupational Therapy for relaxation training and stress management.

EVALUATION

To assess his adaptive level of functioning, evaluation of William's occupational behavior included interviews and a battery of written inventories which included the Interest and Role Checklist and the Activity Record. Range of Motion was also assessed.

Performance

William continued all self-care, daily living, and household tasks including driving a car. He described pain and fatigue as contributory to a decrease in his activity. Measurements showed head rotation limited in active range of motion (L 30%, R 90%) with passive range of motion within normal limits. He could not turn and maintain his head to the left. His back stiffened when leaning back in a chair or lying down.

Transferring from a chair or bed caused pain. He reported that stress and tension increased tightness of his neck muscles.

Occupational History

William completed two years of college which he discontinued due to his inability to stand and talk in front of people; his intent in college was to become a teacher. He described the anxiety caused by practice teaching and other similar experiences as too disabling. After leaving college, he completed two years of military service. The spasmodic tortocollis symptoms appeared for the first time during this period. Upon honorable discharge from the military, he joined a large corporation where he remained for 30 years in personnel work. An exacerbation of symptoms began when he was 35 years old when his position in this company was in jeopardy and again at age 50 when job responsibilities became stressful. The last symptoms were severe enough to necessitate his retirement. Upon retirement, he worked in a real estate office which he found to be a difficult transition time. Gradually, he became self-employed in this area managing his own rental properties. Presently, this is a daily activity but limited to less than one hour a day.

Interest

The modified Interest Checklist (Matsutsuyu, 1967) showed a pattern of maintaining participation in activities in which he had strong interest though the level of interest had diminished in those activities requiring physical coordination and endurance. His interests supported those occupational roles which he valued highly and was presently performing.

Activity Record (ACTRE)

The ACTRE showed time management to be in these proportions:

Household activities	39%
Sleep	34%
Transportation	11%
Rest	6%
Recreation/leisure	5%
Work	4%

Table 5.2 summarizes William's day in terms of human open system components.

Table 5.2.
William's Activity Record Results

		Percent Waking Hours	
		Initial	Discharge
VOLITION SUBSYSTEM			
Personal Causation			
How well the activity was done	very poorly	0	0
	poorly	13	0
	average	53	21
	well	35	79
Interests			
Time in recreation and leisure			
Enjoyment of activities	not at all	6	31
	very little	14	12
	some	50	48
	alot	36	40
Values			
Meaningfulness of activity	not meaningful	0	0
	slightly meaningful	5	0
	meaningful	89	43
	very meaningful	6	57
Value of activities to others	not at all	0	0
	very little	5	0
	some	73	33
	alot	22	64
HABITUATION SUBSYSTEM			
Roles			
Role relating activity			
work		4	18
household activity		39	0
recreation and leisure		5	31
PERFORMANCE SUBSYSTEM			
Skills			
Level of difficulty	very difficult	0	0
	difficult	16	0
	slightly difficult	7.81	11
	not difficult	77	89

Role Checklist

The Role Checklist showed William as having continuous incumbency (that is, he performed the role in the past and present and plans to perform it in the future) in five occupational roles—worker, caregiver, home maintainer, family member, and religious participant, all but home maintainer being considered very valuable. He was not presently performing in the very valuable roles of student and friend but planned to resume these roles in the future.

Values

William's values did not appear to be conflictful. His illness had compromised the goals he presently set for himself and was cause for frustration in his feelings of adequacy in role performance.

He spent less time with his family, retiring early for he felt his presence was depressing to them. He described himself as "getting rid of people," "shucking them off—I just don't feel up to it" whereas previously, the routine of the household was described as "an open-door policy" for friends.

SUMMARY: WILLIAM

William is a retired, middle-aged, married father of three who had reestablished a daily schedule for himself outside of the active work arena but also away from previously valued activities of athletics, family participation and socialization with friends.

Though his spasmodic tortocollis does not exclude work, it does constrain it and heavily inhibits all those activities which William construes as "the good life," in other words, quality of life issues.

TREATMENT GOALS AND STRATEGIES

The objective of treatment was to help William regain a feeling of muscle control in environments where he felt or anticipated tension or stress. The choice of action was to establish realistic treatment goals, teach William relaxation techniques, establish daily practice patterns, identify stressful life situations, and apply relaxation techniques to life situations which he defined as stressful.

REEVALUATION: WILLIAM

Six months after initiation of treatment, the evaluation of William's occupational behaviors were as follows:

Performance Subsystem

Daily activity increased in the area of work by thirteen percent. He no longer finds daily activity difficult (Table 5.2). Pain had decreased.

Subjective reports of increased performance were (a) when feeling less tension, he feels he can keep his head "more centered" when walking; (b) he could turn and maintain control of his head enough to maintain conversation in a group; (c) he sensed that he was walking faster and resumed moderate exercising "with no backlash;" (d) he could sit in his "old chair" and stayed up later with family; (e) his son commented upon an increase in his father's energy; and (f) he described a feeling of inner calm and in his terms "when the insides are calm the muscles are calm." According to the ACTRE, a balance of work/leisure/rest is now in a pattern appropriate for retired individuals.

Habituation Subsystem

Friends have begun to drop in again at the house, his quantifying proof being that he now keeps running out of beer. He has chosen to encounter stressful situations as a father and a friend. In this first instance, choosing to be with his son and actively providing support during a legal matter involving police and lawyers. He began visiting friends, going out to dinner with them—an activity he had relinquished over five years ago because he felt he could not maintain adequate conversation tending to disregard the person on his left due to the head/neck tension.

His increased participation with his family were the instances of application that he related most often, setting new goals in this area over the course of treatment. The family's appreciation for his added time and attention were reported with pride.

Volition Subsystem

William reported resuming activities of previous interest and most notably reported a feeling of control over his daily activities. He indicated participating in very meaningful activities 57 percent of the time (Table 5.1). In choosing to initiate activities, it was no longer predicated on the presence or absence of neck tension. He now entered activities with a feeling that if neck tension began, he had a skill with which to deal with it. He has returned to performing at his previous level of intensity in life roles he considered very valuable and to those activities in which he had a strong interest.

CASE STUDY RHEUMATOID ARTHRITIS*

Sarah

This 37-year-old white female was referred to Rehabilitation Medicine for evaluation and treatment of ongoing activity of daily living problems arising from rheumatoid arthritis of five years standing. Anti-inflammatory medications were prescribed and monitored. She was referred to Occupational Therapy for activities of daily living evaluation, education in energy conservation, and joint protection and hand splints.

In addition to evaluations for upper extremity function a battery of assessments was administered to determine the degree to which Sarah is successfully adapting her occupational lifestyle to the arthritic condition and the impact of her occupational behavior on the arthritis. The complete assessment battery included an arthritis hand evaluation, joint range measurement, occupational history, modified interest checklist, activity record (ACTRE), Table 5.3, and the Role Checklist.

EVALUATION

Upper Extremity Findings and Performance

Joint range is decreased and weakness demonstrated in Sarah's shoulders, wrists, and fingers. Prehension is functionally weak due to synovitis and pain in MCP joints and PIP joints bilaterally. Pain is migratory and primarily involves the hands and feet. She demonstrated difficulty in working with fine tasks and adaptations for eating utensils were provided. Sensation was within normal limits.

Occupational History

Sarah is a credetialed elementary educator who interrupted her career after one year of work to become a full-time homemaker rearing her two children who are now in their early teens. She had planned to

---

*Case study information from Workshop: How the Model of Human Occupation Works: Clinical Application" NIH 1983.

Table 5.3.
Sarah's Activity Record Results

		Percent Waking Hours	
		Initial	Discharge
VOLITION SUBSYSTEM			
Personal Causation			
How well the activity was done	very poorly	0	0
	poorly	19	0
	average	79	83
	well	1	16
Interests			
Recreation/leisure		22	32
Enjoyment of activities	not at all	3	0
	very little	21	0
	some	51	61
	alot	24	39
Values			
Meaningfulness of activity	not meaningtul	8	0
	slightly meaningful	6	0
	meaningful	69	79
	very meaningful	16	23
Value of activities to others	not at all	5	0
	very little	3	0
	some	35	95
	alot	56	5
HABITUATION SUBSYSTEM			
Roles			
Role activities (HHA, WORK, ETC.)		30	44
Habits			
Rest during activity		1	22
PERFORMANCE SUBSYSTEM			
Skills			
Level of difficulty	very difficult	5	0
	difficult	6	0
	slightly difficult	41	46
	not difficult	46	59

return to teaching after the children were grown. Sarah appeared to enter the homemaker role primarily out of a sense of obligation to raise her children full time. While she generally voiced no complaints about the homemaker role, it does not seem that she had found it highly satisfying or important for her self-esteem. Concurrently, with her homemaker role prior to the onset of arthritis, she was an active volunteer in her church, supervising a school program. This volunteer work appeared quite satisfying and important to her. Since the onset of her arthritis, she relinquished the volunteer role and concentrated her efforts on the homemaker and patient role (i.e., compliance with treatment and rest practices for the arthritis which are quite demanding of her time). Sarah currently acknowledges that her children will be gone in the foreseeable future and she will need to find a new life role. She has some vague ideas about returning to teaching as a substitute teacher, but seems both apprehensive and uncertain about her future.

Sarah reported that moderate pain when performing daily living activities interferred with her previous methods of accomplishing tasks but she felt she completed them in a manner and to a level which was acceptable to her personal standards.

Interest Checklist

The modified interest checklist assesses past, present, and desired future interests. Of 80 items Sarah indicated 11 past strong interests in the past 10 years. Currently she maintains a strong interest in only two of those areas, singing and mending. She acquired one new interest, swimming, which she does as "therapy" for her arthritis. She indicated a wide range of activities in which she would like to participate in the future.

Her previous strong interest in bowling which involved both a physical and social component had been discontinued.

Role Checklist

She has been able to maintain continuous friend, family, home maintainer, and religious participant roles. Student and worker roles are no longer viable roles for her nor did she indicate a desire for them in the future. She presently planned to return to the interrupted role of volunteer.

Values

In an interview, Sarah indicated that the fulfillment of external expectations were of high priority to her and her personal satisfaction and self-development were secondary to these. The responsibilities of maintaining her home, caring for her family, and complying to treatment demands for her rheumatoid arthritis overrode her desires for activities which brought her a more personal satisfaction. This may indicate an imbalance of values which could be problematic.

SUMMARY: SARAH

Sarah is a pleasant and intelligent woman who has managed admirably in adjusting to a painful and debilitating disease. She has put considerable effort into arranging her life in order to meet two major obligations: (a) the obligation of conscientiously assuming the role of a chronically disabled person who must manage the disease process, and (b) the role of homemaker. In so doing, it appears, however, that Sarah has left little time for herself. She has undergone a loss of life interests, and her values reflect little attention to self and personal development and pleasure. She does not appear to feel competent, although she has had to make some very difficult adjustments which she managed quite well. Additionally, Sarah is in a period of coming change. With her children soon to be off to school or work, she will have greatly decreased homemaker role demands. At this time it will be important for her to develop a new major life role or roles in order to continue her positive adaptation to the disability.

TREATMENT

The occupational therapist and Sarah mutually explored her changing interest pattern using opportunities to try out new creative activities in the clinic. The findings of the activity record were reviewed with Sarah (Table 5.3). She was given feedback regarding her competent management of her homemaker role and her treatment regimen.

The issue of her feelings of competence were explored with her to ascertain whether she would like to put into her schedule some activities which might serve as a sense of competence. Her daily schedule was studied and revised to incorporate new and developing interests.

She took part in a six week patient education group in energy conservation and joint protection which is based on behavioral objectives. Adaptive aids, hand care, and hand splinting were incorporated in this education program so that health behaviors were defined, established, and supported (Furst, Gerber, & Smith, 1985).

SUMMARY

To summarize, the model of human occupation is based on the open system cycle. The volition subsystem establishes standards of performance and priorities for action. These standards have been developed over time and result from the feedback of interaction with the environment. Habits are the units of behavior that make it possible to structure time and conform to social roles such as homemaker, worker, friend, student, and so on. The skills necessary to enact habits and roles provide the means to facilitate the actions necessary for function. Changes within any subsystem affects the others as well, usually requiring readjustment to maintain adaptive functioning.

If performance standards and priorities remain unchanged, as physical abilities decline, frustration and increasing reluctance to participate in activities is often the result. If the goal of treatment is to facilitate adaptive functioning for the person with musculoskeletal disability, consideration of the factors which influence motivation, role participation, and the mechanics of developing routine behaviors are particularly important to assess. In order to address these areas, it is necessary to determine the status of each subsystem, the environments unique to the individual being evaluated, and the flow of the open system for that person.

ANNOTATED REFERENCE LIST FOR EVALUATION TOOLS

A. Hopkins, H. L., & Smith, H. D. (Eds.). (1978). *Willard and Spackman's occupation therapy* (5th ed., pp. 158–175). Philadelphia: Lippincott. Trombly, C. A., & Scott, A. D. (1977). *Occupational therapy for physical dysfunction*. Baltimore: Williams & Wilkins. Passive and active range of motion, eye-hand/fine-hand coordination, activities of daily living (ADL) evaluations, household activity (HHA) and home evaluations are all basic evaluations of physical capacity. Various forms of these can be found in most rehabilitation or physical medicine departments of hospitals and clinics as well as in the above texts.

B. Melvin, J. L. (1977). *Rheumatic disease: Occupational therapy and rehabilitation* (pp. 97–109). Philadelphia: F. A. Davis. The Rheumatoid Arthritis Hand Assessment evaluates the effect of this disease on the anatomical structures as well as the functional abilities of the hand and wrist.

C. Deniston, O. L., & Jette, A. (1980). A functional status assessment: Validation for an elderly population. *Health Services Research, 15*, 21–34.

Jette, A. M. (1980). Functional status index: Reliability of a chronic disease evaluation instrument. *Arch Phys Med Rehabil, 61*, 395–401. The Functional Status Index is a 20–30 minute interview format assessment of the patient's perception of performance of daily activities. Dependence, difficulty and pain are evaluated regarding performance of 5 categories of activities, including gross mobility, hand activities, personal care, interpersonal activities and home chores.

D. Fries, J. F., Spitz, P., Kraines, R. G., & Holman, H. R. (1980). Measurement of patient outcome in arthritis. *Arthritis and Rheumatism, 23,* 137–144. The Health Assessment Questionnaire (HAQ) is a self-administered assessment which includes an evaluation of performance of daily activities. Consideration of difficulty as well as assistance from others or equipment is included in deriving the disability index.

E. Moorehead, L. (1969). The occupational history. *American Journal of Occupational Therapy, 23,* 239–334. Florey, L., & Michelman, S. (1982). Occupational role history: A screening tool for psychiatric occupational therapy. *American Journal of Occupational Therapy, 32,* 301–308. The Occupational History is an interview used with teens and adults to determine current and past occupational strengths and weaknesses as well as related experiences.

F. National Institutes of Health, Department of Rehabilitation Medicine, Occupational Therapy Service, Building 10 Room 6S235, 9000 Rockville Pike, Bethesda, MD 20892. The Occupational Therapy Functional Screening Tool is a set of interview questions designed to elicit information regarding the status of volition, habituation and performance for adults and older teens. The results are scored on a 5-point scale and are used to determine the need for further, more specific evaluations and/or referral to other services.

G. National Institutes of Health, Department of Rehabilitation Medicine, Occupational Therapy Service, Building 10 Room 65235, 9000 Rockville Pike, Bethesda, MD 20892.
The Activity Record (ACTRE) is a log of activities for each ½ hour of the day for two consecutive weekdays. For each ½ hour, the patient answers questions relating to difficulty, how well done, meaning, value as well as rest, pain and fatigue. This evaluation is used with teens and adults to provide subjective, performance based data about daily behavior. Although not all components of each subsystem are evaluated, the information gained provides unique, patient reported data derived from the problem generating environments. Results are reported in terms of percent of waking hours (i.e., percent of time spent in role activities or percent of time spent meaningfully, etc.).

H. Oakley, F., Kielhofner G., Barris R., & Reichler R. (1986). The role checklist: Development and emperical assessment of reliability. *Occupational Therapy Journal of Research, 6*(3), 157–169. The Role Checklist developed by Oakley is a written instrument grounded in the theoretical framework of the Model of Human Occupation. It assesses an individual's perception of participation in roles with occupational components throughout the lifespan, provides information regarding an individual's capacity to maintain continuity in and a balance among roles, and indicates the degree to which each role is valued. It is appropriate for use with adolescents, adults, and elderly individuals with physical or psychosocial dysfunction. A study of the test/retest reliability indicated that the instrument is satisfactorily stable with a group of normal adults.

I. Schlegel R. P., & Crawford, C. A. (1976). Multidimensionality of internal -external locus of control. *Canadian Journal of Behavioral Science, 8*, 375–387. LeFaut, H. M. (1966). *Locus of control: Current trends in theory and research.* Hillsdale, NJ: Erlbaum (instrument reproduced here). Rotter, J. (1966). Generalized expectancies for internal versus external control of reinforcement. *Psychological Monographs, 80,* 1–28 (original instrument reproduced here). Internal-External (I-E) Scale is a self-administered questionnaire for older adolescents and adults as to belief in control over life events.

J. Morrow, G. R., Chiarello, R. J., & Derogatis, L. R. (1978). A new scale for assessing patients' psychosocial adjustment to mental illness. *Psychological Medicine, 8,* 605–610. Psychosocial Adjustment to Illness Scale-Self Report (PAIS-SR) is a multiple-choice scale to assess a patients psychosocial adjustment to current illness or residual disability. Health care orientation, vocational environment, domestic environment, sexual relationships, extended family relationships, social environment, and psychological distress are each rated on a 4-point scale yielding subtotal and total scores.

K. Meenan, R. R., Yelin, E. H., Nevitt, M., & Epstein, W. V. (1981). The impact of chronic disease: a sociomedical profile of rheumatoid arthritis. *Arthritis and Rheumatism, 24,* 544–549. Meenan, R. F., Anderson, J. J., Kazis, L. E., Egger, M. J., Altz-Smith, M., Samuelson, C. O., Willkens, R. R., Solsky, M. A., Hayes, S. P., Blocka, K. L., Weinstein, A., Guttadauria, M., Kaplan, S. B., & Klippel, J. (1984). Outcome assessment in clinical trials: Evidence for the sensitivity of a health status measure. *Arthritis and Rheu-*

matism, 27(12), 1344–1352. Arthritis Impact Measurement Scale (AIMS) assesses mobility, physical activity, dexterity, household activities (HHA), activities of daily living (ADL) social activity, anxiety, depression, and pain using a self-administered evaluation. The scores (0–10) are grouped into three categories: physical disability, depression, and pain.

L. Matsutsuyu, J. (1967). The interest checklist. *American Journal of Occupational Therapy, 32,* 628–630. The interest checklist is a list of 80 interests for which the patient indicates a casual, strong or no level of interest as well as add interests not on the list. Patients were also asked to describe their leisure activities.

REFERENCES

Bombardier, C., Tugwell, P., Sinclair, A., Dok, C., Anderson, G., & Buchanan, W. W. (1982). Preference for endpoint measures in clinical trials: Results of structured workshops. *Journal of Rheumatology, 9,* 798–801.

Furst, G. P., Gerber, L. H. & Smith, C. B. (1985). *Rehabilitation through learning: Energy conservation and joint protection—A workbook for persons with rheumatoid arthritis* (Stock No. 017-045-00107-4). Washington, DC: United States Government Printing Office.

Gerber, L. H. (1985). Rehabilitation of patients with rheumatic disease. In W. N. Kelley, E. D. Harris, S. Ruddy C. B. Sledge (Eds.), *Textbook of rheumatology* (2nd ed., Vol. *111*, pp. 1771–1172). Philadelphia: W. B. Saunders.

Kelley, W. N., Harris, E. D., Jr., Ruddy, S., & Sledge, C. B. (Eds.). (1985). *Textbook of rheumatology* (2nd ed.). Philadelphia: W. B. Saunders.

Kielhofner, G. (1980a). A model of human occupation, Part 2. Ontogensis from the perspective of temporal adaptation. *American Journal of Occupational Therapy, 34,* 657–663.

Kielhofner, G. (1980b). A model of human occupation, Part 3. Benign and vicious cycles. *American Journal of Occupational Therapy, 34,* 731–737.

Kielhofner, G. (1985). Occupational function and dysfunction. In G. Kielhofner (Ed.), *A model of human occupation: Theory and application* (pp. 63–75). Baltimore: Williams and Wilkins.

Kielhofner, G., & Burke, J. P. (1980). A model of human occupation, Part 1. Conceptual framework and content. *American Journal of Occupational Therapy, 34,* 572–581.

Matsutsuyu, J. (1967). The interest checklist. *American Journal of Occupational Therapy, 32,* 628–630.

Oakley, F. (1982). *The model of human occupation in psychiatry.* Unpublished master's project, Virginia Commonwealth University, Medical College of Virginia, Richmond, VA.

Oakley, F., Kielhofner, G., & Barris, R. (1985). An occupational therapy approach to assessing psychiatric patients' adaptive functioning. *American Journal of Occupational Therapy, 39,* 147–154.

Oakley, F., Kielhofner, G., Barris, R., & Reichler, R. (1986). The role checklist: Development and emperical assessment of reliability. *Occupational Therapy Journal of Research, 6*(3), 157–169.

Rodman, G., Schumacher, M. D., & Zvaifler, N. J. (Eds.). (1983). *Primer on the rheumatic diseases* (8th ed.). Atlanta: Arthritis Foundation.

6

Behavioral Approaches in the Treatment of Inflammatory Arthritis Disability—A Selected Review

Matthew H. Liang
Alison Partridge
Raymond Partridge

Brigham and Women's Hospital
Boston, MA

Over 100 forms of arthritis exist in which joint pain is either the dominant problem or occurs as part of a systemic illness. Of these, about 11 diseases and their subtypes have the potential of causing joint destruction (Decker, 1983). Some of these diseases have known causes and can be cured if treated appropriately. These are, by and large, arthritides caused by infectious agents or crystal deposition. Others have obscure causes or result from partially understood aberrations of the immune system, and have an unpredictable course.

In the United States, inflammatory arthritis affects about 10 million persons. The most prevalent is rheumatoid arthritis, with an estimated 7 million patients. The other inflammatory arthritides and their epidemiology are given in Table 6.1.

This chapter reviews the inflammatory arthritides, a conceptual framework for understanding rheumatic disability, the evidence linking psychosocial variables and disease causes, and the application of selected behavioral techniques in the treatment of these diseases.

THE NATURE OF THE INFLAMMATORY DISEASE PROCESS

Joint inflammation (synovitis) may occur as a result of crystal deposition (monosodium urate, calcium pyrophosphate, hydroxyapatite) infectious agents, immune complex formation, or by other undetermined mechanisms. Joint inflammation may progress inexorably despite treatment, remit (heal spontaneously or by treatment), or heal with ankylosis (bone or fibrous tissue bridging the joint space). The amount of joint damage caused by inflammation is directly related to the degree and duration of inflammation.

Persistent synovitis causes local destruction of cartilage, bone, and ligaments. Joint inflammation in rheumatoid arthritis may also occur with inflammation in other tissues such as blood vessels (vasculitis), which, if severe, can cause symptoms or dysfunction in the organs which the vessels nourish. Thus, in some patients, erosive joint disease may be compounded by vasculitis, causing ischemia of peripheral nerve, skin and muscle, inflammation of serosal surfaces (pleuritis, pericarditis), or by disorders associated with inflammatory disease such as Raynaud's Phenomenon, and the sicca syndrome. Except for infectious arthritis, inflammatory joint diseases take a variable, unpredictable course, ranging from a single attack to an aggressive, progressive course. The commonest pattern is a slowly progressive course punctuated by flares and remissions.

In most inflammatory arthritis, precise pathobiology is unknown. It is likely to be the result of a complex interplay between host, environment and, occasionally, a specific pathogen (infectious arthritis) or chemical substance (the crystalline arthritides). The inheritance of rheumatic disorders is not understood in great detail. Recent developments show a striking prevalence of tissue type HLA B27 in the spondyloarthropathies (ankylosing spondylitis, Reiter's disease, psoriatic arthritis, and inflammatory bowel disease). Specific modes of inheritance are not predictable, thus making genetic counseling impossible.

Table 6.1.
Epidemiology of Selected Forms of Inflammatory Arthritis

	Sex Ratio (women:men)	Race Ratio (black:white)	Estimated Prevalence (per 100)	Estimated Incidence (per 100)	Reference
Rheumatoid arthritis	3:1	1:1	0.3–1.0	0.075	
Ankylosing spondylitis	1:10	?	0.01	?	Masi & Medsger (1979)
Juvenile arthritis	1:5:1	?	0.02–0.10	?	Gewanter, Roghmann & Baum (1983)
Systemic lupus erythematosus	5:1	4:1	0.005	0.007	Masi & Medsger (1979)
Gout	1:7	—	0:3	0.1	Kellgren (1964)
Systemic sclerosis	2:5:1	2:1	?	0.001	Masi & Medsger (1979)
Polymyositis/dermatomyositis	2:1	3:1	?	0.001	Masi & Medsger (1979)

CONCEPTUAL FRAMEWORK FOR UNDERSTANDING DISABILITY

Disability in rheumatic disorders can be understood by building on the conceptual framework of Nagi (1965) who distinguished four aspects of disability. *Pathology* is characterized by a disease or injury which interrupts normal processes and includes the reaction of the body in order to restore it to normality. *Impairment* is defined as an anatomical loss or damage. An impairment may impose *functional limitations*. Unlike impairment, which is a physiological state, *disability* is seen as a form of behavior in reaction to that condition. Disability occurs when the functional limitations imposed by an impairment interfere with normal, expected activities or roles. In the context of work, disability occurs when functional limitations interfere with and interrupt job requirements.

The classification of disability by the World Health Organization (Wood, 1980) builds on Nagi's.

Impairment: any loss or abnormality of psychological, physiological, or anatomical structure or function. Impairments signify that a pathological state is exteriorized. In principle, this represents disturbance at the organ level. Some major subclasses of impairment include intellectual, language, aural, ocular, visceral, skeletal, and disfigurement.

Disability: any restriction or lack (resulting from an impairment) of ability to perform an activity in the manner or within the range considered normal for a human being. Disabilities reflect the consequences of impairment in terms of functional performance and activity. Disabilities represent disturbances at the level of the person, and the principal subclasses are concerned with behaving, communicating, personal care, locomotion, body disposition, and dexterity.

Handicap: any disadvantage for a given individual, resulting from an impairment or a disability, that limits or prevents the fulfillment of a role that is normal (depending on age, sex, and social and cultural factors) for that individual. Handicaps are concerned with interaction with and adaptation to the individual's surroundings, and they represent socialization of an illness experience. Thus, they occur when there is interference with the ability to sustain what may be designated as "survival roles"—orientation, physical independence, mobility, occupation, social integration, and economic self-sufficiency.

Inflammatory disease does not occur in a vacuum, but in a complex host with membership in a race, culture, and society which defines, in part, the illness created by the disease. The model is depicted in Figure 6.1. We believe that each step is reversible and the causal chain is modified by a number of factors, including environmental, social, or

(DISEASE ACTIVITY) x TIME ⇆ IMPAIRMENT ⇄ DISABILITY ⇄ HANDICAP

FIGURE 6.1. Inflammatory Disease Model

behavioral manipulation. The cause(s) of rheumatic diseases are influenced by host phenomena, such as host susceptibility, and possible environmental factors. Uncontrolled inflammatory arthritis leads to pain and limitation of normal joint motion and joint destruction. These elements contribute to inability to perform routines of daily life, self-care, employment, and recreational activities. This progression can be affected by health care (medical, surgical, and/or rehabilitative care). Access to care, health manpower and health-care financing determine, in part, the distribution and quality of help; patient compliance (cooperation in self-management) with a long-term program influences the effectiveness of these interventions. Whether or not inflammatory arthritis is controlled, an individual may suffer considerable social handicap from his or her affliction. Personality as well as environmental factors, for example, the existence of social support, can modulate the expression of social handicap in an individual with an arthritic disability. Strong personal motivation may overcome barriers resulting from structural deficits. Social support can diminish the emotional or psychological impact of chronic disease or make it worse if it is not effective. Cultural attitudes toward those with physical disabilities can increase the stress of having arthritis. The lack of public access to public buildings may increase their social isolation. Financial independence can moderate the effects of work disbility on the one hand, while on the other its absence increases the individual's dependency on society for basic needs.

PROTOTYPES OF RHEUMATIC DISABILITY

Musculoskeletal disease of all types is the leading cause of activity limitation in the United States, affecting 6.3 million individuals (Reynolds, 1978). It is useful to think of four major rheumatic disability prototypes.

Rheumatoid Disability (rheumatoid arthritis, seronegative polyarthritis, juvenile arthritis, psoriatic arthritis, Reiter's disease)

Rheumatoid disability is seen in polyarticular synovitis such as rheumatoid arthritis and juvenile rheumatoid arthritis. Rheumatoid disability is a prototype of disability characterized by polyarticular involvement, chronicity, variability, and occasional systemic symptoms.

Features of rheumatoid disability are affected by the person's age and social role. In children, polyarthritis affects biological, psychological, and social growth development. It may interfere with the attainment of educational and career goals, the acquisition of skills required for job, and family life. In adolescence it may interfere with emancipation from parents, interaction with peers, self-esteem, and body image. The treatment of children with arthritis is aimed toward controlling the basic disease process but needs to be done in a way that does not disrupt the patient's schooling or social development.

Polyarthritis in young adults may affect the critical issues of that stage which are separation from parents and home, training, career choice, achieving economic independence, peer relationships, and finding a mate.

In middle age, polyarthritis may affect career development, the raising of a family, family relationships, or a return to work when children are grown.

Polyarthritis occurring in older persons accentuates the aging process and accelerates physical dependency.

Osteoarthritis Disability

Osteoarthritis with its involvement of the small joints of the hand or of the weight-bearing joints in the lower extremity is characterized by its onset in middle or old age, its lack of systemic symptoms, and its mono or pauci articular involvement.

Osteoarthritis disability unfolds slowly paralleling the aging process and thus its psychosocial impact is not as apparent as rheumatoid disability. Indeed many individuals (and physicians) assume that musculoskeletal symptoms from osteoarthritis are an inevitable part of aging. In old age it is the most common form of chronic arthritis and a major reason for dependence and being homebound (Master et al., 1980).

Spondylitis Disability (ankylosing spondylitis, spondylitis associated with psoriasis, inflammatory bowel disease, juvenile arthritis)

Spondylitis disability is characterized by back stiffness and restrictive movement of the spine with occasional involvement of the peripheral joints, commonly the shoulder, hip, or knee. The disability is characterized by its male predominance, onset in young and middle-aged adults, and by the episodic nature of the peripheral arthritis. Spondylitis disability is compatible with good function except when it involves peripheral joints, in which case it can affect mobility. Occasionally patients may have iritis, aortic insufficiency, or lung disease as a part of the syndrome. Usually physical mobility and independence are maintained.

Spondylitis in young adult males may affect self-esteem, body image, leisure activities, and peer relationships particularly in the exercise and physique conscious milieu of the 1980s.

Systemic Rheumatic Disease Disability

This disability occurs in systemic rheumatic diseases such as systemic lupus erythematosus, scleroderma, polymyositis, vasculitis, and some patients with rheumatoid arthritis. Except for the latter, arthralgias are more common than arthritis and much of the disability is due to other organ involvement such as lung, heart, Raynaud's, sicca syndrome, or from constitutional symptoms such as fatigue and decreased endurance. These disabilities affect work capacity and socialization. Self-esteem and body image may be impaired by medications such as steroids or the disease process itself (such as seen in scleroderma with its tight skin and contractures of the joint). There are additional problems of having a rare disease and the fear and uncertainty of relapse or death.

PSYCHOSOCIAL FACTORS AND THE ETIOLOGY OF INFLAMMATORY RHEUMATIC DISEASE

Since the etiology of most inflammatory rheumatic diseases is unknown, it is not surprising that speculations about the role of psychological and behavioral factors has a long history (Anderson, Bradley, Young, McDaniel, & Wise, 1985; Genest, in press). Three hypotheses relating psychological factors and rheumatoid arthritis have been put forth (Meyerwitz, 1966).

1. Specificity hypothesis: Certain psychological characteristics exist prior to the onset of rheumatoid arthritis.
2. Disease onset hypothesis: Certain psychological characteristics cause rheumatoid arthritis.
3. Disease course hypothesis: Psychologic responses influence the course of rheumatoid arthritis.

Psychological symptoms, particularly anxiety and depression, are common in chronic disease (Cassileth et al., 1984; Liang et al., 1984), but cause and effect cannot be established by cross-sectional studies. Baum has pointed out that responses to questions may be affected by pain the patient is experiencing at the time the test is administered which undermines the validity of the responses when comparison is made with a "normal group" (Baum, 1982). More than a third of the Minnesota Multiphasic Personality Inventory (MMPI) questions are related to painful conditions and may well bias the results towards a neurotic score (Smythe, 1984; Pincus, Callahan, Bradley, Vaughn, & Wolfe, 1986). The diagnosis of rheumatoid arthritis is ill-defined in many studies.

Efforts to demonstrate a personality type in rheumatoid arthritis have been confounded by methodological differences in techniques for assessing psychological and emotional factors and may account for some of conflicting data. In one review of a series of studies it was found that 50 percent of the personality and psychological tests used were ad hoc ones devised by the investigators and not used by others (Baum, 1982).

The rheumatoid personality has been variously described as depressed (Blom & Nicholls, 1954), perfectionist (Robinson, 1957), restricted in emotional experience, and unable to express feelings of anger (Blom & Nicholls, 1954), but the patterns are variable and divergent (Moos, 1963; Ludwig, 1955).

Moos and Solomon (1964) analyzed personality characteristics of patients with rheumatoid arthritis. They failed to find many of the personality profiles previously described including dependency or athletic participation. The patients, however, seem to be more concientious, masochistic, self-sacrificing, and nonhostile than nonaffected siblings and perceived a greater degree of parental rejection than their siblings. Patients with most rapidly progressing disease experienced feelings of ego disintegration and concommitant anxiety and depression, reflecting a decrease in their capacity to maintain previously effective modes of coping.

Other studies show an apparent temporal relationship between major life changes and the onset or exacerbation of symptoms of rheumatoid arthritis (Shochet et al., 1969). Solomon showed that there was a similarity between personality characteristics of patients with RA and of patients with other immunologically mediated diseases such as ulcerative colitis, SLE, multiple sclerosis, and Graves disease (Solomon, 1981). No difference was noted, in another study, in MMPI scores between groups of patients with rheumatoid arthritis, multiple sclerosis, gastric ulcer, and lower back pain (Spergel, Ehrlich, & Glass,

1978), suggesting that a "chronic disease personality" might exist in a wide variety of patients.

When critically studied with well-defined patients and comparison groups, there appears to be no distinctive personality profile unique to rheumatoid arthritis, even in cross-sectional studies (Cassileth et al., 1984; Liang et al., 1984). Vollhardt and colleagues measured mood and psychological symptoms in 68 ambulatory arthritis patients with two standard questionnaires (Vollhardt, Ackerman, Grayzel, & Barland, 1982). Two groups had rheumatoid arthritis, and one group had other forms of arthritis. Patients with rheumatoid arthritis were divided on the basis of seropositivity with erosive disease and seronegativity and nonerosive disease. It was found that with the psychological measures used, the correct classification of the medical diagnosis could be made in 63–100 percent of patients. Among the patients with seropositive rheumatoid arthritis, a close association was found to exist between the psychological variables and a set of clinical characteristics.

A study of 500 patients with RA compared to matched controls by the Empire Rheumatism Council (1950) found no psychological differences between the groups. In a prospective study of early rheumatoid arthritis Crown and his colleagues found that these patients resembled normal controls, more than they did a group of patients with psychoneurosis (Crown & Crown, 1973). Longitudinal studies of rheumatoid arthritis have indicated that psychological disturbances occured when the disease became chronic and severe (Crown & Crown, 1975).

Mindham studied 28 patients with rheumatoid arthritis over the course of one year and found that psychiatric symptoms occured in patients with severe active disease which seriously interfered with daily activities (Mindham, Bagshaw, James, & Swannell, 1981). The study showed the appearance of affective symptoms to be related to the severity of RA in a general way without a specific link between psychiatric complications and any particular symptom or group of symptoms of the rheumatic disorder. A depressive illness in rheumatoid arthritis only occured where the patients were severely ill with pain, active disease, disability, and change in the pathological tests.

Studies in children with juvenile rheumatoid arthritis have also been conflicting. Henoch, Batson, and Baum (1978) studied 88 children with JRA and controls. In the JRA group there was a high incidence of divorce, separation of parents, or death of one parent. The prevalence of adoption was higher in the JRA children. Rimon, Belmaker, and Ebstein (1977) were unable to show any significant family interaction, but noted personality characteristics similar to those in adult RA.

In 1964 Moos described emotional trauma, separation, major surgery, and death in the family that led to the development of rheumatoid arthritis (Moos & Solomon, 1964). Evidence of stress before the onset of disease was found by Meyerowitz as an initiating factor in a study of monozygotic twins discordant for rheumatoid arthritis (Meyerowitz, 1968). The twin who developed the arthritis had the episode of stress prior to the development of arthritis. Rimon described two groups of patients with RA; one group had an acute onset, rapid disease progression, and a negative family history for RA associated with psychological conflict prior to onset; the other group had insidous onset, slow progression, a positive family history for RA that was unassociated with prior psychological stress (Rimon, 1969). Similar findings have been reported in juvenile rheumatoid arthritis although appropriate control groups were lacking (Rimon, Belmaker, & Ebstein, 1977).

Studies in other rheumatic diseases have shown little consistent evidence to support a preexisting "disease-predisposing" personality. In recent years fibrositis or the fibromyalgia syndrome has been an area of intense study. Fibrositis is a clinical syndrome occuring predominantly in younger and middle-aged women characterized by diffuse musculoskeletal pain, multiple painful muscular "trigger points," morning stiffness, sleep disturbance, and severe fatigue. Routine pathological and laboratory evaluation is normal. Many of the patients with these symptoms appear depressed and an association between the syndrome and psychological disorders has been suggested. Carefully controlled studies have given conflicting results from evidence of increased depression and "psychological disturbance" to studies that show no personality disturbances or depression (Bradley, Anderson, Young, & McDaniel, 1985). Again, as in the early studies with rheumatoid arthritis, the lack of a clearly defined set of disease characteristics or markers may result in population differences in the groups studied.

Thus, for rheumatoid arthritis and fibrositis, the best evidence suggests that psychological symptoms and patterns are the result and not the cause of these disorders. Whether stress or other phenomenon can modify the disease or its perception is moot.

Zeitlin has proposed a multicausal hypothesis for some rheumatic diseases such as rheumatoid arthritis that recognizes the role of genetic, infectious, autoimmune, and psychological factors that creates a "predisposition mix" (Zeitlin, 1977). A precipitating event such as psychological emotional change due to a catastrophic event may precipitate arthritis.

Ader and Cohen (1984) recognize that there is a marked interaction between psychological and physiological events in the control of homeostatic mechanisms. This also implies that there is a relationship between behavioral and immune processes, even though the mechanisms are yet to be elucidated. It is postulated that the immune system may be under the control of the central nervous system, although this is denied by some authors (Sell, 1972). A variety of experimental evidence links various immune processes to psychological factors (Rogers, Dubey, & Reich, 1979). Changes in lymphocyte response in stressed animals have been reviewed in a number of studies, particularly in mice. In vitro responses in lymphoid cells to marked stimulation with lipopolysaccharide and parnet show depression of driven lymphocyte proliferation initially and after one month early stimulation and increase in the activity.

Results on in vivo cellular responses have given conflicting results. Pitkin (1965) showed that there was a reduced delayed hypersensitivity response in mice when they were exposed to high temperature. Other studies have shown reduced inflammatory responses to auditory stress (Christian & Williamson, 1958; Funk & Jenson, 1967; Smith, Molomut, & Gottfried, 1960). Electric shock stimulation of guinea pigs, however, showed an increased reactivity in response to a topically applied chemical irritant (Guy, 1952; Meltrop & Visser, 1969). Perhaps the disparity of response in these cases is due to the difference of the test animal.

Alterations in the psychophysiological character of the host resulting from experimental manipulation in early life have been shown to modify immunological reactivity. These include mortality of mice with lymphocytic choriomeningitis virus as related to the nature of mother-young interactions (Hotchin, Benson, & Gardiner, 1970). Rats handled daily between birth and weaning have more pronounced primary and secondary responses to innoculation with Flagellin than do unstimulated controls when tested as adults (Solomon, Levine, & Kraft, 1968). There seems to be evidence that experiential factors such as the quantity and quality of the environmental stimulation, the variety of host factors in the nature of the immunogenic stimulus, and the parameters of immunological reactivity that are chosen for measurement are capable of modifying immune responses in animals. Also important are the temporal relationship between psychological and immunological events, procedural factors, and the differences in the experimental animals that are chosen. Recent research shows that it is possible to psychologically condition suppression of the response of T-cell dependent and T-cell independent antigens and to condition supression of a cell-mediated immune response. The effects of these conditioning studies have not been large, but they have been consistent and independently reproducible and cannot be accounted for simply on the basis of changes in corticosteroid levels.

Connective tissue diseases, particularly rheumatoid arthritis, display significant immunologic changes. Whether these changes in immunological reactivity can be accounted for by behavioral alterations in the afflicted person is uncertain. Results of studies give quite contrary results. Hendrie, Paraskevas, Baragar, and Adams (1971) did not see any differences in life-score changes between RA and controls, but higher life-score changes occured amongst those RA patients who had elevated immunoglobulin levels, perhaps linking psychological stress and an immunological reaction and polyarthritis.

BEHAVIORAL APPROACHES TO THE TREATMENT OF RHEUMATIC DISEASES

The development of behavioral approaches in the treatment of physical illness in recent years has been paralleled by a growing trend among patients to become partners in their health care by being informed; being partners in decision making; and by utilizing techniques which promote a sense of control over their disease and its impact on their lives.

Behavioral techniques used in the treatment of inflammatory rheumatic diseases have had limited application to date. A review of the literature shows studies of biofeedback for the treatment of Raynaud's disease, relaxation for the management of pain, and the enhancement of coping skills through group participation. Of these, only biofeedback has been extensively studied and reported. Studies of the influence of social support on the prevalence and impact of chronic illness, and the evaluation of different coping strategies suggest promising areas for future research (Berkman & Syme, 1979; Bruhn & Philips, 1984; Felton & Revenson, 1984).

Unfortunately more attention has been given to *lack* of social support (for example, divorce, loss of parent or spouse) as a stressor in rheumatic diseases and no study, to our knowledge, has measured the influence or outcome of *positive* social support. Longitudinal studies (Duthie, Brown, Truelove, Baragar, & Lawrie, 1964; Pincus, Callahan, Sale, Brooks, Paynes, & Vaughn, 1984) have tended to measure functional outcome in terms of social functioning by the American Rheumatism Association functional class (Steinbrocker, Traeger, & Balterman, 1949) which depends on a person's ability to engage in normal, light, or no gainful employment. In chronic inflammatory rheumatic disease such as rheumatoid arthritis, ability to remain in work may depend as much on the attitude and flexibility of employer and coworkers as it does on the actual job tasks (Yelin, 1980).

Relaxation

Relaxation techniques are not traditionally a part of the management program. Relaxation therapy can be used (a) to alleviate discomfort when pain cannot immediately be relieved by other measures, (b) to facilitate therapeutic exercise, or (c) to reduce anxiety, for example in children requiring repeated venipuncture or intramuscular injections (Mooney, 1983). Relaxation techniques such as autogenic training, the relaxation response, progressive muscular relaxation, and guided imagery have all been reported to be helpful in arthritis. The preferred technique should depend on the age, personality, and preference of the individual patient.

Few studies exclusively address arthritis pain compared to those addressing low back pain or nonspecific chronic pain. A lack of definition of "chronic pain," lack of objective data to substantiate a complaint of pain (for example, a hot swollen joint), and the variability of arthritis symptoms from day to day confound interpretation of the results. Patients with rheumatoid arthritis are occasionally admitted to chronic pain units but seldom do well. In a review of published psychological studies in the management of arthritis pain, Bradley found studies deficient with regard to small subject sample, inadequate control procedures, and follow-up measurements (Bradley et al., 1984).

In a small study of hemophiliacs with chronic arthritis pain Varni found that self-regulation techniques consisting of progressive muscle relaxation exercises, meditative breathing, and guided imagery resulted in clinically significant decreases in pain intensity (Varni, 1981; Varni & Gilbert, 1982). Linton found that applied relaxation can produce significant decreases in pain in patients experiencing chronic pain from back and joints and that the addition of an operant program did not improve pain reductions although it did improve activity and the need for analgesis (Linton & Gotestan, 1984).

In a study of 111 patients emphasizing relaxation procedures for low back pain, Keefe reported that those who improved most had initially rated their pain more severe, had continuous pain for a few years, and were less likely to be on disability or to have had multiple surgical procedures. This hypothesis might usefully be tested in arthritis patients (Keefe, Block, Williams, & Surwit, 1981).

Groups

A group setting for patients with rheumatic disease and their families provides a supportive milieu to verbalize and share concerns, to learn about the disease, to realize that others have similar experiences and emotional reactions, and to strengthen coping strategies through problem solving. Therapeutic groups for arthritis patients were first described by Henkle (1975). Since that time the outcomes of many groups offering psychological support and education have been reported. Three group models, each with a different emphasis, organization, and leadership exist. All have an educational component and emphasize communication skills, coping strengths, and mutual support but focus more on one than the other. Much of the data reported so far relate to knowledge increase and factors such as improvement in communication and coping are based on clinical impression or patient self-report. One study reported improvement in joint tenderness in groups receiving stress management and mutual support (Shearn & Fireman, 1985).

Psychological Support Group Model. Udelman describes an inpatient psychotherapy group model for patients with RA and spouses that was used by husband and wife co-therapists (Udelman & Udelman, 1978). The goals of the group were educational, social integrational, supportive ventilative, and exploratory dynamic, dealing with underlying conflict and defenses either etiologic or reactive to physical illness.

Schwartz describes a similar group which also had the goal of improving education of physicians concerning the emotional impact of chronic disease. Observed improvement occurred in compliance with treatment, communication with families and physicians, and modified lifestyle (Schwartz, Marcus, & Gordon, 1978). Groups emphasizing psychological support are usually led by psychiatrists, psychologists, social workers, and other health professionals with special group training.

A recent survey evaluated the effectiveness of psychotherapy, group assertion/relaxation training, and no treatment (Strauss et al., 1986). Fifty-seven rheumatoid arthritis patients were randomly assigned to each of the three groups and the dependent variables were standardized items taken from various self-reported measures of satisfaction and physical, psychological, and social function and a physician global evaluation of disease activity. Measures were recorded at baseline, immediately after the interventions and 12 months after baseline. There were few outcome measures for which either treatment resulted in significantly higher scores than seen in the control group, though there was more improvement noted in patients who received conventional group psychotherapy.

Education Support Group Model. In a controlled study of an educational support group for patients with ankylosing spondylitis

(Gross & Brandt, 1981) patients in the experimental group had significant increased knowledge and observed improved compliance with exercise programs. Verbal feedback concerning improved coping abilities was given in most cases. Control patients showed no substantial changes in knowledge or compliance.

The Arthritis Self-Help Course (Lorig, 1985) has had wide dissemination and over 2,000 graduates. A structured eight-session program taught by a trained lay leader combines information about arthritis, its management by medication and exercises, and how to cope with a chronic illness. Behavioral and health status outcomes of this program were measured in two ways: a 4-month randomized experiment and a 20-month longitudinal study. At 4 months, experimental subjects significantly exceeded control subjects in knowledge, recommended behaviors, and lessened pain. These change remained significant at 20 months.

Peer Mutual Support Groups. These groups, usually described as clubs or support groups, may also be disease-specific—for example, arthritis, systemic lupus erythematosus, or scleroderma. Organized by the Arthritis Foundation, the Lupus Foundation, or the Scleroderma Society, they are usually peer groups and have not so far been studied systematically. Mutual support groups may also be formed by patients who have participated in a time-limited group but who still wish to maintain contact with each other.

Raynaud's Disease and Phenomenon

Raynaud's is a clinical syndrome in which there is intermittent vasospasm of the hands and feet which can be induced by cold and/or stress. During a classic attack, the affected area blanches and then may turn cyanotic or hyperemic as vasospasm is relieved. Raynaud's occurs five times more often in women than in men and usually in the first and second decades of life. When the syndrome results from identifiable pathological process such as prior vascular injury from frostbite or in association with connective tissue diseases, it is known as Raynaud's phenomena. The physiology of Raynaud's is not completely understood but has been believed since its original description by Maurice Raynaud that the malady is somehow related to sympathetic reactivity.

Voluntary control of the vasomotor tone and control of peripheral blood flow has been manipulated by a variety of biofeedback and behavioral approaches. Whether these behavioral techniques are effective in the management of Raynaud's is debated but there appears to be marked benefit in some patients. Whether this is mediated through increasing blood flow or through a placebo response may be academic since drug management provides only partial relief, sometimes with considerable side effects and expense.

The literature regarding the efficacy of behavioral techniques in the management of Raynaud's Disease include anecdotes or uncontrolled studies which do not attempt to control for spontaneous remissions induced by warm weather or by natural fluctuations in symptomatology or do not take into account the normal trend of hand temperature to increase after the patients are allowed to sit quietly in a room with comfortable ambient temperature.

Jacobson randomized patients with Raynaud's disease from 2–15 years into biofeedback and relaxation or relaxation only and found that patients were able to increase their skin temperature anywhere from .1°–3.2° and reported improvement up to two years (Jacobson, Manschreck, & Silverberg, 1979).

Surwit and his colleagues used biofeedback techniques in 30 female patients ranging from 23 to 54 years old with idiopathic Raynaud's disease (Surwit, Bradner, Fenton, & Pilon, 1979). The outcome measured was whether patients could demonstrate significant digital skin temperature increases during cold stress. All patients benefited from the training. Subjects with low scores on the alienation scale of a psychological screening inventory had significantly more improvement than subjects with high scores on the scale. In addition older subjects were found to respond better than younger ones to behavioral treatment.

A study of patients with Raynaud's disease who have undergone either autogenic training, biofeedback, or a combination of autogenic training and temperature biofeedback indicated that the mean number of vaso spastic attacks per day at one year after training was approximately equal to the number occurring at the end of the initial training (1.2–1.3 per day) (Keefe, Surwit, & Pilon, 1979). In a similar study, Keefe showed that 21 patients with idiopathic Raynaud's disease responded equally to autogenic training, progressive muscle relaxation, or a combination of autogenic training and skin temperature feedback (Keefe, Surwit, & Pilon, 1980). Patients were instructed in three 1-hour group sessions spaced a week apart. In addition, patients underwent four laboratory cold-stress tests during which they were instructed to maintain digital temperature as the ambient temperature was dropped from 26° to 17° centigrade. All patients improved during the first four weeks of training and the ability of patients to maintain digital temperatures during their cold challenge showed significant improvement from their first to their last test. Symptomatic improvement was maintained by nine weeks after the start of training.

One would posit that—in patients with Raynaud's phenomenon secondary to vascular disease where fixed obstruction to blood flow occurs—behavioral management would have limited efficacy. Several studies address this.

Twenty-four patients with scleroderma and Raynaud's were randomly assigned to receive finger temperature biofeedback, EMG biofeedback, or autogenic training (Freedman, Ianni, & Wenig, 1984). Only those receiving finger temperature feedback showed significant increases in finger temperature during training but no group had significant clinical improvement as evaluated by self-report of symptoms and by ambulatory monitoring of finger temperature.

Twenty-three patients, 11 with Raynaud's and 12 with Raynaud's phenomenon, were retrospectively studied. After finger temperature biofeedback all patients evaluated their baseline temperatures and patients with scleroderma and systemic lupus erythematosus had the greatest improvement (Yocum, Hodes, Sundstrom, & Cleeland, 1985).

SUMMARY

The inflammatory arthritides affect all forms of functioning and have a major psychosocial impact on patients and their families. These effects, although qualitatively different do not occur more in these patients. The link between social factors and disease pathogenesis is circumstantial, although there are tantilizing findings from the field of psychoimmunology that would give possible explanation to some of the observed relationships. Behavioral techniques in regard to self-help groups, psychological counseling, and behavioral approaches to treating manifestations of arthritis, such as pain and Raynaud's, are described. Behavioral techniques have had limited application and evaluation in the rheumatic diseases, although their application has great promise.

REFERENCES

Ader, R., & Cohen N. (1984). Behavior and the immune system. In W. D. Gentry (Ed.), *Handbook of behavioral medicine* (pp. 117–173). New York: Guilford Press.

Anderson, K. O., Bradley, L. A., Young, L. D., McDaniel, L. K., & Wise, C. (1985). Rheumatoid arthritis: Review of psychological factors related to etiology, effects and treatment. *Psychological Bulletin 98*, 358–387.

Baum, J. (1982). A review of the psychological aspects of rheumatic diseases. *Seminars in Arthritis and Rheumatism, 11*, 352–361.

Berkman, L. F., & Syme, S. L. (1979). Social networks, host resistance and mortality. A nine year follow up study of Alameda County residents. *American Journal of Epidemiology, 109*, 186–204.

Blom, G. E., & Nicholls, G. (1954). Emotional factors in children with rheumatoid arthritis. *American Journal of Orthopsychiatry, 24*, 588–601.

Bradley, L. A., Anderson, K. O., Young, L. D., & McDaniel, L. K. (1985). Is psychological disturbance highly associated with primary fibrositis? Evidence that primary Fibrositis is not a form of Psychogenic Rheumatism. *Behavioral Medicine Abstracts, 6*, 145–147.

Bradley L. A., Young, L. D., Anderson, K. O., McDaniel, L. K., Turner, R. A., & Agudelo, C. A. (1984). Psychological approaches to the management of arthritis pain. *Social Science and Medicine, 19*, 1353–1360.

Bruhn, J. G., & Phillips, B. U. (1984). Measuring social support: A synthesis of current approaches. *Journal of Behavioral Medicine, 7*, 151–169.

Cassileth, B. R., Lusk, E.J., Strouse, T. B., Miller, D. S., Brown, L. L., Cross, P. A., & Tenaglia, A. N. (1984). Psychosocial status in chronic illness: A comparative analysis of six diagnostic groups. *New England Journal of Medicine, 311*, 506–511.

Christian, J. J., & Williamson, H. O. (1958). Effect of crowding on experimental granuloma formation in mice. *Proceedings of the Society for Experimental Biology and Medicine, 99*, 385–387.

Crown S., & Crown, J. M., (1973). Personality in early rheumatoid disease, *Journal of Psychosomatic Research, 17*, 189–196.

Crown, S., Crown, J. M., & Fleming, A. (1975). Aspects of the psychology and epidemiology of rheumatoid disease. *Psychological Medicine, 5*, 291–299.

Decker, J. L. (1983). American Rheumatism Association nomenclature and classification of arthritis and rheumatism. *Arthritis and Rheumatism, 26*, 1029–1032.

Duthie, J. J. R., Brown, P. E., Truelove, L. H., Baragar, F. D., & Lawrie, A. J. (1964). Course and prognosis in rheumatoid arthritis. A further report. *Annals of the Rheumatic Diseases, 23*, 193–204.

Empire Rheumatism Council. (1950). A controlled investigation into the etiology and clinical features of rheumatoid arthritis. *British Medical Journal, 1*, 799–805.

Felton, B. J., & Revenson, T. A. (1984). Coping with chronic illness: A study of illness controllability and the influence of coping strategies on psychological adjustment. *Journal of Consulting and Clinical Psychology, 52*, 343–353.

Freedman, R. R., Ianni, P., & Wenig, P. (1984). Behavioral treatment of Raynaud's phenomenon in Scleroderma. *Journal of Behavioral Medicine, 7*, 343–353.

Funk, G. A., & Jenson, M. M. (1967). Influence of stress and granuloma formation. *Proceedings of the Society for Experimental Biology and Medicine, 124*, 653–655.

Genest, M. (1989). The relevance of stress to rheumatoid arthritis. In R. W. J. Neufeld (Ed.), *Advances in the investigation of psychological stress* (pp. 343–366). New York: Wiley.

Gewanter, H. L., Roghmann, K. J., & Baum, J. (1983). The prevalence of juvenile arthritis. *Arthritis and Rheumatism, 26*, 599–603.

Gross, M., & Brandt, K. D. (1981). Educational support groups for patients with ankylosing spondylitis: A preliminary report. *Patient Counselling and Health Education, 3*, 6–12.

Guy, W. B., (1952). Neurogenic factors in contact dermatitis. *Archives fur Dermatologie und Syphilis, 66*, 1–8.

Hendrie, H. C., Paraskevas, F., Baragar, F. D., & Adamson, J. D. (1971). Stress, immunoglobulin levels and early polyarthritis. *Journal of Psychosomatic Research, 15*, 337–342.

Henkle, C. (1975). Social groupwork as a treatment modality for hospitalized people with rheumatoid arthritis. *Rehabilitation Literature, 36*, 334–341, 354.

Henoch, M. J., Batson, J. W., & Baum, J. (1978). Psychological factors in juvenile rheumatoid arthritis. *Arthritis and Rheumatism, 21*, 229–233.

Hotchin, J., Benson, L., & Gardiner, J. (1970). Mother-infant interaction in lymphocytic choriomeningitis virus infection of the newborn mouse; the effect of maternal health on mortality of offspring. *Pediatric Research, 4*, 194–200.

Jacobson, A. M., Manschreck, T. C., & Silverberg, E. (1979). Behavioral treatment of Raynaud's disease: A comparative study with long-term follow-up. *American Journal of Psychiatry, 136*, 844–846.

Keefe, F. J., Block, A. R., Williams, R. B., & Surwit, R. S. (1981). Behavioral treatment of chronic low back pain: Clinical outcome and individual differences in pain relief. *Pain, 11*, 221–231.

Keefe, F. J., Surwit, R. S., & Pilon, R. N. (1979). A one-year follow-up of Raynaud's patients treated with behavioral therapy techniques. *Journal of Behavioral Medicine, 2*, 385–391.

Keefe, F. J., Surwit, R. S., & Pilon, R. N. (1980). Biofeedback, autogenic training, and progressive relaxation in the treatment of Raynaud's disease: A comparative study. *Journal of Applied Behavior Analysis, 13*, 3–11.

Kellgren, J. H. (1964). The epidemiology of rheumatic diseases. *Annals of the Rheumatic Diseases, 23*, 109–122.

Liang, M. D., Rogers, M., Larson, M., Eaton, H. M., Murawski, B. J., Taylor, J. E., Swafford, J., & Schur, P. H. (1984). The psychological impact of systematic lupus erythematosus and rheumatoid arthritis. *Arthritis and Rheumatism, 27*, 13–19.

Linton, S. J., & Gotestan, K. G. (1984). A controlled study of the effects of applied relaxation and applied relaxation plus operant procedures in the regulation of chronic pain. *British Journal of Clinical Psychology, 23*, 291–299.

Lorig, K., Lubeck, D., Kraines, R G., Seleznick, M., Brown, B. W., & Holman, H. R. (1985). Outcomes of self help education for patients with arthritis. *Arthritis and Rheumatism, 28*, 680–685.

Ludwig, A. O. (1955). Psychiatric considerations in rheumatoid arthritis. *Arthritis and Rheumatism, 6*, 166–171.

Masi, A. T., & Medsger, T. A. (1979). Epidemiology of the rheumatic diseases. In D. McCarty (Ed.), *Arthritis and allied conditions* (9th ed., pp. 11–35). Philadelphia: Lea & Febiger.

Master, R. J., Feltin, M., Jainchill, J., Mark, R., Kavesh, W., Rabkin, M., Turner, B., Bachrach, S., & Lenox, S. (1980). A continuum of care for the inner city. *New England Journal of Medicine, 302*, 1434–1440.

Mettrop, P. J., & Visser, P. (1969). Exteroceptive stimulation as a contingent factor in the induction and elicitation of delayed-type hypersensitivity reactions to 1-chloro-2-4, dinitrobenzene in Guinea pigs. *Psychophysiology, 5*, 385–388.

Meyerwitz, S. (1966). The continuing investigation of psychosocial variables in rheumatoid arthritis. In A. G. Hill (Ed.), *Modern trends in rheumatology* (2nd series, pp. 92–105). New York: Appleton-Century Crofts.

Meyerowitz, S., Jacox, R. F., & Hess, D. W. (1968). Monozygotic twins discordant from rheumatoid arthritis. *Arthritis and Rheumatism, 11*, 1–21.

Mindham, R. H. S., Bagshaw, A., James S. A., & Swannell, A. J. (1981). Factors associated with the appearance of psychiatric symptoms in rheumatoid arthritis. *Journal of Psychosomatic Research, 25*, 429–435.

Mooney, N. E. (1983). Coping with chronic pain in rheumatoid arthritis. *Rehabilitation Nursing, 8*, 20–25.

Moos, R. H. (1963). Personality factors associated with rheumatoid arthritis: a review. *Journal of Chronic Diseases, 17*, 41–55.

Moos, R. H., & Solomon, G. F. (1964). Personality correlates of the rapidity of progression of rheumatoid arthritis. *Annals of the Rheumatic Diseases, 23*, 141–151.

Nagi, S. (1965). Some conceptual issues in disability and rehabilitation. In M. B. Sussman (Ed.), *Sociology and rehabilitation* (pp. 100–113). Washington, DC: American Sociological Association.

Pincus, T., Callahan, L. F., Sale, W. G., Brooks, A. L., Paynes, L. E., & Vaughn, W. K. (1984). Severe functional declines, work disability, and increased mortality in seventy five rheumatoid arthritis patients studied over nine years. *Arthritis and Rheumatism, 27*, 864–872.

Pincus, T., Callahan, L. F., Bradley, L. A., Vaughn, W. K., & Wolfe, F. (1986). Elevated MMPI scores for hypochondriasis, depression and hysteria in patients with rheumatoid arthritis reflect disease rather than psychological states. *Arthritis and Rheumatism, 29*, 1456–1466.

Pitkin, D. H. (1965). Effect of psychological stress on the delayed hypersensitivity reaction. *Proceedings of the Society for Experimental Biology and Medicine, 120*, 350–351.

Reynolds, M. D. (1978). Prevalence of rheumatic diseases as causes of disability and complaints by ambulatory patients. *Arthritis and Rheumatism, 21*, 377–382.

Rimon, R. A. (1969). A psychosomatic approach to rheumatoid arthritis. A clinical study of 100 female patients. *Acta Rheumatologica Scandinavica, 13*, 1–154.

Rimon, R., Belmaker, R. H., & Ebstein, R. (1977). Psychosomatic aspects of juvenile rheumatoid arthritis. *Scand Journal of Rheumatology, 6*, 1–10.

Robinson, C. E. (1957). Emotional factors and rheumatoid arthritis. *Canadian Medical Association Journal, 77*, 344–345.

Rogers, M. P., Dubey, D., & Reich, P. (1979). The influence of the psyche and the brain on immunity and disease susceptibility: A critical review. *Psychosomatic Medicine, 41*, 147–164.

Schwartz, J. H., Marcus, R., & Gordon, R. (1978). Multidisciplinary group therapy for rheumatoid arthritis. *Psychosomatics, 19*, 289–293.

Sell, G. (1972). *Immunology, immunopathology and immunity*. Hagerstown, PA: Harper.

Shearn, M. A., & Fireman, B. H. (1985). Stress management and mutual support groups in rheumatoid arthritis. *The American Journal of Medicine, 78*, 771–775.

Shochet, B. R., Lisansky, E. T., Schubart, A. F., Fiocco, V., Kurland, S., & Pope, M. (1969). A medical-psychiatric study of patients with rheumatoid arthritis. *Psychosomatics, 10*, 271–279.

Smith, L. W., Molomut, N., & Gottfried, B. (1960). Effect of subconclusive audiogenic stress in mice on turpentine induced inflammation. *Proceedings of the Society for Experimental Biology and Medicine, 103*, 370–372.

Smythe, H. A. (1984). Problems with the MMPI. *Journal of Rheumatology, 11*, 417–418.

Solomon, G. F. (1981). Emotional and personality factors in the onset and course of autoimmune disease, particularly rheumatoid arthritis. In R. Ader (Ed.) *Psychoneuroimmunology* (pp. 159–182). New York: Academic Press.

Solomon, G. F., Levine, S., & Kraft, J. K. (1968). Early experience and immunity. *Nature, 220*, 821–822.

Spergel, P., Ewrlich, G. E., & Glass, D. (1978). The rheumatoid arthritis personality a psychodiagnostic myth. *Psychosomatics, 19*, 79–86.

Steinbrocker, O., Traeger, C. H., & Batterman, R. C. (1949). Therapeutic criteria in rheumatoid arthritis. *Journal of the American Medical Association, 140*, 659–662.

Strauss, G. D., Spiegel, J.S., Daniels, M., Spiegel, T., Landsverk, J., Roy-Byrne, P., Edelstein, C., Ehlhardt, J., Falke, R., Hindi, L., & Zackler, L. (1986). Group therapies for rheumatoid arthritis: A controlled study of two approaches. *Arthritis and Rheumatism, 29*, 1203–1209.

Surwit, R. S., Bradner, M. N., Fenton, C. H., & Pilon, R. N. (1979). Individual differences in response to the behavioral treatment of Raynaud's disease. *Journal of Consulting Clinical Psychology, 47*, 363–367.

Udelman, H., & Udelman, D. L. (1978). Group therapy with rheumatoid arthritic patients. *American Journal of Psychotherapy, 32*, 288–299.

Varni, J. W. (1981). Self-regulation techniques in the management of chronic arthritis pain in hemophilia. *Behavioral Therapy, 12*, 185–194.

Varni, J. W., & Gilbert, A. (1982). Self regulation of chronic arthritic pain and longterm analgesic dependence in a hemophiliac. *Rheumatology and Rehabilitation, 21*, 171–174.

Vollhardt, B. R., Ackerman, S. H., Grayzel, A. I., & Barland, P. (1982). Psychologically distinguishable groups of rheumatoid arthritis patients: a controlled single blind study. *Psychosomatic Medicine, 44*, 353–361.

Wood, P. H. N. (1980). Appreciating the consequences of disease: The international classification of impairments, disabilities and handicaps. *WHO Chronicle, 34*, 376–380.

Yelin, E., Meenan, R., Nevitt, M., & Epstein, W. (1980). Work disability in Rheumatoid Arthritis: Effects of disease, social and work factors. *Annals of Internal Medicine, 43*, 551–556.

Yocum, D. E., Hodes, R., Sundstrom, W. R., & Cleeland, C. S. (1985). Use of biofeedback training in treatment of Raynaud's disease and phenomenon. *Journal of Rheumatology, 12*, 90–93.

Zeitlin, D. J. (1977). Psychological issues in the management of rheumatoid arthritis. *Psychosomatics, 18*, 7–14.

7

Electromyographic Biofeedback and Musculoskeletal Disorders

Glenn R. Caddy

Nova University
Ft. Lauderdale, FL

Trudy Block

Clinical Psychology Institute
Ft. Lauderdale, FL

INTRODUCTION

Given that the striate musculature comprises slightly more than 40 percent of the overall body mass, inevitably this system and dysfunctions associated with it have a major impact on human functioning. Muscular activity is obviously linked to survival skills and adaptation. Primitive humans were equipped physiologically with a brain and a neuromusculature which, in the evolutionary process, developed to permit special responding during emergency circumstances. In the contemporary human, many of the physiological mechanisms that served only emergency requirements in the primitive ancestor appear to be continuously, or at least chronically, activated in adjusting to the complexities of the present day stresses of living. Thus, mechanisms that evolved to respond to short-term stressors or crises are now consistently operating to "protect" the organism from the demands placed upon it by life in a modern society. It is not surprising, therefore, that various systems within the human organism malfunction and produce conditions such as anxiety, neuromuscular disorders, headache, and vascular disturbance, among others. (For a thorough discussion of these physiological malfunctions, see Malmo, 1975.) Direct and controlling linkages exist between the brain and the muscloskeletal system. Given the extent to which this system is complex, modifiable by learning, responsive to internal injuries and internal and external stressors, it is not surprising that dysfunction is one of the consequences of the individual interacting ineffectively with an increasingly complex environment.

Muscular tension, anxiety-related disorders, insomnia, head and facial pain (including dental disorders), and a whole range of other neuromuscular conditions clearly all have substantial psychological components. All the preceding disorders have had special significance in the emergence of the field of behavioral medicine.

The development of biometrics (see Cromwell, Weibell, Pfeiffer, & Usselman, 1973) and more specifically, the application of electromyographic (EMG) biofeedback technology (Budzinski, Stoyva, Adler, & Mullaney, 1973) have greatly furthered understanding of both the nature of and implications for intervention in the muscular and neuromuscular disorders. The procedures that have been developed from the use of EMG-based technology have been powerfully directed to the treatment of chronic and acute anxiety and panic disorders through an extension of the relaxation paradigm, to the treatment of tension-based head and facial pain, to the adjunctive management of dental conditions such as bruxism and to the growing field of neromuscular reeducation/rehabilitation. Peripherally, EMG biofeedback also has been applied experimentally, with some success, in the management of disorders such as dysmenorrhea, stuttering, and diabetes.

GENERAL RELAXATION PROCEDURES

Anxiety Disorders

A variety of biofeedback-based procedures have been employed in the treatment of anxiety disorders. All of these procedures have addressed one or more symptoms commonly associated with the experience of anxiety (i.e., increased heart rate, peripheral vasoconstriction, abrupt changes in rate and depth of respiration, and muscle tension). The rationale for employing these various biofeedback procedures stems from the general hypothesis that anxiety can be decreased when the autonomically mediated physiological arousal, concomitant with subjective reports of anxiety, can be reduced and/or regulated. As a general rule, research studies addressing the efficacy of biofeedback in reducing anxiety have employed biofeedback exclusively in order to assess its specific effect (Raskin, Bali, & Peeke, 1980). It is for this reason, perhaps, that well-controlled studies have generally not shown biofeedback per se to be particularly effective in alleviating anxiety disorders. In the clinical setting, however, the management strategies for anxiety reduction have extended beyond the exclusive use of biofeedback. Clinicians typically are less concerned with demonstrating the efficacy of a particular strategy. Rather, they favor the use of a variety of procedures integrated to produce presumably optimal treatment gains. In such a context, EMG and other biofeedback approaches may be best conceptualized as ancillary or complementary elements (assertiveness training, desensitization procedures, social skills training, and cognitive approaches, for example), in the overall treatment of the condition.

It is well documented that muscular tension often occurs during stressful situations and deep muscle relaxation has been a primary aspect of many treatment packages for the alleviation of anxiety (Jacobsen, 1938; Schultz & Luthe, 1959). As deep muscle relaxation and anxiety states cannot mutually coexist, or so it has been assumed, it has been hypothesized that EMG training may be effective in the management of anxiety (Budzinski, 1973), and a number of studies to be discussed have shown this to be the case. It also must be acknowledged, however, that muscular tension need not always be present during episodic or chronic anxiety states. There are those patients who evidence primarily a galvanic skin response or a gastrointestinal response to stress inducing stimuli while showing little or no significant muscular contractions. Despite the fact that muscle tension is not the sine qua non of anxiety, EMG-assisted relaxation training has produced substantial benefit in the treatment of anxiety disorders.

Townsend, House, and Addario (1975) compared EMG biofeedback (individually administered) to group "psychotherapy," a somewhat questionable control procedure, in a treatment study with chronically anxious patients. The results obtained immediately after treatment indicated that subjects in the biofeedback condition significantly decreased their EMG levels in comparison to control subjects. Further, experimental subjects evidenced improvement in mood states, trait anxiety measures, and to a lesser extent, a measure of state anxiety. No such decreases were noted in the control subjects. At a six month follow-up, data were available on only two experimental subjects who had continued self-practice procedures and the use of instructional tapes. These subjects reportedly maintained improvement. Clearly while the problem of significant subject loss and other concerns must color any acceptance of Townsend et al.'s interpretation of success, it is noteworthy that the experimental subjects attained the level of improvement reported, especially given that the instructional set administered to them consisted of neutral statements regarding the likelihood of a treatment outcome.

LeBoeuf and Lodge (1980), in a study which is less subject to criticisms associated with internal and external validity than the one by Townsend et al., utilized a frontalis EMG biofeedback group and a progressive relaxation group. While subjects in the biofeedback group achieved significant reductions in frontal EMG levels, no differences were noted between subjects in the two groups with respect to measures of anxiety symptomatology. (This finding of no difference is not surprising, given that reduction in autonomic arousal is an element that comes with successful training in both the procedures studied.) LeBoeuf and Lodge's conclusion regarding the study are perhaps obvious but worth stating: Namely, that EMG biofeedback is very unlikely to represent a panacea in the treatment of anxiety, for anxiety would appear to be multidimensional in its nature and likely to require a variety of procedures to be applied to the successful management in the individual case.

Increasingly, some of the more recent research employing EMG feedback has integrated the technique with other more cognitively oriented self-control strategies. Such an approach seems to have developed from the conceptualization that there are two relatively independent types of anxiety—cognitively mediated anxiety and somatically mediated anxiety. Davidson and Schwartz (1976) suggested that physiological interventions may not impact on the cognitive aspects of the anxiety and vice versa. If one accepts the aforementioned proposition, it would appear crucial that effective assessment procedures be utilized in order to differentiate anxiety patients along the physiological/cognitive dimensions, thereby enabling appropriate treatment strategies to be implemented in the individual case.

Weinman, Semchuk, Saebe, and Mathew (1983) examined the effects of frontalis EMG feedback and relaxation training on a group of 20 patients classified either as high-stress or low-stress subjects. It had been hypothesized that for high-stress individuals the sense of control over one's circumstances can lead to a sense of mastery, thus permitting an alteration in one's perception of symptoms (Stern, Miller, Ewy, & Grant, 1980). While Weinman et al. found no differences in frontalis EMG scores at the initiation of treatment, following 10 sessions of biofeedback-assisted relaxation, and at a 6-week follow-up, subjects classified in the high-stress group showed changes on EMG, state and trait anxiety measures, depression scores, and anxiety symptomatology. Over the same time period the low-stress subjects did not show notable improvement. Moreover, when subjects were asked what made it possible for them to use the feedback effectively, 70 percent of the high-stress subjects stated the belief that they were in control of their minds and bodies; and 67 percent of the low-stress subjects described their success in achieving maximal muscle relaxation as a function of the amount of effort they put into the task. Further, most of the high-stress subjects (60%) stated the EMG feedback procedure to be the most important element in the treatment. Low-stress subjects, on the other hand, most frequently rated the trainees as most important to their success in the program.

The implications of the Weinman et al. study, as well as the work of Lazarus (1975) and Meichenbaum (1976) relate to the notion that individuals who attain a sense of responsibility for their own well-being and consequently seek a sense of mastery over their symptomatology and circumstances, tend to achieve a more consistently successful treatment outcome than do subjects who depend on factors external to them to reduce their symptoms. Successful EMG feedback training may be instrumental in the development of relaxation skills in order to counteract both cognitive and physiological arousal and concomitantly reinforce the sense of perceived mastery and competence over anxiety inducing stimuli and circumstances.

Insomnia

Individuals with chronic sleep disturbances comprise a heterogeneous population with difficulties ranging from sleep onset latency, sleep dissatisfaction, somnambulism, frequency of awakenings, nightmares, and early awakenings. With respect to insomnia, the incidence of the condition in the general population has been estimated to be between six percent and 15 percent (Karacan, Williams, Littell, & Salis, 1973).

Insomnia is often related to various forms of high arousal. Delay of sleep onset may be related to physiological arousal (Monroe, 1967; Robinson, 1969), although not always (Friedman & Papsdorf, 1976), to cognitive activity (Baekeland & Hoy, 1971; Roth, Kramer, & Lutz, 1976; Starker & Hassenfeld, 1976) and/or to emotional arousal such as anxiety and depression (Coursey, Buchsbaum, & Frankel, 1975; Kales, Caldwell, Preston, Healey, & Kales, 1976). Some studies have suggested that therapeutic interventions for sleep onset insomnia might best be directed to reducing such arousal. Drugs such as muscle relaxants, hypnotics, and CNS depressants have been prescribed but the side effects, including their potential for dependence and their possible impact on the quality of the sleep, have led to the increased use of nonpharmacologic approaches.

Montgomery, Perkins and Wise (1975) and Ribordy and Denney (1977) have reviewed the literature on the therapeutic alternatives to pharmacologic interventions in insomnia. While some of the studies in this essentially behavioral literature have been conducted with insomniacs selected from the general population (Borkovec, Steinmark, & Nau, 1973; Hinkle & Lutker, 1972; Nicassio & Bootzin, 1974), the majority have studied more youthful university students who met the criteria defining poor sleepers, though their condition may not have been as chronic as in the more "clinical" subjects (Borkovec, Kaloupek, & Slama, 1975; Freedman & Papsdorf, 1976; Gershman & Clouser, 1974; Kahn, Baker, & Weiss, 1968).

Montgomery and Besner (1975) examined the efficacy of EMG biofeedback and relaxation training on latency of sleep onset, subjects' attitudes regarding difficulty in fall asleep, and the degree of restfulness the sleep provided. During treatment the subjects attended laboratory-based 20-minute frontalis EMG training sessions twice weekly, for three weeks, and weekly thereafter for a further 13 weeks. Relaxation training was initiated in the laboratory and then practice was transferred to the home environment. The results indicated that following the training these subjects significantly decreased their muscle tension, slept more restfully, and perceived themselves to have less difficulty in falling asleep. This last finding is of particular interest, especially given the findings of Schwartz, Guilbaud, and Fishgood (1963), who reported that as many as 50 percent of insomniacs show a normal amount of sleep according to polygraph records but believe, nevertheless, that they sleep very little.

In a subsequent and more ambitious investigation, Besner (1975) sought to control for placebo and other effects utilizing four experimental and three control conditions. No significant differences between insomnia groups were found but there were significant reductions in the measured sleep indices. Further, although there was no significant change in sleep duration reported, there was an overall positive change in the subjects' attitudes toward sleep. It appeared that, as in the previous study, some change in the subjects' perceptions of their sleep patterns occurred, perhaps as a by-product of their participation in the treatment programs.

Similar findings were reported in a treatment study by Hauri (1978), who noted that although subjects perceived and reported an improvement in their sleeping patterns, this was not reflected in their EEG measures. In a subsequent study, noteworthy for its methodological sophistication, Hauri (1981) selected a group of insomniacs and randomly assigned them to one of four conditions: (a) Frontalis EMG biofeedback, (b) frontalis EMG followed by theta biofeedback, (c) feedback of sensory motor rhythm, (SMR), and (d) a control condition. Subjects in all groups received laboratory sleep evaluations as well as a comprehensive psychological testing phase at the conclusion of the treatment sequence and again nine months thereafter. Hauri reported that all subjects improved their sleeping patterns to at least some degree including the controls, and some subjects improved their sleeping patterns quite markedly. In the EMG feedback group, subjects with higher initial tension (defined by baseline EMG and anxiety scores) attained greater benefit from EMG biofeedback. Similar findings also were obtained from subjects in the theta/EMG group. It has been noted that feedback is most effective when it is simple and provided in only one modality which could explain the results for the combined EMG/SMR group. The pattern was reversed for subjects in the SMG group where, on 4 of the 6 sleep variables, tense subjects were less likely to benefit from the SMR training. Further, according to data from the home sleep logs, subjects, who, based upon baseline muscle tension levels, qualified for EMG relaxation training, lengthened their total sleep time by an average of 38 minutes while muscularly tense subjects who received SMR training slept an average of 18 minutes less following SMR biofeedback. Similarly, for subjects in both the EMG relaxation and SMR groups, appropriate biofeedback decreased the number of awakenings at home during the night while inappropriate feedback increased such awakenings. Results of laboratory sleep analyses indicated similar changes. Clearly, different types of biofeedback effected different subjects in unique and specific ways. Important, too, is that inappropriate feedback may produce effects detrimental to the quality of the patients' sleep (see Hauri, Percy, Hellekson, Hartmann, & Russ, 1982). An important implication of such findings is that for treatment to be maximally effective it must be patient-specific and prescribed and implemented only following a detailed assessment of the unique requirements of the individual case.

Localized Muscle Tension

Under certain conditions muscle tension may be concentrated within a given musculature and lead to severe and, in some instances, chronic syndromes such as muscle contraction headaches, preorbital facial muscle tension, and hypertonicity associated with tardive dyskinesia. Some of the aforementioned occur as a function of environmental stressors, while others appear to be related to neurological conditions.

Muscle Contraction Headache

Tension headache is usually described as a steady, dull pain located in the occiput or posterior region, often extending around to the forehead. This pain may be reported as located on one side of the head but often it is presented as having a "band-like" quality with pressure from all sides. Appenzeller (1973) estimated that 80–85% of all patients seen at headache clinics suffer from tension headache or other psychologically associated stress conditions resulting in some form of headpain (see also Dalessio, 1972). Tension headache is believed to be largely a product of sustained contraction of the skeletal muscles of the face, scalp, neck, and shoulders (Martin, 1966; Phillips, 1977; van Boxtel & van der Ven, 1978; Hutchings & Reinking, 1976) though vasoconstriction of extracranial blood vessels also may play a significant role (Tunis & Wolff, 1954; Dalessio, 1972).

Budzinski, Stoyva, and Adler (1970) and Budzinski, Stoyva, Adler, and Mullaney (1973) first investigated the application of frontalis EMG feedback for the treatment of muscle tension headache. These investigators reported such encouraging results that they have provided a foundation for subsequent research which has been voluminous.

Budzinski and his colleagues reported that (a) Frontal EMG feedback training produced lower EMG levels in trained subjects than in subjects who received no feedback or noncontingent feedback; (b) while all subjects were required to practice relaxation twice daily, only those who received accurate feedback showed a significant reduction in headache activity. Most feedback subjects, though not all, showed clinically meaningful reductions in headache activity with two sessions per week over an 8-week training period; (c) Subjects appeared to go through several stages of progress while undergoing training; (d) Regular home-practice in relaxation appeared to be a crucial aspect in the continued reduction in headache after termination of biofeedback.

Given the aforementioned findings of the efficacy of EMG feedback as a viable treatment strategy for tension headache, confirming evidence was ultimately provided by a number of independent researchers (Wickramasekera, 1972, 1973; Raskin, Johnson, & Rondestvedt, 1973). In the latter research the findings of headache reduction were incidental to its main goal of anxiety reduction through EMG frontalis biofeedback. Nevertheless, anxiety patients reported a reduced frequency and intensity of headache as a by-product of the EMG training.

Thereafter, research in this area has attempted a component analysis in order to determine the essential and unique determinants of treatment success and/or has studied the role of relaxation training and practice in headache reduction. Wickramasekera (1973) noted that the use of relaxation training prior to EMG feedback facilitated reduction in headache intensity during the training phase. Epstein, Hersen, and Hemphill (1974) in a single case study showed EMG feedback to reduce frontalis tension and headache intensity but lasting improvement was achieved only when the patient employed yoga techniques when he felt tense.

There have been a number of studies employing EMG feedback in combination with autogenic training, transcendental meditation, alpha feedback, progressive relaxation, yoga, and other similar procedures (see, for example, Bernstein & Borkcovec, 1973; Chesney & Shelton, 1976; Janssen, 1983; McKenzie, Ehrisman, Montgomery, & Barnes, 1974; Montgomery & Ehrisman, 1976; Schultz & Luthe, 1959; Tasto & Hinkle, 1973). A major result of this research has been to address the issue of the relative efficacy and unique contribution of EMG biofeedback in the treatment of muscle contraction headache as opposed to the general relaxation components that may be inherent in such procedures. A number of investigations directed at the comparative efficacy of EMG biofeedback, various relaxation procedures, and combinations thereof (see, for example, Chesney & Shelton, 1976; Cox, Freundlich, & Meyer, 1975; Haynes, Griffin, Mooney, & Parise, 1975; Hutchings & Reinking, 1976) have produced contradictory results leading Nuechterlein and Holyroyd (1980) to conclude that "biofeedback and verbal relaxation training are equally effective and no special advantage accrues from the combination of these modalities" (p. 871). Given that the human body is controlled by central regulating mechanisms and that the relaxation of a given set of musculature may impact the autonomic nervous system via such regulating mechanisms, these conclusions are not at all surprising.

Recent research employing somewhat more sophisticated methodology has continued to examine the differential efficacy of EMG biofeedback versus other procedures in the treatment of tension headache as well as to examine the integrity of these procedures in maintaining their effects over time. Janssen (1983), for example, studied the potency of EMG feedback and combined EMG feedback and relaxation instructions in 18 tension headache patients assigned to one of three conditions: a waiting list, an EMG training procedure, and an EMG feedback and progressive relaxation procedure. Patients in the treatment conditions received 12 training sessions scheduled twice weekly and returned three months after treatment for a follow-up session. Janssen noted no consistent differences between EMG feedback and the combined treatment procedures nor did the placement of the electrodes (neck or frontalis) result in treatment differences, though both procedures resulted in a reduction of symptomatology.

Germane to this entire general area of investigation is the question, to what extent are gains made in the course of therapy maintained over an extended time course? In reviewing the literature one find that relatively few studies report follow-up that is long-term with 3–4 months or less being the most frequently cited follow-up data, if any such data is reported at all (see, for example, Daly, Donn, Galliher, & Zimmerman, 1983, McKenzie et al., 1974; Wickramasekera, 1973). The Epstein et al. (1974) study, on the other hand, involved a follow-up of up to seven months. In this single-case ABAB design the patient maintained improvement only while the feedback continued except that a series of yoga exercises were credited with maintaining the low incidence of headache at seven months. Montgomery and Ehrisman (1976) followed their 13 subjects for 6 and 36 months. The treatment phase incorporated autogenic training, progressive relaxation, and Silver's controlled relaxation procedure together with auditory-based alpha training administered over 10 sessions. They showed substantial reductions of severity and frequency in their subjects' symptomatic patterns. This improvement was largely maintained throughout the course of their follow-up.

Reinking and Hutchings (1981) focused specifically on follow-up data at 3, 6, and 12 months posttreatment where subjects during treatment were exposed to one of three treatment strategies: (a) verbal instruction in relaxation, (b) frontalis EMG feedback, or (c) a combined procedure. At each follow-up interval subjects were asked to complete headache activity and medication charts covering a 7-day period prior to the follow-up contact. Of the original 30 subjects, follow-up data were obtained from 23, 20, and 18 subjects respectively, at the 3 follow-up periods. Results indicated that the type of treatment administered was relevant only in explaining the initial successes. Again, the continued practice of relaxation appeared more significant in accounting for the longer-term positive therapeutic outcomes.

Libo and Arnold (1983) noted similar outcomes in a follow-up study which extended over a period of 1 to 5 years. Of those patients who continued to practice relaxation techniques following treatment, 86 percent improved with respect to headache activity. However, 50 percent of those subjects who had ceased relaxation practice improved as well. Improvement appeared unrelated to regular or frequent practice of the relaxation techniques, in that occasional practice following therapy was sufficient to sustain the treatment gains over a long period of time.

DENTAL DISORDERS

Bruxism

Bruxism has been defined as a nonfunctional grinding of the teeth and, although it has been primarily seen as a dental phenomenon, research literature is providing increasing evidence for the position that it is a psychophysiologic disorder. As such, it is subject to intervention from a psychological/behavioral perspective. The disorder reportedly occurs with equal frequency among males and females (Bober, 1958) and among children and adults (Lindqvist, 1971). The reported incidence ranges from approximately 5 percent to 21 percent (Meklas, 1971; Reding, Rubright, & Zimmerman, 1966). The grinding produces conditions which ultimately lead the patient to seek treatment and includes the following: (a) abnormal wear of the teeth (Scharer, 1974); (b) damage to the temperomandible joint (Glickman, 1972); (c) damage to the structures surrounding the teeth (Glickman, 1972); (d) facial pain (Vestergaard, 1967); and (e) headache (Schwartz & Chayes, 1968). Psychologically oriented theories most often have established a link between anxiety and bruxism (Lindqvist, 1972; Thaller, 1960; Vernallis, 1955). The treatment approaches for bruxism have encompassed dental treatments, psychodynamically based approaches, classical or avoidance conditioning based studies, massed practice, tension reduction strategies, and EMG biofeedback.

Biofeedback technology assumes that this training will enable the individual to discriminate muscle tension levels and—consequently—upon experiencing high tension, initiate relaxation responses that then serve to inhibit tension and subsequently eliminate grinding of the teeth. Casas, Beemsterboer, & Clark (1982) compared stress reduction, behavioral counseling, and contingent nocturnal EMG biofeedback on nighttime bruxism. These investigators assigned 16 subjects to four treatment conditions (stress reduction, behavioral counseling, nocturnal biofeedback, and a waiting list control group). The behavioral counseling group received cognitively oriented treatment procedures outlined by Beck (1976), Goldfried (1979), and Meichenbaum (1974). The EMG biofeedback group was trained in the use of a portable EMG unit that awakened the subject with an audible tone when the biting force reached a predetermined level. Behavioral counseling sessions were conducted during 4 weekly meetings of 60 minutes each and individually administered. Their focus was on the alteration of maladaptive cognitive responses where bruxism was attributed to specific cognitions and/or self-statements rather than to a variety of stimuli and dispositions. This group did, however, receive EMG training although it was presented as monitoring rather than as a treatment strategy. No significant differences between the groups were noted but the authors concluded (somewhat questionably, we suggest, given the sample sizes and the confounded methodology which characterized this study), that the results favored the group which learned cognitively based stress reduction skills.

The results reported by Clark, Beemsterboer, and Rugh (1981) were clearer and more easily attributable to the intervention strategy. Clark et al. recorded masseter muscle activity of 10 heavy bruxists before and after EMG biofeedback training. The subjects received an auditory feedback signal when they clenched their teeth with moderate force and had to perform an arousal task each time the signal occurred. Nine of their ten subjects significantly reduced EMG activity as a function of the contingent feedback signal. There was also a decrease in the number of awakenings, suggesting a general reduction in bruxism. At a 3-month follow-up, seven subjects responded to the questionnaire and six of these seven respondents had maintained the treatment results (see also Piccione, Coates, George, Rosenthal, & Karzmark, 1982). Clearly, additional clinical research employing various behavioral medicine strategies in the management of bruxism would appear desirable.

NEUROMUSCULAR REHABILITATION

Muscular dysfunction can be associated with hypertrophy, atrophy, or lack of coordinated movement. Central (cerebral) injury as occurs following stroke or other head trauma and/or spinal cord injuries commonly produce impairment in the neural pathways which may result in paralysis or limitations in the use of the muscles. The establishment of neural linkages or the strengthening of existing but greatly impaired connections frequently involves EMG biofeedback techniques administered adjunctive to other neuromuscular or muscular retraining procedures. The goal of such treatment strategies is to enable the patient to acquire or strengthen voluntary control over neural systems and/or muscle groups whose functions are limited by the injury. The usefulness of EMG feedback in the rehabilitative process has been amply demonstrated in patients who have sustained injuries due to trauma such as spinal cord injuries, cerebrovascular accidents, or strokes. Basmajian, Kukulka, Narayan, and Takebe (1975) randomly assigned hemiplegic subjects to either therapeutic exercise or therapeutic exercise supplemented by EMG feedback. The results clearly favored the group receiving the combined procedure. Despite some methodological as well as statistical limitations, this research encouraged other investigators to demonstrate the efficacy of EMG biofeedback in increasing range of motion, motor power, gait, and general usage of muscles, in hemiplegic and hemiparetic patients (Baker, Regenos, Wolf, & Basmajian, 1977; Lee, Hill, Johnston, & Smiehorowski, 1976; Middaugh, 1978; Shahani, Connors, & Mohr, 1977).

A variety of feedback techniques, including the use of EMG feedback, have been employed in the treatment of Cerebral Palsy (Finley, Niman, Standley, & Wansley, 1977, 1976; Wooldridge & Russell, 1976). There is considerable evidence that a fine degree of motor control, equivalent to that of normal subjects, can be achieved by cerebral palsy patients, particularly if the treatment is tailored to the individual case and uses an interdisciplinary treatment model (Batshaw & Haslam, 1976). The major difficulties in treating such patients appear to be related to a lack of maintenance of treatment gains beyond the experimental setting (Wooldridge & Russell, 1976) or over a long-term follow-up (Finley et al., 1977). The Finely et al. study noted improvement in the speech and motor skills of cerebral palsy children during frontal EMG training and "electrophysiologic behavior modification." However, at a six-week follow-up, treatment gains had deteriorated although reinstitution of the treatment strategy produced reacquisition of lowered frontal EMG scores and recovery of speech and motor function.

Spasmodic torticollis is viewed as a disturbance in the control of the posture of the head such that the head is drawn to one side and the patient typically looks over one shoulder. Although this position tends to be sustained, there are frequently spasms and headjerks which are superimposed upon the deviated head position. Treatments have consisted of chemotherapy, surgery, and psychotherapy. The behavioral treatments have included massed negative practice (Agras & Marshall, 1965), relaxation training and systematic desensitization (Meares, 1973), and some form of feedback for torticollis movements (Bernhardt, Hersen, & Barlow, 1972). A number of studies have reported the successful use of EMG biofeedback techniques with torticollis patients where feedback is provided for reduction of muscle activity in the hyperactive muscles.

Investigators have employed EMG biofeedback alone (Brudny, Grynbaum, & Korein, 1974; Brudny et al., 1974; Jankel, 1978; Jones, Massong, & Buckley, 1983) while others have used EMG and electric shock feedback with torticollis patients (Cleeland, 1973; Russ, 1975). Although many of the research outcomes can be criticized due to lack of methodological rigor and reliance on case studies, there is, nevertheless, considerable evidence that EMG feedback for sternocladomastoid muscle activity can be considered an effective treatment for the reduction of torticollis symptoms where patients voluntarily maintained a neutral (forward-looking) head position. Furthermore, several researchers have demonstrated that these gains can be maintained over follow-ups ranging from 3 months to 40 months (Brudny et al., 1974; Cleeland, 1973; Jones, Massong, & Buckley, 1983; Russ, 1975). Similarly, EMG biofeedback was applied to treat blepharospasms or eye tics, a disorder that involves the involuntary clonic and tonic spasms of the eyelid and the muscles surrounding the eyes (Ballard, Doerr, & Varni, 1972; Peck, 1977; Stephenson, 1976). Treatment gains ranging from complete absence of spasms to what appears as an ordinary eye blink, were maintained through as long as a nine-month follow-up. However, the treatment sessions required to achieve such results consist of as many as 60 sessions (Stephenson, 1976). It may, thus, be rather difficult to maintain sufficient patient motivation to achieve such results. Given the aforementioned, there can be no question but that there are factors other than those associated with the treatment techniques themselves that influence results.

OTHER APPLICATIONS

Since the discovery that a number of responses thought to be exclusively under autonomic nervous system control can be influenced volitionally, researchers have worked diligently to increase the armamentarium of biofeedback techniques in the treatment of disorders that fall under the rubric of autonomically mediated conditions. Thus, for example, investigators studying the application of EMG biofeedback have examined treatments for conditions as diverse as diabetes (Fowler, Budzinski, & Vandenbergh, 1976; Seeburg & DeBaer, 1980), dermatological conditions such as eczema (Schandler, 1978), and even hyperhydrosis (massive palmar sweating in response to emotional stimuli or changes in temperature; Rickles, 1978). While further study of these and other conditions may appear warranted, the early findings of the diabetes research are particularly intriguing. In both of the diabetes studies referenced above, EMG biofeedback was employed as a central component in two single case studies and both reported an increase in subjective well-being and at least some reduction in the level of daily insulin required. These studies raised considerable concern regarding the need to provide close medical monitoring of insulin levels for patients as there appeared a considerable instability of these levels. Neither study involved any control procedures designed to reduce placebo or other experimenter related effects.

Other areas of application have included the attempted control of stuttering (Alexander, 1975; Craig & Cleary, 1982; Guitar, 1975; Hanna, Wilfling, & McNeill, 1975; Lanyon, 1978; Lanyon, Barrington, & Newman, 1976), dysmenorrhea and menstrual distress (Ballick, Elfner, May, & Moore, 1982; Clayman & Simkins, 1975; Dietvorst & Osborne, 1978; Hatch, 1981; Schneider & Culver, 1977; Sedlacek & Heczey, 1977; Tubbs & Carnahan, 1976), and urinary incontinence (Pearne, Zigelbaum, & Peyser, 1977; Suhel & Satler, 1977). The aforementioned literature has pointed to the relevance of EMG as both an adjunctive procedure in the control of bodily responses to stress and anxiety which interfere with more normative bodily functioning, and as a focal procedure in specific instances such as stuttering, where specific muscle tension reduction may offer an opportunity to ameliorate the condition. Again, however, while much of this research offers hope for clinical utility, it still suffers from a lack of rigor and a general failure to employ experimental designs that permit the teasing out of components that may be incidental to, or critical to, the overall outcome.

Ultimately, the real issue in this entire field is the question of whether biofeedback per se is the sine qua non of success in the modification of the muscular/vascular responses which result in symptomatology and in the maintenance of treatment gains attained during the training process. This is not to say that biofeedback technology has value simply because of its placebo effect. The argument of Holroyd and his colleagues has particular relevance here. These investigators argue that biofeedback may be effective not because it directly controls the physiological responses experienced in the case of headache sufferers, but because it indirectly induces these individuals to modify the methods by which they deal with headache symptomatology and the related stressors (Coyne & Holroyd, 1982; Holroyd, 1979; Holroyd & Lazarus, 1982). Furthermore, it is inconceivable to assume that the individual in the process of biofeedback training does not engage in cognitive activity that aids in the interpretation and integration of the biofeedback experience while acquisition of the response is occurring and during the transfer of this training to the day-to-day environment. In fact, such cognitive activity may be of central importance in facilitating such transfer of training. Convincing data may presently not offer an assurance of the relative contribution of the specific biofeedback technology versus the more general cognitive process associated with it. It is, nevertheless, almost inevitably the case that cognitive components associated with EMG-related therapy must be seen to be of substantial significance to the overall process, and in fact the recent literature is especially focused on this perspective.

Holroyd and Andrasik (1982), for example, studied the relative efficacy of the treatment of chronic tension headache sufferers who completed either a stress-coping training sequence or an EMG biofeedback training program. Over the course of a two-year follow-up, subjects who had received the cognitive therapy reported that they continued to use the strategies they had been taught, and that they were still significantly improved in their reported headache symptomatology. Of the biofeedback subjects, approximately half reported substantial improvement immediately following treatment with the remainder reporting only minor improvement or no change. A similar pattern of such mixed outcome in this latter group was evident at the two-year follow-up.

In two single-case design experiments also with headache sufferers, Kremsdorf, Kochanowicz, and Costell (1981) showed that biofeedback training influenced their subjects' mean frontalis EMG readings but that such changes were not associated specifically with concomitant reductions in headache activity. Rather, it was the presence or absence of cognitive skills training that determined whether each subject reported changes in his headache activity.

Stern and Berrenberg (1977) noted that subjects following biofeedback training exhibited a shift from an external to an internal locus of control on the Rotter I-E scale while those subjects who received false feedback or no feedback experienced no such shifts. Subjects frequently report a greater sense of personal control following biofeedback treatment, suggesting a process that is not measurable by EMG levels alone. Biofeedback may simply be one of a multitude of strategies which facilitate the attainment of coping skills that may or may not be under the deliberate influence of the investigators. What has often been relegated to the influence of placebo, in fact, may be the impact of self-generated cognitive strategies which contribute to relief in symptomatology and maintenance of gains at follow-up. Certainly, methodologies that incorporate and study the contribution of cognitive factors are becoming more prevalent in the literature and may offer alternative or perhaps more adequate explanations of the biofeedback strategies in the treatment of psychophysiological disorders.

REFERENCES

Agras, S., & Marshall, C. (1965). The application of negative practice to spasmodic torticollis. *American Journal of Psychiatry, 122,* 579–582.

Alexander, P. T. (1975). Effects of electromyographic feedback conditioning on the severity of stuttering. *Dissertation Abstracts International, 35*(7B), 3653B–3654B.

Appenzeller, O. (1973). Getting a sore head from banging it on the wall. *Headache, 13,* 131–132.

Baekelund, F., & Hoy, P. (1971). Reported vs. recorded sleep characteristics. *Archives of General Psychiatry, 24,* 548–551.

Baker, M., Regenos, E., Wolf, S. L., & Basmajian, J. V. (1977). Developing strategies for biofeedback: Applications in neurologically handicapped patients. *Physical Therapy, 57,* 402–408.

Ballick, L., Elfner, L., May, J., & Moore, J. D. (1982). Biofeedback treatment of dysmenorrhea. *Biofeedback and Self-Regulation, 7,* 499–520.

Ballard, P., Doerr, H., & Varni, J. (1972). Arrest of disabling eye disorder using biofeedback. *Psychophysiology, 9,* 271.

Basmajian, J. V., Kukulka, C. G., Narayan, M. G., & Takebe, K. (1975). Biofeedback treatment of foot-drop after stroke compared with standard rehabilitation technique: Effects of voluntary control and strength. *Archives of Physical Medicine & Rehabilitation, 56,* 231–236.

Batshaw, M. L., & Haslam, R. H. (1976). Multidisciplinary management of dystonia misdiagnosed as hysteria. In I.R. Eldridge & S. Fahn (Eds.), *Advances in neurology* (Vol. 4). Dystonia, NY: Raven Press.

Beck, A. T. (1976). *Cognitive therapy and the emotional disorders.* New York: International University Press.

Bernhardt, A. J., Hersen, M., & Barlow, D. H. (1972). Measurement and modification of spasmodic torticollis: Analysis. *Behavior Therapy, 3,* 294–297.

Bernstein, D. A., & Borkovec, T. D. (1973). *Progressive Relaxation training: A manual for the helping professions.* Champaign, IL: Research Press.

Besner, H. F. (1975). *A comparison of selected biofeedback Techniques in treating chronic onset insomnia.* Unpublished doctoral dissertation, Nova University, Ft. Lauderdale, FL.

Bober, H. (1958). Cause and treatment of bruxism and bruxomania. *Dental Abstracts, 3,* 658–659.

Borkovec, T. D., Kaloupek, D. G., & Slama, K. M. (1975). The facilitative effect of muscle tension–release in the relaxation treatment of sleep disturbance. *Behavior Therapy, 6,* 301–309.

Borkovec, T. D., Steinmark, S. W., & Nau, S. D. (1973). Relaxation training and single-item desensitization in the group treatment of insomnia. *Journal of Behavior Therapy & Experimental Psychiatry, 4,* 401–403.

Brudny, J., Grynbaum, B. B., & Korein, J. (1974). Spasmodic torticolla: Treatment by feedback display of the EMG. *Archives of Physical Medicine & Rehabilitation, 55,* 403–408.

Brudny, J., Korein, J., Levidow, L., Grynbaum, B. B., Lieberman, A., &

Friedman, L. W. (1974). Sensory feedback therapy as a modality of treatment in central nervous system disorders of voluntary movement. *Neurology, 24,* 925–932.

Budzynski, T. H. (1973). Biofeedback procedures in the clinic. *Seminars in Psychiatry, 5,* 537–547.

Budzinski, TY. H., Stoyva, J. M., & Adler, C. S. (1970). Feedback-induced muscle relaxation: Application to tension headache. *Behavior Therapy & Experimental Psychiatry, 1,* 205–211.

Budzinski, T. H., Stoyva, J. M., Adler, C. S., & Mullaney, D. J. (1973). EMG biofeedback and tension headache: A controlled outcome study. *Psychosomatic Medicine, 35,* 484–496.

Casas, J. M., Beemsterboer, P., & Clark, G. T. (1982). A comparison of stress–reduction behavioral counseling and contingent nocturnal EMG feedback for the treatment of bruxism. *Behaviour Research & Therapy, 20,* 9–15.

Chesney, M. A., & Shelton, J. L. (1976). A comparison of muscle relaxation nd electromyogram biofeedback treatments for muscle contraction headache. *Journal of Behavior Therapy & Experimental Psychiatry, 7,* 221–226.

Clark, G. T., Beemsterboer, P., & Rugh, J. D. (1981). The treatment of nocturnal bruxism using contingent EMG feedback with an arousal task. *Behaviour Research & Therapy, 19,* 451–455.

Clayman, K. K., & Simkins, L. (1975). *The relationship of temperature control to menstrual distress.* Paper presented at the Sixth Annual Meeting of the Biofeedback Research Society.

Cleeland, C. S. (1973). Behavioral techniques in the modification of spasmodic torticollis. *Neurology, 23,* 1241–1247.

Coursey, R., Buchsbaum, M., & Frankel, B. L. (1975). Personality measures and evoked responses in chronic insomniacs. *Journal of Abnormal Psychology, 84,* 239–249.

Cox, D. J., Freundlich, A., & Meyer, R. G. (1975). Differential effectiveness of EMG feedback, verbal relaxation instructions and medication placebo with tension headaches. *Journal of Consulting & Clinical Psychology, 43,* 892–898.

Coyne, J., & Holroyd, K. (1982). Stress, coping, & illness: A transactional perspective. In T. Million, C. Green, & R. Meagher (Eds.), *Handbook of health care clinical psychology.* New York: Plenum.

Craig, A. R., & Cleary, P. J. (1982). Reduction of stuttering by young male stutterers using EMG Feedback. *Biofeedback and Self-Regulation, 7,* 241–255.

Cromwell, L., Weibell, F. J., Pfeiffer, E. A., & Usselman, L. B. (1973). *Biomedical instrumentation & measurement.* Englewood Cliffs, NJ: Prentice-Hall.

Dalessio, J. (1972). *Wolff's headaches and other head pain.* New York: Oxford University Press.

Daly, E. J., Donn, P. A., Galliher, M. J., & Zimmerman, J. S. (1983). Biofeedback applications to migraine and tension headaches: A double-blind outcome study. *Biofeedback & Self-Regulation, 8,* 135–152.

Davidson, R. J., & Schwartz, G. E. (1976). The psychobiology of relaxation & relaxed states: A multiprocess theory. In D.I. Mostofsky (Ed.), *Behavior control and modification of physiological activity.* Englewood Cliffs, NJ: Prentice-Hall.

Dietvorst, T. F., & Osborne, D. (1978). Biofeedback assisted relaxation training for primary dysmenorrhea: A case study. *Biofeedback and Self-Regulation, 3,* 301–305.

Epstein, L. H., Hersen, M., & Hemphill, D. P. (1974). Music feedback in the treatment of tension headache: An experimental case study. *Journal of Behavior Therapy & Experimental Psychiatry, 5,* 59–63.

Finley, W. W., Niman, C. A., Standley, J., & Wansley, R. A. (1977). Electrophysiologic behavior modification of frontal EMG in cerebral palsied children. *Biofeedback & Self-Regulation, 2,* 59–79.

Fowler, J. E., Budzinski, T. H., & Vandenbergh, R. L. (1976). Effects of an EMG biofeedback relaxation program on the control of diabetes: A case study. *Biofeedback & Self-Regulation, 1,* 105–112.

Friedman, R., & Papsdorf, L. (1976). Biofeedback and progressive relaxation treatment of sleep-onset insomnia: A controlled, all-night investigation. *Biofeedback & Self-Regulation, 1,* 253–271.

Gershman, L., & Clouser, R. A. (1974). Treating insomnia with relaxation and desensitization in a group setting by an automated approach. *Journal of Behavior Therapy & Experimental Psychiatry, 5,* 31–35.

Glickman, I. (1972). *Clinical Periodontology* (4th eds.). Philadelphia, PA: Saunders.

Goldfried, M. R. (1980). Psychotherapy as coping skills training. In M.J. Mahoney (Ed.), *Psychotherapy process: Current issues and future directions.* New York: Plenum.

Guitar, B. (1975). Reduction of stuttering frequency using analog electromyographic feedback. *Journal of Speech & Hearing Disorders, 40,* 270–273.

Hanna, R., Wilfling, F., & McNeill, B. (1975). A biofeedback treatment for stuttering. *Journal of Speech & Hearing Disorders, 40,* 270–273.

Hatch, J. P. (1981). Voluntary control of sexual responding in men and women: Implications for the etiology and treatment of sexual dysfunctions. *Biofeedback & Self-Regulation, 6,* 191–205.

Hauri, P. (1978). Biofeedback techniques in the treatment of chronic insomnia. In R.L. Williams & I. Karacan (Eds.), *Sleep disorders: Diagnosis & Treatment.* New York: John Wiley.

Hauri, P. (1981). Treating psychophysiologic insomnia with biofeedback. *Archives of General Psychiatry, 38,* 752–758.

Hauri, P. J., Percy, L., Hellekson, C., Hartmann, E., & Russ, D. (1982). The treatment of psychophysiologic insomnia with biofeedback: A replication study. *Biofeedback & Self-Regulation, 7,* 223–235.

Haynes, S. N., Griffin, P., Mooney, D., & Parise, M. (1975). Electromyographic biofeedback and relaxation instructions in the treatment of muscle contraction headaches. *Behavior Therapy, 6,* 672–678.

Hinkle, J. E., & Lutker, E. R. (1972). A new approach. *Psychotherapy: Theory, Research & Practice, 9,* 236–237.

Holroyd, K. A. (1979). Stress, coping, and the treatment of stress related illness. In J.R. McNamara (Ed.), *Behavioral approaches in medicine: Application analysis.* New York: Plenum.

Holroyd, K. A., & Andrasik, F. (1982). Do the effects of cognitive therapy endure? A two-year follow-up of tension headache sufferers treated with cognitive therapy or biofeedback. *Cognitive Therapy & Research, 6,* 325–334.

Holroyd, K. A., & Lazarus, R. S. (1982). Stress, coping and somatic adaption. In L. Goldberger & J. Breznitz (Eds.), *Handbook of stress.* New York: Free Press.

Hutchings, D. F., & Reinking, R. H. (1976). Tension headaches: What form of therapy is most effective? *Biofeedback & Self-Regulation, 1,* 183–190.

Institute of Medicine. (1979). *Report of a study: Sleeping pills, insomnia, and medical practice.* Washington, DC: National Academy of Sciences.

Jacobsen, E. (1938). *Progressive relaxation.* Chicago: University of Chicago Press.

Jankel, W. R. (1978). *EMG feedback in spasmodic torticollis.* Paper presented at the ninth annual meeting of the Biofeedback Society of America, Albuquerque, NM.

Janssen, K. (1983). Differential effectiveness of EMG feedback versus combined EMG-feedback and relaxation instructions in the treatment of tension headache. *Journal of Psychosomatic Research, 27,* 243–253.

Jones, G. E., Massong, S. R., & Buckley, M. F. (1983). Treatment of spasmodic torticollis through spasm control and muscle reeducation: A case study. *Behavior Therapy, 14,* 178–184.

Kahn, M., Baker, B. L., & Weiss, J. M. (1968). Treatment of insomnia by relaxation training. *Journal of Abnormal Psychology, 73,* 556–558.

Kales, A., Caldwell, A. B., Preston, T. A., Healey, S., & Kales, J. D. (1976). Personality patterns in insomnia. *Archives of General Psychiatry, 33,* 1128–1134.

Karacan, I., Williams, R., Littell, R., & Salis, P. (1973). Insomniacs: Unpredictable and idiosyncratic sleepers. In W.P. Koella & P. Levin (Eds.), *Sleep: Physiology, biochemistry, psychology, pharmacology: Clinical implications.* Basel: Karger.

Kremsdorf, R. B., Kochanowicz, N. A., & Costell, S. (1981). Cognitive skills training versus EMG biofeedback in the treatment of tension headaches. *Biofeedback and Self-Regulation, 6,* 93–102.

Lanyon, R. I. (1978). Behavioral approaches to stuttering. In M. Hersen, R.M. Eisler, & P. M. Miller (Eds.), *Progress in behavior modification* (Vol. 6). New York: Academic Press.

Lanyon, R. I., Barrington, C.C., & Newman, A. C. (1976). Modification of stuttering through EMG biofeedback: A preliminary study. *Behavior Therapy, 7,* 96–103.

Lazarus, R. S. (1975). A cognitively oriented psychologist looks at biofeedback. *American Psychologist, 30,* 553–561.

LeBoeuf, A., & Lodge, J. (1980). A comparison of frontalis EMG feedback training and progressive relaxation in the treatment of chronic anxiety. *British Journal of Psychiatry, 137,* 279–284.

Lee, K. H., Hill, E., Johnson, R., & Smiehorowski, T. (1976). Biofeedback for muscle retraining in hemiplegic patients. *Archives of Physical Medicine & Rehabilitation, 57,* 588–591.

Libo, L. M., & Arnold, G. E. (1983). Relaxation practice after biofeedback therapy: A long-term follow-up study of utilization and effectiveness. *Biofeedback & Self-Regulation, 8,* 217–227.

Lindqvist, B. (1971). Bruxism in children. *Odontologisk Revy, 22,* 413–424.

Lindqvist, B. (1972). Bruxism and emotional disturbance. *Odontologisk Revy, 23,* 231–242.

Lindqvist, B. (1973). Occlusal interferences in children with bruxism. *Odontologisk Revy, 24,* 141–148.

Malmo, R. B. (1975). *On emotions, needs, and our archaic brain.* New York: Holt, Rinehart, & Winston.

Martin, M. J. (1966). Tension headache, a psychiatric study. *Headache, 6,* 47–54.

McKenzie, R. E., Ehrisman, W. J., Montgomery, P. S., & Barnes, R. H. (1974). The treatment of headache by means of electroencephalographic biofeedback. *Headache, 13,* 164–172.

Meares, R. (1973). Behavior therapy and spasmodic torticollis. *Archives of General Psychiatry, 28,* 104–107.

Meichenbaum, D. (1974). *Cognitive behavior modification.* Morristown, NJ: General Learning Press.

Meichenbaum, D. (1976). Cognitive factors in biofeedback therapy. *Biofeedback & Self-Regulation, 1,* 201–216.

Meklas, J. F. (1971). Diagnosis and treatment. *Journal of the Academy of General Dentistry, 19,* 31–36.

Middaugh, S. (1978). EMG feedback as a muscle re-education technique: A controlled study (Paper presented at the annual meetings of the Society for Psychophysiological Research, San Diego, CA, October 1976). *Physical Therapy, 58,* 15–22.

Monroe, L. J. (1967). Psychological and physiological difference between good and poor sleepers. *Journal of Abnormal Psychology, 72,* 255–264.

Montgomery, D. D., & Besner, H. F. (1975). Reduction of chronic onset insomnia through electromyographic relaxation training. *The Journal of Biofeedback, 2,* 28–32.

Montgomery, P. S., & Ehrisman, W. J. (1976). Biofeedback alleviated headaches: A follow-up. *Headache, 16,* 64–65.

Montgomery, I., Perkin, G., & Wise, D. (1975). A review of behavioral treatments for insomnia. *Journal of Behavioral Therapy & Experimental Psychiatry, 6,* 93–100.

Nicassio, P., & Bootzin, R. A. (1974). A comparison of progressive relaxation and autogenic training as treatments for insomnia. *Journal of Abnormal Psychology, 83,* 253–260.

Nuechterlein, K. H., & Holroyd, J. C. (1980). Biofeedback in the treatment of tension headache: Current status. *Archives of General Psychiatry, 37,* 866–873.

Pearne, D. H., Zigelbaum, S. D., & Peyser, W. P. (1977). Biofeedback assisted EMG relaxation for urinary retention and incontinence. *Biofeedback & Self-Regulation, 2,* 213–217.

Peck, D. F. (1977). The use of EMG feedback in the treatment of a severe case of blepharospasm. *Biofeedback & Self-Regulation, 2,* 273–279.

Phillips, C. (1977). The modification of tension headache pain using EMG biofeedback. *Behaviour Research & Therapy, 15,* 119–129.

Piccione, A., Coates, T. J., George, J. M., Rosenthal, R., & Karzmark, P. (1982). Nocturnal biofeedback for nocturnal bruxism. *Biofeedback & Self-Regulation, 7,* 405–419.

Raskin, M., Johnson, G., & Rondestvedt, S. W. (1973). Chronic anxiety treated by feedback-induced muscle relaxation. *Archives of General Psychiatry, 28,* 263–267.

Raskin, M., Bali, L. T., & Peeke, H. V. (1980). Muscle biofeedback and transcendental meditation. *Archives of General Psychiatry, 37,* 83–97.

Reding, G. R., Rubright, W. C., & Zimmerman, S. O. (1966). Incidence of bruxism. *Journal of Dental Research, 45,* 1198–1204.

Reinking, R., & Hutchings, D. (1981). Follow-up to "Tension headaches: What form of therapy is most effective?" *Biofeedback & Self-Regulation, 6,* 57–62.

Ribordy, S. C., & Denney, D. R. (1977). The behavioral treatment of insomnia: An alternative to drug therapy. *Behaviour Research & Therapy, 15,* 39–50.

Rickles, W. (1978). Treatment of a case of hyperhydrosis with vapor pressure feedback. *Annual Proceedings of the Biofeedback Society of America,* pp. 92–93.

Robinson, T. (1969). *Presleep activity and sleep quality of good and poor sleepers.* Unpublished doctoral dissertation, University of Chicago, Chicago, IL.

Roth, T., Kramer, M., & Lutz, T. (1976). The nature of insomnia: A descriptive summary of a sleep clinic population. *Comprehensive Psychiatry, 17,* 217–220.

Russ, K. L. (1975). *EMG biofeedback of spasmodic torticollis: A case study.* Annual Proceedings of the Biofeedback Research Society.

Schandler, S. (1978). *Use of muscle biofeedback relaxation in the treatment of eczema.* Annual Proceedings of the Biofeedback Society of America.

Scharer, P. (1974). Bruxism. *Frontiers of Oral Physiology, 1,* 293–322.

Schneider, C., & Culver, D. (1977). *Group and individual biofeedback treat-*

ment for dysmenorrhea: A pilot study. Paper presented at the Annual Meeting of the Rocky Mountain Psychological Association, Albuquerque, NM.

Schultz, J. H., & Luthe, W. (1959). *Autogenic training: A psychophysiological approach in psychotherapy.* New York: Grune & Stratton.

Schwartz, B., Guilbaud, G., & Fishgood, H. (1963). Etudes electroencephalographiques sur le sommeil de muit. 1. To Linsomme chronique. *Presse Medicale, 71,* 1474–1476.

Schwartz, L., & Chayes, C. M. (1968). *Facial pain and mandibular dysfunction.* Philadelphia, PA: Saunders.

Sedlacek, K., & Heczey, M. (1977). A specific biofeedback treatment for dysmenorrhea. *Biofeedback & Self-Regulation, 2,* 294 (Abstract).

Seeburg, K. N., & DeBoer, K. F. (1980). Effects of EMG biofeedback on diabetes. *Biofeedback & Self-Regulation, 5,* 289–293.

Shahani, B. T., Connors, L., & Mohr, J. P. (1977). Electromyographic audiovisual feedback training effect on the motor performance in patients with lesions of the central nervous system. *Archives of Physical Medicine & Rehabilitation, 58.*

Starker, S., & Hasenfeld, R. (1976). Daydream styles and sleep disturbance. *Journal of Nervous and Mental Disease, 163,* 391–400.

Stephenson, N. L. (1976). Successful treatment of blepharospasm with relaxation and biofeedback. (Paper presented at the seventh annual meeting of the Biofeedback Society of America, Colorado Springs, March 1976). *Biofeedback & Self-Regulation, 1,* 33 (Abstract).

Stern, G. S., & Berrenberg, J. D. (1977). Biofeedback training in frontalis muscle relaxation and enhancement of belief in personal control. *Biofeedback & Self-Regulation, 2,* 173–182.

Stern, G. S., Miller, R. C., Ewy, H. W., & Grant, P. S. (1980). Perceived control: Bogus pulse rate feedback and reported symptom reduction for individuals with accumulated stressful life events. *Biofeedback & Self-Regulation, 5,* 37–49.

Suhel, P., & Satler, J. (1977). Use of biological feedback in correction of urinary incontinence. *Urologia Internationalis, 32,* 238–246.

Tasto, D. L., & Hinkle, J. E. (1973). Muscle relaxation treatment for tension headaches. *Behaviour Research & Therapy, 11,* 347–349.

Thaller, J. L. (1960). The use of the Cornell Index to determine the correlation between bruxism and the anxiety state. *Journal of Periodontology, 31,* 138–140.

Townsend, R. E., House, J. F., & Addario, D. A. (1975). A comparison of biofeedback mediated relaxation and group therapy in the treatment of chronic anxiety. *American Journal of Psychiatry, 132,* 598–601.

Tubbs, W., & Carnahan, C. (1976). Clinical biofeedback for primary dysmenorrhea: A Pilot. *Biofeedback & Self-Regulation, 1,* 323 (Abstract).

Tunis, M. M., & Wolff, H. G. (1954). Studies on headache: Cranial artery vasoconstriction and muscle contraction headache. *Archives of Neurology & Psychiatry, 71,* 425–435.

van Boxtel, A., & van der Ven, J. R. (1978). Differential EMG activity in subjects with muscle contraction headaches related to mental effort. *Headache, 17,* 233–237.

Vernallis, F. F. (1955). Teeth-grinding: Some relationships to anxiety, hostility, and hyperactivity. *Journal of Clinical Psychology, 11,* 389–391.

Vestergaard, C. L. (1967). Facial pain from the masticatory system induced by experimental bruxism. *Tandlaegelbladt, 71,* 1171–1181.

Weinman, M. L., Semchuk, K. M., Gaebe, G., & Mathew, R. J. (1983). The effect of stressful life events on EMG biofeedback and relaxation training in the treatment of anxiety. *Biofeedback & Self-Regulation, 8,* 191–205.

Wickramasekera, I. (1972). Electromyographic feedback training and tension headache: Preliminary observations. *American Journal of Clinical Hypnosis, 15,* 83–85.

Wickramasekera, I. (1973). Temperature feedback for the control of migraine. *Journal of Behavior Therapy & Experimental Psychiatry, 4,* 343–345.

Wooldridge, C. P., & Russell, G. (1976). Head positioning training with the cerebral palsied child: An application of biofeedback techniques. *Archives of Physical Medicine & Rehabilitation, 57,* 407–414.

III

PAIN

8

Psychological Assessment of Chronic Pain

Stanley L. Chapman

Director of Psychology
Pain Control and Rehabilitation Institute of Georgia
Decatur, Georgia
and
Clinical Assistant Professor of Rehabilitation Medicine
Emory University
Atlanta, Georgia

Appreciation of the role of psychological and emotional factors in pain dates back at least to Aristotle, who described pain as a "passion of the soul." For many centuries, pain then was seen in Western cultures largely in a religious context, as a punishment for sins or as a manifestation of God's will. In the 17th century, Descartes proposed that medical difficulties could be studied scientifically and resided either in the body or in the mind, which he viewed as being quite separate from each other. Sensory physiologists in the 19th century saw pain as being reflective of direct transmission of sensory information from the pain receptors through the spinal cord into the brain, where these impulses were registered as pain. Cognitive and emotional factors frequently were relegated to a secondary role and viewed as mere "reactions to pain;" however, the sensory theory did not explain many cases in which pain complaints did not fit with pathology or were not removed with physical interventions.

A primary role for psychological and emotional factors in the pain experience was restored in Melzack and Wall's (1965) "gate-control" model of pain, which viewed pain perception as resulting from the interaction of sensory, affective, and evaluative components. According to this theory, somatic input is modulated through a central control mechanism before it evokes pain perception. Psychological methods that affect cognitive and affective processes thus may prevent, remove, or reduce the perceived intensity of pain. Asserting that somatic and psychological factors interact at every level along the spinal cord, the gate-control theory contradicted Descartes' notion that the body and mind are quite separate and independent of each other.

Empirical support for the interaction of body and mind comes from research in many areas. For example, research in biofeedback has demonstrated that physiological functions can be altered systematically through training of emotional and behavioral responses, and research in hypnosis has suggested that some individuals are able systematically to alter their perception of pain through selective attention processes. Moreover, cognitive variables such as expectancy, perceived control, catastrophic thinking, and the meaning of the situation in which pain is experienced have been found to affect pain reports significantly when measured in volunteers exposed to painful stimuli or in a naturalistic setting (e.g., Beecher, 1959; Bobey & Davidson, 1970; Genest, Meichenbaum, & Turk, 1977; Kanfer & Goldfoot, 1966). Nevertheless, the Cartesian idea that human experience belongs either to the realm of body or mind has persisted, and many physicians and mental health professionals mistakenly assume that a psychiatric diagnosis should be applied in individuals with chronic pain because physical findings are absent. Because the body and the mind dynamically interact with each other constantly, pain better can be looked at as being 100 percent organic and 100 percent psychological.

PSYCHOLOGICAL AND ENVIRONMENTAL FACTORS IN CHRONIC PAIN

Evidence for emotional dysfunction in chronic pain patients is seen in psychological test results, which frequently include elevations on many clinical scales of the MMPI (particularly the Hypochondriasis, Depression, and Hysteria scales) and a high Neuroticism score on the Eysenck Personality Inventory (Woodforde & Merskey, 1972a). There has been much controversy about whether the psychological dysfunctions precipitate or predispose an individual to chronic pain, or primarily are reactions to the chronic pain experience. A better understanding of the relationship awaits epidemiological research in which a population at risk for chronic pain can be studied longitudinally.

The role of depression in chronic pain patients has aroused particular controversy. There is little doubt that many individuals with chronic pain report similar symptoms as those who are clinically depressed, such as a low energy level, difficulty getting started, difficulty sleeping, and feelings of being demoralized and unable to enjoy life (e.g., Pinsky, 1979). Blumer and Heilbronn (1982) hypothesized that chronic pain is a variant of depressive disease, which they labeled "the pain-prone disorder." They cited as evidence studies revealing that chronic pain patients show the same frequency of early escape from dexamethasone and abnormal REM latency as patients with a major affective disorder; the frequent presence of bodily aches and pains among depressives; frequent family histories of depression, alcoholism, and other behavioral problems in chronic pain patients; and the frequency of pain relief with antidepressant medication (e.g., Blumer, Heilbronn, & Pedraza, et al., 1980; Blumer, Zorick, & Heilbronn, 1982; Blumer & Heilbronn, 1984).

A number of critics have questioned the conceptualization of chronic pain as a depressive equivalent, citing a variety of conceptual and methodological weaknesses in the argument and some nonconfirmatory data (Rosenbaum, 1982; Turk & Salovey, 1984). For example, France and Krishnan (1985) found that only 14 or 80 chronic back pain patients showed evidence of a positive dexamethasone suppression test. Their finding that all 45 patients who did not show symptoms of a major depressive disorder also did not show suppression of dexamethasone did not fit with any supposition that they might have a depressive illness but were masking the symptoms. Dessonville, Reeves, Thompson, and Gallagher (1984) divided items of the Beck Depression Inventory into those items describing somatic, affective, and cognitive aspects of depression and found that chronic back pain patients tended to endorse many somatic items but not many cognitive and affective items. They suggested that depression is a multidimensional syndrome, only some of which is shared by chronic pain patients. Moreover, Loeser (1979) suggested that the beneficial effects of tricyclic antidepressants in treating chronic pain may be attributable to their effect on restoring normal circadian rhythms rather than to any effect on an underlying affective disorder. He observed that symptoms of depressed activity as well as disturbances in circadian rhythm might be common in pain patients because of their frequent reliance on narcotic and sedative-hypnotic medications. Finally, Brena and Chapman (1985) described many symptoms of depression found in chronic pain patients as being common results of a syndrome of physical inactivity. These include psychomotor depression, cognitive stagnation, and sleep disturbances.

It is a widely held belief that chronic pain is not so much a product of depression, but rather that it often results from stress and muscle tension. It has been proposed that repeated muscular hyperactivity may lead to ischemia or oxygen depletion at the affected site and subsequently to the release of pain-eliciting substances such as bradykinin. Pain then can act as an additional stressor, leading to a cycle of increasing pain and tension (Craig, 1984). Though relaxation therapies are almost universally employed at multidisciplinary pain centers and have been found to be rated as helpful by patients (Chapman, 1983), several reviewers have summarized data questioning the strength of the relationship between muscle tension and either back pain (Turk & Flor, 1984) or headaches (Philips, 1978; Holmes & Burish, 1983). Documentation of the role of stress and tension in chronic pain syndromes thus awaits further research.

The pioneering work of Wilbert Fordyce in the 1960s and 1970s highlighted the role of learning in chronic pain (Fordyce, 1974, 1976a, 1976b; Fordyce, Fowler, Lehmann, & DeLateur, 1968). Fordyce emphasized that chronic pain can be conceptualized in terms of observable behaviors typically found in chronic pain sufferers. Examples of such "pain behaviors" might include verbal complaining of pain, limping, grimacing, taking prescribed medications for pain, and remaining inactive and unemployed. Fordyce wrote that these behaviors are not just simply results of physical injury or disease, but rather that they can be highly influenced by basic processes of learning, including operant conditioning, or systematic reward contingent on these behaviors. Examples of such rewards might include financial compensation, attention from significant others, withdrawal from responsibility or stress, or direct relief of anxiety or pain through behaviors such as taking medication or keeping a painful limb immobile. While direct evidence for the importance of operant conditioning in the *development* of a chronic pain syndrome is lacking, there is ample evidence that pain behaviors can be modified by changing contingencies in such a way that such behaviors are ignored and/or alternative "health behaviors" are rewarded (e.g., Cairns & Pasino, 1977; Doleys, Crocker, & Patton, 1982; Fordyce, 1976a; Fordyce, Fordyce, & DeLateur, 1968; Keefe, 1982; Sanders, 1979). Block, Kremer, and Gaylor (1980) found that pain patients with nonsolicitous spouses reported higher levels of pain to a ward clerk than to their spouse, while those with solicitous spouses reported more pain in the presence of the spouse than the ward clerk. Similarly, White and Sanders (1985) demonstrated higher pain behavior when drugs were offered on an as-needed basis rather than on a time-contingent basis.

Other basic processes of learning besides operant conditioning which might play a role in conditioning pain behaviors include classical (or respondent) conditioning and social modeling. Classical conditioning refers to a process by which a previously neutral stimulus can elicit a response through repeated pairing with an "unconditioned" stimulus which has the innate capability of eliciting this response. In the acute situation, pain behaviors can be looked at as responses which are elicited by organic changes associated with injury or dysfunction. These organic changes are paired with a multitude of stimuli, such as the physical setting, the presence of other people and, perhaps, the presence of self-generated thoughts such as "I wonder if this pain will ever go away." One can argue that through repeated pairing with the physical injury, these stimuli can become conditioned to elicit the same behaviors as originally occurred contingent on the presence of the physical injury. Thus, the presence of the pill bottle on the table next to the couch, for example, could come to elicit increased pain behavior or perception. While there is ample evidence to demonstrate that many autonomically mediated reflex responses can be conditioned to occur in the presence of previously neutral environmental stimuli (Brady, 1979; Whitehead et al., 1979), there is an absence of data to document the significance of classical conditioning of pain behavior.

Social modeling refers to the acquisition of a response based on observation of the response in others. Indirect evidence of its importance in chronic pain has come from findings of clear cultural differences in pain responses (Zborowski, 1969), and findings that pain complaints tend to run in families (Apley, 1975; Gentry, Shows, & Thomas, 1974; Violon & Giurgen, 1984). Apley studied 1100 English schoolchildren with chronic abdominal pains. He found that those children without clear medical evidence to account for the pain came from families who visited physicians with medical complaints far more often than did those children with clear medical evidence for abdominal pain. He inferred that children complaining of pain in the absence of physical evidence had learned to focus on pain through observation of behavior in their families. Gentry et al. revealed that major medical problems are common in histories of chronic low back pain patients while Violon and Giurgen found a family history of chronic pain in 78 percent of a mixed group of chronic pain sufferers in comparison with 44 percent of controls with chronic illness in the absence of pain. Though both sets of authors pointed to social modeling processes as being the most likely contributants to their findings, the data also could be interpreted as supporting the theory that a genetic predisposition for pain could be present. Other authors have revealed directly that pain behaviors in experimental situations can be altered depending on the behavior of relevant models and its consequences (Craig & Prkachin, 1978; Thelen & Frye, 1981).

THE ASSESSMENT PROCESS

In order to fully assess variables affecting psychological dysfunction, data from a psychological/behavioral assessment need to be integrated with evidence from medical and physical assessments. Just as physicians and physical therapists need to be aware of their limitations in interpreting psychological and behavioral data, so also do psychologists and other mental health professionals need to be aware of their limitations in interpreting medical and physical data. Even when comprehensive data are available, interpretation can be quite difficult; "state-of-the-art" testing procedures are far from perfect and the etiology of many pains is not well understood.

Behavioral-Psychological Interviewing

One of the best sources of assessment data is a comprehensive psychological interview. An interview permits direct observation of affect, mental status, and cognitive status and also allows in-depth exploration of identified problem areas. It also provides a direct sample of the patient's handling of a particular interpersonal situation. Limitation of interview data lies in the subjective nature and reliance on self-report. The value of such data may depend on many factors, such as the skill of the interviewer in pursuing important areas, the rapport between interviewer and interviewee, and the patient's perception about what the interviewer wants to hear or how he or she will use the data provided (Block et al., 1980; Cairns & Pasino, 1977). Thus, it is important to correlate interview data with objective measures whenever possible, and to gather information from multiple sources. Interviewing the spouse (or other person(s) who may be living with the patient) separately not only provides a reliability check for the information provided by the patient, but also yields important data regarding interpersonal relationships and problems in the way in which significant other(s) respond to the patient's pain behaviors. Comprehensive assessment also may necessitate interviewing others who can provide important information regarding the nature and history of the pain problem and related behavior, such as previous physicians, employers, and/or the patient's attorney and rehabilitation counselor.

Table 8.1 provides a summary of information to be sought in a psychological assessment interview. It is often wise to ask questions regarding the pain and its patterns first, as the patient may be resistant to answer questions relating to psychopathology until some rapport is established. Pain complaints that are diffuse, vaguely described, and do not fit with expectations based on medical data may reflect influences of learning. Information regarding the circumstances surrounding the onset of pain help to explain its etiology. Hirschfeld and Behan (1963) have written, for example, that job-

Table 8.1.
Outline for Psychological/Behavioral Interviewing

I. Pain Complaints.
   A. Location, description, patterns of occurrence.
   B. Onset.
   C. History of treatments, including medications.
   D. Previous history of pain-related illnesses.
   E. Nonverbal pain behavior observed.
II. Physical, Social and Recreational Activities.
   A. Level, average day's schedule.
   B. Changes, restrictions since onset of pain.
   C. Attempts to return to restricted activities.
   D. Pacing, consistency of activities.
III. Work.
   A. Employment, disability, and financial status.
   B. Work history and performance.
   C. Attempts to return to work; perceived restrictions.
   D. Emotional and cognitive responses regarding work and disability status.
IV. Sleep Disturbances: Nature and History.
V. Social Relationships.
   A. Previous and current social reinforcement patterns.
   B. Modeling of illness or pain behavior.
   C. Sexual disturbances.
   D. Family attitudes and expectancies.
VI. Emotional Status.
   A. Previous and current affective or behavioral disturbances.
   B. Mental status.
   C. Treatment history for psychological difficulties.
VII. Cognitive-Attitudinal Factors.
   A. Beliefs regarding nature of pain problem.
   B. Expectancies of outcome.
   C. Openness toward rehabilitation approach.
   D. Perceived meaning of pain.

related "accidents" frequently occur during times of high job stress or significant problems in the worker's life. Pain behavior that starts during periods of stress may be respondent to anxiety and/or may be operantly conditioned through resulting escape from stress or responsibility.

Patterns of occurrence in pain behavior also can provide important information. Pain behavior that varies depending upon the attentiveness or support of the observer may be operant; pain complaints that are particularly severe at the end of a stressful day of work are more likely to be respondent in nature; patterns of pain behavior that fit closely with medical data, such as worsening arthritic pain in the morning, suggest the importance of organic factors.

The history and evolution of pain complaints also provide significant clues to underlying processes and mechanisms. There are some preliminary data to show that particular types of early problems in life can be associated with particular types of pain. For example, Haber and Roos (1984) found a history of sexual or spouse abuse to be particularly common in women with abdominal or vaginal pain of unknown etiology. Ascertaining the presence, etiology, and pattern of other previous health problems and pain behaviors can provide clues about factors such as tendencies to develop illnesses under stress or tendencies toward somatization.

The treatment history for the current pain complaint also can yield important psychological information. Pain behaviors can persist despite multiple previous medical treatment because underlying psychological issues were not addressed; Chapman and Brena (1982) showed, for example, that chronic low back pain patients with environmental reinforcers contingent on pain complaints and high pain behaviors were less likely to respond favorably to sympathetic nerve blocks than were patients showing minimal evidence of learned pain behaviors. Many pain behaviors, such as those associated with depressed mood, can be iatrogenic in nature, reflecting adherence to suggestions from health professionals to continue to take habit-forming depressant medications and/or remain inactive.

Patterns of past and present medication use also need to be ascertained. The opportunity to take drugs that induce anxiety relief can be a powerful reinforcer for pain behavior. When medications are effective in relieving pain, or if dependency or addiction is present, cessation of their use can be very aversive. In addition, there is some evidence to suggest that pain can sometimes be respondent to medications originally designed to counteract it (e.g., Kudrow, 1982; Saper, 1983).

The interviewer also should note the frequency of verbal and non-verbal pain behaviors (such as complaining, groaning, wincing, rubbing a painful area, postural abnormalities, and shifts) and assess the degree to which these fit with expectations based on organic pathology or may be attention seeking. Sometimes these behaviors are in conflict with verbal statements, as in the case of the patient who claims he or she cannot sit for more than 20 minutes without having to get up, yet sits for an hour-long interview. Inconsistencies such as these need to be explored further to ascertain their meaning.

Questions regarding participation in physical activities also are critical to a behavioral/psychological assessment. Pain behaviors can be respondent to overactivity, underactivity, poor choice of activities, inconsistent activity patterns, and difficulties in pacing activities well. Restrictions in activity levels are less likely to be conditioned by relief from stress or responsibility if the patient was active prior to the onset of pain, has made many attempts to return to previous activities, has restricted selectively those activities most affected by his or her physical condition, and has not selectively restricted aversive activities. Participation in social activities can be a fruitful area of inquiry, particularly because these activities may be less directly influenced by a pain-related physical dysfunction than physical activities. Difficulty in starting all activities, particularly if associated with a low energy level, can be one sign of depression.

To ensure maximum reliability, questions regarding the patient's work status and history may need to be directed to a variety of sources, including the spouse and employer. Where available, objective data regarding work ratings and history, job absenteeism, and financial benefits are important to gather. Relief from work stress and responsibility is much less likely to be a reinforcer for pain behavior for the pain-disabled worker if he or she has a stable work history, enjoyed the previous work, saw himself or herself as competent, received good work ratings, is receiving significantly reduced income compared to when working, has made efforts to return to work, and shows clear medical evidence for being unable to fulfill job responsibilities. Research evidence reveals that particularly in the middle ranges of organic pathology, return to work can generally be looked at as a *decision* that is made based on a host of economic, social, and psychological variables (Berkowitz, Johnson, & Murphy, 1976). Table 8.2 lists many of the commonly observed obstacles for failure of chronic pain patients to decide to return to work and for failure of employers to offer employment. Disincentives inherent in some disability systems also are summarized in Table 8.2.

Table 8.2.
Frequent Reasons for Failure of Chronic Pain Patients to Return to Work

I. Patient's Perspective.
   A. Risk of losing disability income and/or seniority.
   B. Loss of self-confidence.
   C. Difficulty of adapting to new work.
   D. Difficulty of managing pain while working.
   E. Fear of re-injury.
   F. Lack of availability of suitable employment.
II. Employer's Perspective.
   A. Expense of job or schedule modifications.
   B. Expense of re-training.
   C. Perceived fairness of special provisions.
   D. Risk of encouraging pain behavior in other workers.
   E. Risk of absenteeism or repeated injury.
   F. Lack of availability of suitable employment.
III. Disincentives of Disability/Legal Systems.
   A. No partial compensation for lighter-duty work.
   B. No trial work periods.
   C. Long waiting times.
   D. Uncertainty of outcome, frequent reversals on appeal.
   E. No limit of liability of employer for subsequent re-injury.
   F. Disability income compares favorably with income available through work.

Sleep disorders are frequently reported by patients with chronic pain and can affect their daily ability to function and cope with pain and stress. Failure to get to sleep at night can reflect underlying anxiety or difficulty distracting oneself from painful input, while frequent awakening throughout the night can be a response to the increase in pain associated with sleeping posture or stiffness. Patients highly dependent on medications may awaken with pain to take another dose. Early morning awakening is one symptom of a possible underlying depression. Obviously, sleeping difficulties can be produced by a host of factors, and valid conclusions about their etiology can only be made from an integration of multiple pieces of evidence.

Pain complaints often have high social stimulus value, as they communicate powerful messages to others and when intense, frequently evoke emotional arousal in others. A psychological assessment thus needs to investigate the character of social relationships presently and historically, and particularly the response of significant others in the patient's environment to pain behaviors. The potential for operant conditioning is enhanced if the patient shows a history of failure to achieve significant social reinforcement in the absence of pain behaviors, demonstrates such behaviors in a highly visible way, and/or receives sympathy, attention, or social support contingent on the expression of such behaviors. In some cases, pain behavior can serve to avoid negative social consequences. Examples might include a patient whose spouse resists placing social or sexual demands, expressing anger, or even filing for divorce contingent on continuation of pain behaviors. Social isolation and alienation are commonly seen in pain patients, and can exacerbate states of depression and dysfunction. Questioning of the spouse and/or significant others might include their learning history and the extent to which they might find the caregiving role as being reinforcing. Turk, Meichenbaum, and Genest (1983) have described a diary for the spouse to complete which includes ratings or descriptions of such variables as the severity of pain, its interference with the patient's and family's life, and the spouse's feelings and reactions when pain behavior is observed.

Investigation of emotional dysfunctions and their temporal relationship with pain behaviors can be important in several respects. Certainly, failure in ability to achieve significant rewards through "well" (i.e., nonpain) behavior enhances the likelihood that rewards available through pain behavior can compete favorably. Furthermore, because emotional and physical functioning are interwoven, failures in emotional function can result in physical dysfunction associated with the experience of pain. Though there is little evidence to suggest a high frequency of delusional chronic pain complaints, the presence of psychotic features certainly can impede self-care and coping. Evidence for characterological disturbances may suggest the likelihood of pain behavior contingent on direct environmental reinforcers or of inaccuracies in self-report data.

A final important area of inquiry is the patient's cognitive self-statements regarding his or her pain problem. Important cognitive variables to assess may include self-image, expectancy, perceived control, attention to pain and bodily cues, and the perceived meaning of the pain in the patient's life (Turk et al., 1983; Weisenberg, 1977). Self-statements might reveal the underpinnings of emotional dysfunction as well as the presence of cognitive distortions. Lefebvre (1981) reported that cognitive distortions about the nature of pain are very common in chronic low back pain patients.

Analysis of Interview Data: Case Example

Both Sanders (1979) and Lake (1981) have suggested the utility of classifying behaviors into three types (overt, covert, and physiological) and listing the antecedents and consequences of each. For the purpose of this analysis, "behavior" is defined broadly so as to include covert and physiological events. "Overt" behavior refers to that which can be observed and includes, for example, verbal statements, posture and motor behavior, and drug use. "Covert" behavior refers to emotions and thoughts which can be inferred from the patient's statements and other overt behaviors. Relevant examples might include expectancies regarding pain, perceived control over pain, feelings of depression, worries, and so on. "Physiological" behavior refers to that which can be detected through observation or testing of medical/physiological functioning, such as heart rate, blood pressure, electromyographic recordings, and so forth. "Antecedents" and "consequences," respectively, refer to relevant stimuli and responses which precede and follow pain behaviors. A meaningful behavioral analysis of pain can look at antecedents and consequences in two ways: over very short periods time such as a few minutes, hours, or days to describe periods of exacerbation or episodic occurrence of pain behavior, or, in the long term, to describe relevant stimuli and responses prior to and since the onset of pain.

These behavioral data can be organized in a table such as Table 8.3, which can aid in identifying important behavioral relationships and in designing treatments. The case of a 35-year-old woman with recurrent headaches can be used as an example. The major pain behaviors observed or reported during a headache episode, as identified by the patient and her husband, are as follows:

- *Overt*: remaining in bed in a dark room, high intensity verbal complaints of pain, taking eight Fiorinal tablets with codeine, missing a day of work.
- *Covert*: focus on the severity of pain, fear that pain will not go away soon, thoughts that the pain cannot be tolerated another minute, distress about falling behind with work and household duties.
- *Physiological*: vomiting, throbbing in the temporal artery, high EMG levels in the frontalis and cervical muscles.

Table 8.3.
Assessment of Pain Behaviors

	Antecedents	Behaviors	Consequences
Overt			
Covert			
Physiological			

Relevant antecedents are as follows:

- *Overt*: kept long hours at work with few breaks, little physical exercise, missed a meal, made up for lost sleeping time during the weeks by oversleeping on the weekend, drank six cups of coffee daily, took two Fiorinal and two aspirin per day as headache preventatives, argued with husband about her failure to do some household tasks.
- *Covert*: felt anxious, worried that daughter's upcoming marriage might not work out, felt angry towards spouse, worried that she might not complete work assignments on time.
- *Physiological*: cold hands and feet, sustained high EMG levels in cervical and frontalis muscles, high blood pressure, sweaty palms.

The consequences of the headache attack include:

- *Overt*: no arguments with husband, who completed household tasks and suggested relaxation for a day to recover from the headache; return to work after missing one day, verbalized how terrible the pain had been and how fearful she was of its occurrence, increased Fiorinal use to four per day, returned after one day to the customary life habits noted under "antecedents."
- *Covert*: Increased worry about falling behind in work assignments, increased fear of headache recurrence, relief to have one day to recover from the headache, greater sense of helplessness regarding the headache problem.
- *Physiological*: some relaxation of muscle tightness, reduction in blood pressure, decrease in perspiration in hands and coldness of hands and feet for one day before these functions returned to customary levels noted under "antecedents."

This analysis reveals a number of respondent stimuli which are likely to have contributed to the headache episode, including chronic worry and anxiety, anger toward the husband, inadequate pacing and stress management, and inconsistent eating and sleeping habits. The caffeine intake from coffee, analgesic use, and Fiorinal is likely to be contributing to the anxiety. While less clear, the possibility of an operant component is enhanced because her husband's ceasing arguments and helping with the housework, and the patient's being able to spend one day in a more relaxed way, were contingent on the occurrence of pain behavior. The increased worry and helplessness and increased drug use that followed the headache also could serve as respondent stimuli for a subsequent headache episode brought on by physiological and emotional instability. It is likely that successful treatment would have to address multiple areas, including medication changes, stress management, cognitive therapy to alter maladaptive self-statements, counseling to change lifestyle, and possibly biofeedback therapy and family intervention.

MEASURES OF PAIN BEHAVIORS

Use of standardized questionnaires are an important part of the assessment process, as resultant data can provide objective comparison of important aspects of the patient's behavior with that of other patients; data found from research with similar patients can be used as a guide for treatment decisions. The need to gather data in a standardized way is highlighted by a study by Harris and Monaco (1978). They found that respondents reported over three times the number of headaches when asked, "Do you get headaches frequently, and if so, how often?" than when asked, "Do you get headaches occasionally and, if so, how often?" Unfortunately, clinicians have assessed important pain behaviors in so many ways that meaningful comparisons often are not possible. The following section will review some of the most commonly employed diaries, questionnaires, and assessment guides.

Measures of Pain Intensity

A variety of different questionnaires or scales have been devised to measure subjective pain intensity. Because pain cannot be measured directly, all of these scales really represent ways of structuring a patient's self-report of his or her pain experience.

Category scales. Budzynski, Stoyra, Adler, and Mullaney, (1973) devised a 6-point rating scale, with each point represented by a different adjective describing a different pain level. The six adjectives empoyed (no pain, mild, discomforting, distressing, horrible, excruciating) subsequently were found by Melzack (1975) to constitute an equal-interval scale, and thus to allow for more powerful statistical techniques (including addition, subtraction, and calculation of averages) to be used on data than would otherwise be the case; however, Heft and Parker (1984) found that the intervals between such adjectives are not always equal in terms of intensity. Turk et al. (1983) have suggested incorporating the 0-to-5 scale using these adjectives into a more comprehensive pain diary in which the patient rates his pain level several times per day and compares it with variables such as time, place, activity, drug intake, interpersonal situation, and thoughts, images, and feelings. Though such diary keeping can bring important patterns of subjective pain intensity into clear focus, many patients have been found to be noncompliant in making multiple daily pain ratings during an 8-week period (Collins & Thompson, 1979). A standardized extension of category scaling is the Wisconsin Brief Pain Questionnaire (Daut, Cleeland, & Flanery, 1983), which includes category scales that measure not only the subjective description of pain but also its impact on normal life.

Visual analog scaling. Another method for assessing subjective pain intensity is through a visual analog scale (VAS). This scale consists of a 10 cm. line with end points labeled "no pain" and "excruciating pain" or "pain as bad as it could be." The subject/patient is instructed merely to make a mark along the line at the point that most accurately corresponds to his or her pain level. There are several versions of this scale in use; in some, the words "light," "moderate," and "severe" are evenly spaced beneath the line, while in others the line is divided into equal units based on Hardy et al.'s (Hardy, Wolff, & Goodell, 1952) finding of 20-to-21 just-noticeable-difference intervals in experimental pain. Visual analog scales have been found to be reliable on test-retest (Huskisson, 1974; Scott & Huskisson, 1976, 1979) and to correlate well with word descriptor scales (Downie et al., 1978; Elton, Burrows, & Stanley, 1979; Ohnhaus & Adler, 1975; Scott & Huskisson, 1976) and with verbal pain intensity ratings (Woodforde & Merskey, 1972b). Price, McGrath, Rafii, and Buckingham (1983) also found that chronic pain patients are consistent in recording their ratings of different levels of experimental thermal pain on a VAS and comparing such levels with their clinical pain. Joyce, Zutish, Hrubes, and Mason (1975) and Sriwatanakul et al. (1983) revealed that patients prefer VAS over word descriptor or category scales and that the VAS is sensitive to changes in pain intensity.

The main advantages of VAS lie in its sensitivity, reliability, simplicity, and efficiency; it takes only a few moments to fill out. Potential disadvantages or limitations include its susceptibility to influence from the attitudes of the experimenter/clinician who administers it (Huskisson, 1982) and its measurement of pain along only one dimension; it often is unclear whether patients' ratings are influenced by affective dimensions. Statistical handling of VAS results also can be problematic. Though Price, McGrath, Rafii, and Buckingham's data on VAS scaling of controlled experimental thermal pain suggested that the VAS has properties of a ratio scale, Chapman (1976) claimed that because clinical ratings of pain cannot be compared to objective measurements, the VAS cannot even be assumed to be an interval scale. An additional statistical problem lies in the finding that VAS ratings in chronic pain patients do not have a normal distribution (Huskisson, 1982).

Many authors have suggested ways by which the VAS can be used or modified for various purposes. These have included taking repeated measures over time to measure clinical changes, rating sensory and affective aspects of the pain experience separately, and rating present and worst pain separately (Gracely, 1980; Gracely & Dubner, 1981). Because past memories of pain behavior often are not reliable (Carlsson, 1983; Linton & Gotestam, 1983), it is hazardous to gather pain intensity data retroactively.

"Pain density". "Density" is a construct of pain measurement which is particularly useful in describing episodic pain (Philips, 1977). It can be derived from scores from category or analog scales. "Density" refers to a mean intensity level over a day's time or over waking hours and can be calculated as a product of intensity and frequency. For example, pain rated at a 50 percent intensity level which is present during half the waking hours can be assigned a density level of 25 percent.

The McGill Pain Questionnaire. A major limitation of both the VAS and the use of verbal categories as methods of scaling pain experience is that both methods measure only one dimension of pain experience. The McGill Pain Questionnaire (MPQ) (Melzack, 1975) represents an attempt to measure pain experience across different dimensions. One part of this questionnaire consists of 78 adjectives merged into 20 different categories that represent different dimensions of pain experience. Within each category, 2-to-6 words are listed in order from those that represent the least to the most intense pain experience. These rankings were based on ratings made by physicians, patients, and students (Melzack & Torgerson, 1971). The patient is instructed to select only those categories that contain a word descriptive of his/her pain and to circle the most descriptive word within that category. From these selections, one can derive the number of words chosen, the average rank value of the words, and the sum of the ranks represented by each word. Melzack referred to the latter as the Pain Rating Index.

The MPQ was derived theoretically to conform with Melzack's (1973) model of pain as having three different major components: a sensory component representing sheer perception of sensory information, an affective component reflecting the emotional or autonomic nervous system response to painful input, and an evaluative component reflecting an appraisal of pain intensity. Thus, 10 of the categories were formulated to represent sensory components, 5 to represent affective components, and 1 to represent the evaluative component. (The other 4 categories are classified as "miscellaneous.")

The validity of this division of pain experience into three major dimensions has been assessed through a variety of correlational and factor analytic studies. Exploratory factor analysis generally has been supportive of Melzack's 3-factor model (e.g., Byrne et al., 1982; Prieto et al., 1980; Reading, 1979; Reading, Everett, & Stedmere, 1982); however, Crockett et al. (1977) and Levitt, Garron, Whisler, and Sheinkop (1978) found that more than three factors could be identified and suggested that classifiction of verbal pain descriptors is more complex than Melzack originally proposed. In addition, the existence of a distinct evaluative component has failed to emerge consistently from several studies (Crockett, Prkachin, & Craig, 1977; Leavitt et al., 1978; Reading, 1979).

Recently, Turk, Rudy, and Salovey (1985) applied a test of "confirmatory" factor analysis, which represents a direct attempt to confirm Melzack's postulated factor model. This method can be differentiated from "exploratory" factor analysis, which is based on no a priori theoretical formulation. Results with diverse pain populations did yield three components of pain experience; however, the three components were found to be highly intercorrelated and thus did not display adequate discriminant validity.

Despite questions regarding the ability of the MPQ to discriminiate three clear dimensions of pain, its validity for measuring treatment outcome and for describing different aspects of the pain experience has been demonstrated in over 60 validity studies (Turk et al., 1985). Scores on the affective dimension have been found to correlate significantly with other measure of the overall affective states of chronic pain patients (Kremer & Atkinson, 1981) and to change specifically with the use of a drug designed to modify affect (Gracely, McGrath, & Dubner, 1978). In addition, different patterns of response on the MPQ have been found to correlate with different types of pain, including low back pain, labor and childbirth, cancer pain, and arthritis (e.g., Dubuisson & Melzack, 1976).

In summary, the MPQ represents a well-researched and -validated tool for quantitative assessment of the quality and intensity of the pain experience. Though it is fairly brief and easy to administer, it is limited to English-speaking subjects, and those with limited vocabularies are likely to have difficulty with some of the words, such as "searing" or "lancinating." Though scoring is easy, the Pain Rating Index is somewhat imprecise because of the uneven pain intensities represented by words of a given rank. Charter and Nehemkis (1983) have advocated scoring each word according to its own intensity rather than according to its rank.

Measurement of Overt Pain Behaviors

Because important goals of pain control centers generally include modifying patients' activity levels while decreasing their reliance on habit-forming medications (Aronoff, Evans, & Enders, 1983; Chapman, 1983), diaries have been devised to assess these variables. Fordyce (1976a, 1976b) measured activity in terms of "uptime," or the amount of time spent with both feet on the floor, while other authors have measured the amount of time patients spend on their feet and moving (e.g., Brena & Unikel, 1976; Chapman, Brena, & Bradford, 1981); however, these self-report measures may not be valid. Sanders (1983) and Kremer, Block, and Gaylor (1981), respectively, found that patients underreported activities in comparison with measures from an automated recording device or in comparison with staff observations. Ready, Sarkis, and Turner (1982) noted that patients' reported medication use was significantly less than their actual free use of medications in a hospital setting. For this reason, self-report data on these behaviors need to be paired with information from automated measures, from significant others in the patients' environment, and/or from direct observation whenever possible. Automated systems developed to measure pain behaviors directly have included measures of time spend standing or walking (Cairns & Pasino, 1977; Sanders, 1980), pedometers, exercycles, and a system employing microswitches under a patient's mattress for measurement of time in bed (Cairns & Pasino, 1977; Cairns, Thomas, Mooney, & Pace, 1976).

A number of systems have been developed for coding staff and family observations of relevant aspects of patient behavior. These systems have encompassed a large number relevant variables, including not only activity level and drug intake, but also a wide variety of measures of physical and psychological function (e.g., Cinciripini & Floreen, 1982; Fordyce, 1976a; Gottlieb et al., 1977; Richards, Nepomuceno, Riles, & Suer, 1982; Shealy & Shealy, 1976; Swanson, Swenson, Maruty, & McPhee, 1976). They generally have included frequency counts as well as ratings along numerical scores with clear descriptive criteria.

Keefe and Block (1982) developed an observational system to measure and rate 5 motor behaviors in low back pain patients, including guarded movement, pain-avoidant posturing (i.e., bracing), rubbing or touching a painful area, grimacing, and sighing. They demonstrated that such ratings met criteria for reliability and validity and could be stnadardized from a structured physical examination. Interestingly, Keefe and his colleagues (Keefe, Wilhins, & Cook, 1984) demonstrated that the number of total pain behaviors observed per minute correlated positively with a measure of subjective pain intensity (r = .53) and was highly related to measure of medical status such as surgical history and positive medical test findings.

The ability to assess and quantify pain behaviors objectively is important for diagnosis and treatment planning and also for providing a way to gauge treatment outcome and patient progress. High levels of pain behavior can be significant for their potential elicitation of solicitous responses from others and for their effect on clinical decisions. However, interpretation of levels of pain behavior can be quite difficult. As Turk et al. (1983) have noted, it is difficult to differentiate between pain behaviors which may be designed to seek attention versus behaviors (such as rubbing a painful area or changing postures) designed to reduce pain experience. In addition, these behavioral measures cannot be separated from the context in which they are being measured and have been found to be related to demand characteristics (Cinciripini & Floreen, 1983), verbal reinforcement (Cairns & Pasino, 1977), financial compensation (Block et al., 1980), anxiety (Beecher, 1972), and ethnicity (Tursky & Sternbach, 1967).

ASSESSMENT OF PSYCHOLOGICAL FUNCTIONING

Brief Screening Tests

Four brief screening tests have been devised to assess the likelihood that psychological factors may be important contributants to chronic pain behavior. One is the Pain Drawing (Ransford, Cairns, & Mooney, 1976), in which the patient is given a blank drawing of the back and front of the body and asked to use different symbols to mark areas in which different feelings of pain (such as numbness, pins and needles, burning, and stabbing) are experienced. The authors presented a rather arbitrary scoring system to assess poor anatomic localization, "expansion or magnification"of pain, and additional unsolicited markings on the page. Though they found a high correlation between scores on the Pain Drawing and those on the Hypochondriasis and Hysteria scores on the MMPI, von Baeyer, Bergstrom, Brodwin, and Brodwin (1983) failed to replicate these results with a new sample and pointed out that the original results were based on the same sample on which the test was validated. While a drawing may be useful to assess clearly the areas of pain complaints and to allow comparison with expectations based on medical findings, there is little evidence that the Pain Drawing screens well for psychopathology.

The Back Pain Classification Scale (Leavitt, 1983) consists of 13 adjectives from the MPQ. The patient merely circles which adjectives apply to his pain experience. The intent of the instrument is to discriminate between back pain patients with primarily organic versus psychological conditioning for pain complaints. Several studies have supported the concurrent validity of the instrument (Leavitt, 1983; Leavitt & Garron, 1979a, 1979b, 1980; Leavitt et al., 1978; Sanders, 1985). Hendler's Ten-Minute Screening Test (Hendler, Viernstein, Gucer, & Long, 1979) is another screening battery designed to differentiate between "functional" and "organic" back pain. It is scored according to responses to 15 questions from a medical interview, and has been found to correlate significantly with objective medical findings and to predict responses to surgery and other pain-relieving modalities (Hendler et al., 1979). Though these instruments deserve further study, the assumption that back pain can be divided into functional and organic categories appears very simplistic.

A fourth test, the Modified Somatic Pain Questionnaire (Main, 1983) was designed primarily to measure somatic indications of anxiety in back pain patients. It consists of a list of 13 symptoms for which the subject is asked to rate the degree of frequency. Main reported some initial validity data suggesting some sensitivity in identifying psychological distress in chronic low back pain subjects, but little additional validity data are available.

Minnesota Multiphasic Personality Inventory

The MMPI is probably the most commonly used instrument for assessing overall psychological functioning in chronic pain patients (Keefe & Bradley, 1984). It was developed in the 1930s and consists of 550 true-false questions which score on a variety of scales designed to measure abnormal personality syndromes, personality traits, or the validity of the test results. Items were assigned to scales measuring personality abnormalities statistically according to whether they differentiated patients with given psychiatric diagnoses from a normal population.

Many clinicians use the first 400 items only, which allows scores on all of the basic scales to be derived.

Much of the early MMPI research with chronic pain patients was designed to differentiate "organic" versus "functional" profiles. Perhaps because such a clear dichotomy is illusory, results were rather unimpressive, with some authors nothing higher scores from "functional" patients on the Hypochondriasis, Depression, and Hysteria scales (Calsyn, Louks, & Freeman, 1976; Freeman, Calsyn, & Louks, 1976; Hanvik, 1951; Louks, Freeman, & Calsyn, 1978; McCreary, Turner, & Dawson, 1977; Turner & McCreary, 1978), and others failing to find such differences (Bradley, Prieto, Hopson, & Prokop, 1978; Cox, Chapman, & Bonica, 1978; Fordyce, Brena, DeLateur, Holcombe, & Loeser, 1978; Liebeskind & Paul, 1977; McCreary, Turner, & Dawson, 1981; Sternbach, Wolf, Murphy, & Akeson, 1973; Woodforde & Merskey, 1972a). Conflicting results likely were attributable to differences in patient selection and to varying criteria in assessing whether pain was "functional." In many cases, this assessment was made by nonpsychiatric physicians.

Another major area of research inquiry with chronic pain patients has been prediction of treatment outcome based on MMPI findings. Again, results have been equivocal. Several authors noted that elevations on the Hypochondriasis scale correlate with poor treatment outcome on a variety of measures, such as posttreatment or follow-up activity levels, subjective pain intensities, or the use of subsequent medical treatment (McCreary, Turner, & Dawson, 1979; Strassberg, Reimherr, Ward, Russell, & Cole, 1981; Turner, Robinson, & McCreary, 1983); however, correlations generally were rather low, and certainly not high enough to form a basis for clear clinical decisions. In addition, Trief and Yuan (1983) found no relationship between the Hypochondriasis scale and a variety of treatment outcome measures.

Because clinical interpretation of the MMPI is based on scale patterns and configurations rather than merely on the elevation of each scale, research that includes some kind of pattern analysis may be more useful and valid. Sternbach (1974) provided descriptive data suggesting that particular patterns such as dual elevations on Hypochondriasis and Hysteria or a peak elevation on Psychopathic Deviance suggested overall poorer outcome than did a peak elevation on Depression; however, McGill, Lawlis, Selby, Mooney, and McCoy, (1983) performed cluster analysis on MMPIs of patients with chronic low back pain and found that different clusters failed to show different outcomes at posttreatment. Pemberton (1985) divided large numbers of chronic low back pain patients into different narrowly defined clusters, each of which was associated with distinct clinical interpretation.

Each cluster was defined in such a way that each subject within that cluster showed very similar basic patterns of elevations of scales. Posttreatment and 4-year follow-up data revealed few significant differences between clusters on subjective pain intensity, activity level, and drug use patterns; however, patients with elevations above a T-score of 80 on both Hypochondriasis and Hysteria reported higher levels of subjective pain intensity at follow-up than did patients with elevations on these two scales in the 70 to 80 range, or those with no elevations exceeding a T-score of 70 on any clinical scale.

When one considers the large number of medical and psychosocial factors that can influence self-report of treatment outcome, these generally negative results should not be surprising. If positive results are to be found, future research on the prognostic value of the MMPI likely will require analysis of outcomes of specific treatments and control of contaminating subject variables such as medical status.

Cluster analyses and comparisons of pain patients with other populations clearly have revealed the presence of multiple MMPI profiles among pain patients (e.g., Armentrout, Moore, Parker, Hewett, & Feltz, 1982; Bradley, Prokop, Margolis, & Gentry, 1978; Louks, Freeman, & Calsyn, 1978; McGill et al., 1983; Naliboff, Coken, & Yellen, 1982). Clinical interpretation of these diverse profiles necessitates a high degree of caution. The clinician must remember that the MMPI does not consider medical data, has numerous psychometric flaws associated with the original establishment of the scales, and was normed on a psychiatric sample, not on chronic pain sufferers. In fact, some items which score on certain psychiatric scales such as the Schizophrenia scale are frequent correlates of chronic musculoskeletal pain. Examples include "I have numbness in one or more regions of my skin," "I have little or no trouble with my muscles twitching or jumping," and "I have never been paralyzed or had any unusual weakness in any of my muscles." Thus, interpretation of elevations on scales highly influenced by pain complaints or by the use of pain medications (particularly Hypochondriasis, Depression, Hysteria, and Schizophrenia) are particularly subject to distortion when conventional guidebooks based on data from psychiatric patients are used. For example, the present author has noted that 38 percent of hundreds of diverse chronic pain patients tested at the Emory Pain Control Center showed a T-score elevation of 70 or more on the Schizophrenia scale, which would be likely to generate interpretations of possible psychotic features and/or organic brain dysfunction; however, virtually none of these patients showed confirmatory evidence of such features.

Recognizing the difficulty of conventional MMPI interpretation in chronic pain patients, Fordyce (1979) suggested a more behavioral guide to interpretation. For example, he predicted that patients high on Hypochondriasis and Hysteria and low on Depression would show high pain behavior with little accompanying worry and concern and a higher-than-average likelihood of operant conditioning of pain behaviors; those with high elevations on the Mania scale would be likely to find activities to be reinforcing, and thus might be more likely to have difficulty in pacing activities. Little research has been performed on behavioral correlates of MMPI elevations on pain patients. Until such work is done, it is suggested that clinicians eschew computerized interpretations and use MMPI data to generate hypotheses about possible psychological problems, which then can be tested from interview and other assessment data. Analysis of individual items within elevated scales can be particularly useful to generate such hypotheses.

Advantages of the MMPI include well-developed validity scales which can aid assessment of the way in which the patient might approach psychological treatment, the comprehensiveness of the questions, and the test's long research history. These advantages need to be counterbalanced with considerations of the above-noted limitations, as well as the questionnaire's length, and the possibility of patient anger or anxiety in answering many invasive questions that screen for major psychological disturbance.

Other Personality Inventories

The Eysenck Personality Inventory is another time-honored test normed on psychiatric patients. It has been used fairly extensively in pain centers in Europe and Australia (Sanders, 1979). Normative data on chronic pain patients have been presented, and the test has been found to discriminate such patients from medically or psychiatrically impaired populations (Lynn & Eysenck, 1961; Woodforde & Merskey, 1972a); however, its specific usefulness in the behavioral assessment of chronic pain remains unproven.

A more recently developed test normed on a psychiatric population is the SCL-90, which includes a list of 90 physical and emotional symptoms, which patients endorse on a 5-point intensity scale according to the degree to which that symptom bothers them. Answers are scored on 9 clinical scales relating to particular syndromes and 3 general scales designed to measure the overall number and intensity of symptoms. Though results provide a good summary of self-reported difficulties, the meaning of the scale elevations in chronic pain patients has not been well researched. The Somatization scale is almost always elevated, and the test has been described as being insensitive in differentiating personality variables among chronic pain patients (Main, 1983).

Questionnaires Designed for Medical Populations

Several questionnaires which have been designed for medical populations have been used to assess chronic pain patients:

Millon Behavioral Health Inventory (MBHI). The MBHI (Millon, Green, & Meagher, 1979) is a 150-item true-false questionnaire. It provides measurement of both overt and covert behavior patterns important in physical ailments in which behavioral or emotional components play a significant role. The focus is not on general personality, but rather on a variety of specific personality dimensions, attitudes, events, and cognitions (such as cooperativeness, recent stress, pessimism, chronic tension, somatic anxiety, etc.) that affect the development of physical illness and/or compliance or prognosis in medical treatment programs. One scale is designed specifically to predict outcome in a multidisciplinary chronic pain program. The MBHI was carefully designed from theoretical formulations, internal structural analyses, and studies of relationships of items and scales to external criterion variables. While its utility appears promising, few validity studies have been performed with a chronic pain sample. In fact, the test scoring is continually undergoing changes based on new data and the manual is very sketchy in providing interpretive guidance. Thus, computer scoring and interpretation is almost a requirement. Another limitation is that scale scores are expressed in relationship to base rates rather than according to mean and standard deviations and thus are hard to assess statistically.

Illness Behavior Questionnaire. The Illness Behavior Questionnaire is a 62-item true-false instrument designed to delineate patterns of abnormal illness behavior (Pilowsky & Spence, 1975). Its theoretical basis is largely psychoanalytic in nature. Several scales developed from factor analysis were labeled as General Hypochondriasis, Disease Conviction, Psychological versus Somatic Perception of Illness, Affective Inhibition, Affective Disturbance, Denial, and Irritability. Other scales were based on second-order factor analysis or discriminant analysis designed to assess the likelihood of a "conversion disorder." Validity studies have revealed different patterns of scores among pain patients, psychiatric patients, and acute medical cases and positive correlations with other measures of personality or affective disturbance (Pilowsky & Spence, 1983). There is a need for cross-validation of the original factor analysis used to scale responses and for testing the psychoanalytic interpretations of scale elevations.

Other instruments. The Sickness Impact Profile (Bergner, Bobbitt, Carter, & Gilson, 1981) is a 136-item questionnaire designed specifically to measure physical, psychosocial, work and recreational dysfunction associated with chronic illness. Follick, Smith, and Ahern (1985) have found that this test correlates substantially with activity level and with emotional distress, and that it is sensitive as a dependent measure of treatment outcome in a pain rehabilitation program.

Another test designed to measure fairly specific dimensions that are likely to be relevant to chronic pain is the Multidimensional Health Locus of Control Scale (MHLC) (Wallston & Wallston, 1978). This 18-item test measures the extent to which one sees his or her health as being attributable to one's own behavior, the behavior of powerful others such as physicians, or fate. Locus of control has been found to be a personality dimension which can predict behavior in a variety of health care settings in which patient compliance with suggested treatment is important (e.g., Wallston & Wallston, 1978).

A final scale derived for medical populations which has been used for chronic pain patients is the Cornell Medical Index (CMI), a 195-item true-false questionnaire developed in the 1940s as a screening device in doing initial assessment interviews; however, the scales are not well standardized, and as with the MHLC, few validity studies with chronic pain patients have been performed.

Tests Designed Specifically for Chronic Pain Patients

With the recent proliferation of specialized centers for management of chronic pain patients, multidimensional batteries are being developed specifically for use with such patients. Three examples are the Psychosocial Pain Inventory (Heaton et al., 1982) the Chronic Pain Battery (Levitt, 1983) and the West Haven-Yale Multidimensional Pain Inventory (WHYMPI) (Kerns, Turk, & Rudy, 1986). The Psychosocial Pain Inventory is a quantification from a standard interview of many aspects of pain behavior, including drug taking, activity level, social reinforcement, work and medical history, disability status, and family history of illness. Normative data for chronic patients are available. Unfortunately, the scoring of responses is rather arbitrary, which may limit the utility of the instrument.

The Chronic Pain Battery is a self-administered set of multiple choice and true-false questions designed to compile and describe medical, psychological, behavioral, and social data. Unlike many tests, this battery includes assessment of patient expectations and goals. A narrative computer report can be generated.

The WHYMPI is a 52-item self-administered inventory divided into three sections. One section measures five important dimensions of the pain experience, including pain severity and suffering, interference with function, appraisal of support from others, perceived life control, and affective distress. Two other sections relate to specific responses to pain in significant others and to social, recreational, and physical activities. This battery was developed using factor analysis and careful item analysis to establish the validity of the items and scales. The authors pointed out the need for cross-validation on new subjects besides the original sample. Because of its psychometric sophistication and evaluation of many areas of psychosocial impact, this test may prove very useful for assessment of social, psychological, and behavioral factors; however, it is not designed to measure medical aspects of pain.

PHYSIOLOGICAL RESPONSES IN PAIN ASSESSMENT

While considerable data have been collected, particularly with headache patients, the role of particular measurable physiological responses in pain assessment remains quite controversial. Headaches and other pain problems do not seem to bear a simple clear relationship to such physiological measures as baseline levels of frontalis EMG, hand temperature, skin conductance, EEG, or heart rate; however, relationships may become clearer as methods of quantifying physiological responses on a 24-hour basis in the patient's normal environment are developed and used, and as more specific relationships are studied. Meaningful psychological assessment of physiological aspects of pain may need to include multiple physiological functions at different sites and under a variety of stimulus conditions, such as during movement and during personally relevant stressful conditions as well as during rest (Gannon, Haynes, Safranek, & Hamilton, 1981; Philips & Hunter, 1982; Sutton & Belar, 1982; Thompson & Adams, 1984; Wolf, Nacht, & Kelly, 1982). There are some data to suggest that subjects who are found to show high correlations between EMG levels and pain are more likely to respond to biofeedback treatment (Large, 1985). In the absence of clear research support for significant correlation (let alone causation) between pain and physiological measures derived from biofeedback diaries, interpretation of physiological assessments must be made cautiously and be supported by other confirmatory data.

SUMMARY

In summary, psychological assessment of pain must be based on an integration of information from multiple sources. There is no single battery or instrument that can adequately assess a pain patient in terms of the nature of his or her psychological difficulties or in terms of recommendations for psychological treatment. As more and more information becomes available, simplistic concepts or assumptions about chronic pain are proving inadequate. Examples include ideas that pain is either organic or functional, that depression, anxiety, or muscle tension are sufficient explanations of many individuals' pain complaints, and that pain behavior which does not fit with expectations based on medical data must be psychologically based. Pain patients clearly do not fit with easy categorization of types and may be better described in terms of their diversity than in terms of their commonality. Psychological assessment thus must be systematic and comprehensive, and data must be integrated carefully with that available through other relevant medical and physical evaluations.

REFERENCES

Apley, J. (1975). *The child with abdominal pains.* Oxford: Blackwell.

Armentrout, D., Moore, J., Parker, J., Hewett, J., & Feltz, C. (1982). Pain-patient MMPI subgroups: The psychological dimensions of pain. *Journal of Behavioral Medicine, 5*, 201–211.

Aronoff, G. M., Evans, W. O., & Enders, P. L. (1983). A review of follow-up studies of multidisciplinary pain units. *Pain, 16*, 1–11.

Beecher, H. K. (1959). *Measurement of subjective responses: Quantitative effects of drugs.* New York: Oxford.

Beecher, H. K. (1972). The placebo effect as a non-specific force surrounding disease and the treatment of disease. In R. Janzen, W. D. Keidel, & A. Herz, et al. (Eds.), *Pain: Basic principles, pharmacology, therapy.* Stuttgart, West Germany: Geosythieme.

Bergner, M., Bobbitt, R. A., Carter, W. B., & Gilson, B. S. (1981). The Sickness Impact Profile: Development and final revision of a health status measure. *Medical Care, 19*, 787–805.

Berkowitz, M., Johnson, W., & Murphy, E. (1976). *Public policy toward disability.* New York: Praeger.

Block, A., Kremer, E., & Gaylor, M. (1980). Behavioral treatment of chronic pain: The spouse as a discriminative cue for pain behavior. *Pain, 9*, 243–252.

Blumer, B., Zorick, F., Heilbronn, M., & Roth, T. (1982). Biological markers for depression in chronic pain. *Journal of Nervous and Mental Disease, 170*, 425–428.

Blumer, D., & Heilbronn, M. (1982). Chronic pain as a variant of depressive disease: The pain-prone disorder. *Journal of Nervous and Mental Disease, 170*, 381–394.

Blumer, D., & Heilbronn, M. (1984). "Chronic pain as a variant of depressive disease": A rejoinder. *Journal of Nervous and Mental Disease, 172*, 405–407.

Blumer, D., Heilbronn, M., & Pedraza, E., (1980). Systematic treatment of chronic pain with antidepressants. *Henry Ford Hospital Medical Journal, 28*, 15–21.

Bobey, M. J., & Davidson, P. O. (1970). Psychological factors affecting pain tolerance. *Journal of Psychosomatic Research, 14*, 371–376.

Bradley, L. A., Prokop, C. K., Margolis, R., & Gentry, W. D. (1978). Multivariate analyses of the MMPI profiles of low back pain patients. *Journal of Behavioral Medicine, 1*, 253–272.

Bradley, L. A., Prieto, E. J., Hopson, L., & Prokop, C. K. (1978). Comment on "Personality organization as an aspect of back pain in a medical setting." *Journal of Personality Assessment, 42*, 573–578.

Brady, J. V. (1979). Learning and conditioning. In O. F. Pomerlean & J. P. Brady (Eds.), *Behavioral medicine: Theory and practice*. Baltimore: Williams & Wilkins.

Brena, S. F., & Chapman, S. L. (1985). Acute versus chronic pain states: "The Learned Pain Syndrome." In S. F. Brena & S. L. Chapman (Eds.), *Clinics in anaesthesiology. Chronic pain: Management principles*. London: Saunders.

Brena, S. F., & Unikel, I. P. (1976). Nerve blocks and contingency management in chronic pain states. In J. J. Bonica & D. Albe-Fessard (Eds.), *Advances in pain research and therapy* (Vol. 1). New York: Raven.

Budzynski, T. H., Stoyva, J. M., Adler, C. S., & Mullaney, D. J. (1973). EMG biofeedback and tension headache: A controlled outcome study. *Seminars in Psychiatry, 5*, 397–410.

Byrne, M., Troy, A., Bradley, L. A., Marchisello, P. J., Van der Keide, L. H., & Prieto, E. J. (1982). Cross-validation of the factor structure of the McGill Pain Questionnaire. *Pain, 13*, 193–201.

Cairns, D., & Pasino, J. A. (1977). Comparison of verbal reinforcement and feedback in the operant treatment of disability due to chronic low back pain. *Behavior Therapy, 8*, 621–630.

Cairns, D., Thomas L., Mooney, V., & Pace, J. (1976). A comprehensive treatment approach to chronic low back pain. *Pain, 2*, 301–308.

Calsyn, D. A., Louks, J., & Freeman, C. W. (1976). The use of the MMPI in low back pain patients with a mixed diagnosis. *Journal of Clinical Psychology, 32*, 532–536.

Carlsson, A. M. (1983). Assessment of chronic pain. I. Aspects of the reliability and validity of the visual analogue scale. *Pain, 16*, 87–101.

Chapman, C. R. (1976). Measurement of pain: Problems and issues. In J. J. Bonica & D. G. Albe-Fessard (Eds.), *Advances in pain research and therapy* (Vol. 1). New York: Raven.

Chapman, S. L. (1983). Behavior modification. In S. F. Brena & S. L. Chapman (Eds.), *Management of patients with chronic pain*. New York: SP Medical & Scientific Books.

Chapman, S. L., & Brena, S. F. (1982). Learned helplessness and responses to nerve blocks in chronic low back pain patients. *Pain, 14*, 355–364.

Chapman, S. L., Brena, S. F., & Bradford, L. A. (1981). Treatment outcome in a chronic pain rehabilitation program. *Pain, 11*, 255–268.

Charter, R. A., & Nehemkis, A. M. (1983). The language of pain intensity and complexity: New methods of scoring the McGill Pain Questionnaire. *Perceptual and Motor Skills, 56*, 519–537.

Cinciripini, P. M., & Floreen, A. (1982). An evaluation of a behavioral program for chronic pain. *Journal of Behavioral Medicine, 5*, 375–389.

Cinciripini, P. M., & Floreen, A. (1983). An assessment of chronic pain behavior in a structured interview. *Journal of Psychosomatic Research, 27*, 117–123.

Collins, F. L., & Thompson, J. K. (1979). Reliability and standardization in the assessment of self-reported headache pain. *Journal of Behavioral Assessment, 1*, 73–86.

Cox, G. B., Chapman, C. R., & Bonica, J. J. (1978). The MMPI and chronic pain: The diagnosis of psychogenic pain. *Journal of Behavioral Medicine, 1*, 437–443.

Craig, K. D., & Prkachin, K. M. (1978). Social modeling influences on sensory decision theory and psychophysiological indexes of pain. *Journal of Personality and Social Psychology, 36*, 805–815.

Craig, K. D. (1984). Emotional aspects of pain. In P. D. Wall & R. Melzack (Eds.), *Textbook of pain* (pp. 153–161). Edinburgh: Churchill Livingstone.

Crockett, D. J., Prkachin, K. M., & Craig, K. (1977). Factors of the language of pain in patient and volunteer groups. *Pain, 4*, 175–182.

Daut, R. L., Cleeland, C. S., & Flanery, R.C. (1983). Development of the Wisconsin Brief Pain Questionnaire to assess pain in cancer and other diseases. *Pain, 17*, 197–210.

Dessonville, C. L., Reeves, J. L., Thompson, L. W., & Gallagher, D. (1984, September 3). *The pattern of depressive symptomatology in geriatric normals, depressives, and chronic pain patients*. Presentation at the Fourth World Congress on Pain, Seattle, WA.

Doleys, D. M., Crocker, M., & Patton, D. (1982). Response of patients with chronic pain to exercise quotas. *Physical Therapy, 62*, 1111–1114.

Downie, W. W., Leatham, P. A. Rhind, V. M., Wright, V., Branco, J. A., & Anderson, J. A. Studies with pain rating scales. *Annals of Rheumatic Disease, 37*, 378–381.

Dubuisson, D., & Melzack, R. (1976). Classification of clinical pain descriptions by multiple group discriminant analysis. *Experimental Neurology, 51*, 480–487.

Elton, D., Burrows, G. D., & Stanley, G. V. (1979). Clinical measurement of pain. *Medical Journal of Australia, 1*, 109–111.

Follick, M. J., Smith, T. W., & Ahern, D. K. (1985). The Sickness Impact Profile: A global measure of disability in chronic low back pain. *Pain, 21*, 67–76.

Fordyce, W. E. (1974). Pain as learned behavior. In J. J. Bonica (Ed.), *Advances in neurology* (Vol. 4). New York: Raven.

Fordyce, W. E. (1976a). Behavioral concepts in chronic pain and illness. In P. Davidson (Ed.), *The behavioral management of anxiety, depression, and pain*. New York: Brunner/Mazel.

Fordyce, W. E. (1976b). *Behavioral methods for chronic pain and illness*. St. Louis: Mosby.

Fordyce, W. E. (1979). Use of MMPI in the assessment of chronic pain. In J. Butcher, G. Dahlstrom, M. Gynther, & W. Schofield (Eds.), *Clinical notes on the MMPI*. Nutley, NJ: Hoffmann-La Roche.

Fordyce, W. E., Brena, S. F., DeLateur, B., Holcombe, S., & Loeser, V. (1978). Relationship of patient semantic 43 pain descriptors to physician diagnostic judgments, activity level measures and MMPI. *Pain, 5*, 293–303.

Fordyce, W. E., Fowler, R., & DeLateur, B. (1968). An application of behavior modification technique to a problem of chronic pain. *Behaviour Research and Therapy, 6*, 105–107.

Fordyce, W. E., Fowler, R., Lehmann, J., & De Lateur, B. (1968). Some implications of learning in chronic pain. *Journal of Clinical Diseases, 21*, 179–190.

France, R. D., & Krishnan, K. R. R. (1985). The dexamethasone suppression test as a biologic marker of depression in chronic pain. *Pain, 21*, 49–55.

Freeman, C., Calsyn, D., & Louks, J. (1976). The use of the Minnesota Multi-Phase Personality Inventory with low back patients. *Journal of Clinical Psychology, 32*, 294–298.

Gannon, L. R., Haynes, S. N., Safranek, R., & Hamilton, J. (1981). A psychophysiological investigation of muscle-contraction and migraine headache. *Journal of Psychosomatic Research, 25*, 271–280.

Genest, M., Meichenbaum, D. H., & Turk, D. C. (1977, December). *A cognitive-behavioral approach to the management of pain*. Paper presented at the 11th annual convention of the Association for Advancement of Behavior Therapy, Atlanta, GA.

Gentry, W. D., Shows, W. D., & Thomas, M. Chronic low back pain: A psychological profile. *Psychosomatics* (1974), *15*, 174–177.

Gottlieb, H., Strite, L., Koller, R., Madorsky, A., Hockersmith, V., Kleeman, M., & Wagner, J. (1977). Comprehensive rehabilitation of patients having chronic low back pain. *Archives of Physical Medicine and Rehabilitation, 58*, 101–108.

Gracely, R. H. (1980). Pain measurement in man. In L. K. Y. Ng & J. J. Bonica (Eds.), *Pain, discomfort and humanitarian care*. Amsterdam: Elsevier/North Holland.

Gracely, R. H., & Dubner, R. (1981). Pain assessment in humans—A reply to Hall. *Pain, 11*, 109–120.

Gracely, R. H., McGrath, P., & Dubner, R. (1978). Validity and sensitivity of ratio scales of sensory and affective verbal pain descriptors: Manipulation of affect by diazepam. *Pain, 5*, 19–29.

Haber, J., & Roos, C. (1984, September 4). *Effects of spouse abuse and/or sexual abuse in the development and maintenance of chronic pain in women.* Presentation at the Fourth World Congress on Pain, Seattle, WA.

Hanvik, L. J. (1951). MMPI profiles in patients with low back pain. *Journal of Consulting Psychology, 5*, 350–353.

Hardy, J., Wolff, H., & Goodell, H. (1952). *Pain sensations and reactions.* Baltimore: Williams & Wilkins.

Harris, R., & Monaco, G. (1978). Psychology of pragmatic implications: Information processing between the lines. *Journal of Experimental Psychology: General, 107*, 1–22.

Heaton, R. K., Getto, C. J., Lehman, R. A. W., Fordyce, W. E., Brauer, E., & Groban, S. E. (1982). A standardized evaluation of psychosocial factors in chronic pain. *Pain, 12*, 165–174.

Heft, M. W., & Parker, S. R. (1984). An experimental basis for revising the graphic rating scales for pain. *Pain, 19*, 153–161.

Hendler, N., Viernstein, M., Gucer, P., & Long, D. (1979). A preoperative screening test for chronic back pain patients. *Psychosomatics, 20*, 801–808.

Hirschfeld, A. H., & Behan, R. C. (1963). The accident process. I. Etiological considerations of industrial injuries. *Journal of the American Medical Association, 186*, 193–199.

Holmes, D. S., & Burish, T. G. (1983). Effectiveness of biofeedback for treating migraine and tension headaches: A review of the evidence. *Journal of Psychosomatic Research, 27*, 515–532.

Huskisson, E. C. (1974). Measurement of pain. *Lancet, ii*, 1127–1131.

Huskisson, E. C. (1982). Measurement of pain. *Journal of Rheumatology, 9*, 768–769.

Joyce, C. R., Zutish, D. W., Hrubes, V., & Mason, R. M. (1975). Comparison of fixed interval and visual analogue scales for rating chronic pain. *European Journal of Clinical Pharmacology, 8*, 415–420.

Kanfer, F. H., & Goldfoot, D. A. (1966). Self-control and tolerance of noxious stimulation. *Psychology Reports, 18*, 79–85.

Keefe, F. J. (1982). Behavioral assessment and treatment of chronic pain: Current status and future trends. *Journal of Consulting and Clinical Psychology, 50*, 896–911.

Keefe, F. J., & Block, A. R. (1982). Development of an observational method for assessing pain behavior in chronic low back pain patients. *Behavior Therapy, 13*, 363–375.

Keefe, F. J., & Bradley, L. A. (1984). Behavioral and psychological approaches to the assessment and treatment of chronic pain. *General Hospital Psychiatry, 6*, 49–54.

Keefe, F. J., Wilkins, R. H., & Cook, W. A. (1984). Direct observation of pain behavior in low back pain patients during physical examination. *Pain, 20*, 59–68.

Kerns, R. D., Turk, D. C., & Rudy, T. E. (1985). The West Haven-Yale Multidimensional Pain Inventory (WHYMPI). *Pain, 23*, 345–356.

Kremer, E., & Atkinson, J. H. (1981). Pain measurement: Construct validity of the affective dimension of the McGill Pain Questionnaire with chronic benign pain patients. *Pain, 11*, 93–100.

Kremer, E. F., Block, A. J., & Gaylor, M. S. (1981). Behavioral approaches to treatment of chronic pain: the inaccuracy of patient self-report measures. *Archives of Physical Medicine and Rehabilitation, 62*, 188–191.

Kudrow, L. (1982). Paradoxical effects of frequent analgesic use. *Advances in neurology, 33*, 335–341.

Lake, A. E. (1981). Behavioral assessment considerations in the management of headache. *Headache, 21*, 170–178.

Large, R. G. (1985). Prediction of treatment response in pain patients: The illness self-concept repertory grid and EMG feedback. *Pain, 21*, 279–288.

Leavitt, F. (1983). Detecting psychological disturbance using verbal pain measurement: The back pain classification scale. In R. Melzack (Ed.), *Pain measurement and assessment.* New York: Raven.

Leavitt, F., & Garron, D. C. (1979a). Psychological disturbance and pain report differences in both organic and non-organic low back pain patients. *Pain, 7*, 187–195.

Leavitt, F., & Garron, D. C. (1979b). The detection of psychological disturbance in patients with low back pain. *Journal of Psychosomatic Research, 23*, 149–154.

Leavitt, F., & Garron, D. C. (1980). Validity of a back pain classification scale for detecting psychological disturbance as measured by the MMPI. *Journal of Clinical Psychology, 36*, 186–189.

Leavitt, F., Garron, D. C., Whisler, W. W., & Sheinkop, M. B. (1978). Affective and sensory dimensions of back pain. *Pain, 4*, 273–281.

Lefebvre, M. F. (1981). Cognitive distortion and cognitive errors in depressed psychiatric and low back pain patients. *Journal of Consulting and Clinical Psychology, 49*, 517–525.

Levitt, S. R. (1983). *Chronic pain battery.* Durham, NC: Pain Resource Center.

Liebeskind, J. C., & Paul, L. A. (1977). Psychological and physiological mechanisms of pain. In M. R. Rosenzweig & L. W. Porter (Eds.), *Annual review of psychology* (Vol. 28). Palo Alto, CA: Annual Reviews, Inc.

Linton, S. J., & Gotestam, K. G. (1983). A clinical comparison of two pain scales: Correlation, remembering chronic pain and a measure of compliance. *Pain, 17*, 57–65.

Loeser, J. D. (1979). Letter to the editor: Re: "Effects of Doxepin on Perception of Laboratory-induced Pain in Man." *Pain, 6*, 241–242.

Louks, J. L., Freeman, C. W., & Calsyn, D. H. (1978). Personality organization as an aspect of back pain in a medical setting. *Journal of Personality Assessment, 42*, 151–158.

Lynn, A., & Eysenck, H. J. (1961). Tolerance for pain extraversion, and neuroticism. *Perceptual and Motor Skills, 12*, 161–162.

Main, C. J. (1983). The modified somatic perception questionnaire (MSPQ). *Journal of Psychosomatic Research, 27*, 503–514.

McCreary, C., Turner, J., & Dawson, E. (1977). Differences between functional and organic low back pain patients. *Pain, 4*, 73–78.

McCreary, C., Turner, J., & Dawson, B. (1979). The MMPI as a predictor of response to conservative treatment for low back pain. *Journal of Clinical Psychology, 35*, 278–284.

McCreary, C., Turner, J., & Dawson, E. (1981). Principal dimensions of the pain experience and psychological disturbance in chronic low back pain patients. *Pain, 11*, 85–92.

McGill, J. C., Lawlis, G. F., Selby, D., Mooney, V., & McCoy, C. E. (1983). The relationship of Minnesota Multiphasic Personality Inventory (MMPI) profile clusters to pain behaviors. *Journal of Behavioral Medicine, 6*, 77–92.

Melzack, R. (1973). *The puzzle of pain*. Harmondsworth, England: Penguin.

Melzack, R. (1975). The McGill Pain Questionnaire: Major properties and scoring methods. *Pain, 1*, 277–299.

Melzack, R., & Torgerson, W. S. (1971). On the language of pain. *Anesthesiology, 34*, 50–59.

Melzack, R., & Wall, P. (1965). Pain mechanisms: A new theory. *Science, 50*, 971–979.

Millon, T., Green, C. J., & Meagher, R. B. (1979, August). The MBHI: A new inventory for the psychodiagnostician in medical settings. *Professional Psychology*, pp. 529–539.

Naliboff, B. D., Cohen, M. J., & Yellen, A. N. (1982). Does the MMPI differentiate chronic illness from chronic pain? *Pain, 13*, 333–341.

Ohnhaus, E. E., & Adler, R. (1975). Methodological problems in the measurement of pain: A comparison between the verbal rating scale and the visual analogue scale. *Pain, 1*, 379–384.

Pemberton, J. S. (1985). *Personality variables and prediction of response to treatment of chronic low back pain*. Unpublished doctoral dissertation, Georgia State University, Atlanta, GA.

Philips, C. (1977). A psychological analysis of tension headache. In S. Rachman (Ed.), *Contributions to medical psychology* (Vol. 1). New York: Pergamon.

Philips, C. (1978). Tension headache: Theoretical problems. *Behaviour Research and Therapy, 16*, 249–261.

Philips, H. C., & Hunter, M. S. (1982). A psychophysiological investigation of tension headache. *Headache, 22*, 173–179.

Pilowsky, I., & Spence, N. D. (1975). Patterns of illness behaviour in patients with intractable pain. *Journal of Psychosomatic Research 19*, 279–287.

Pilowsky, I., & Spence, N. D. (1983). *Manual for the Illness Behaviour Questionnaire (IBQ)* (2nd ed.).

Pinsky, J. J. (1979). Aspects of the psychology of pain. In B. L. Crue (Ed.), *Chronic pain: Further observations from City of Hope Medical Center.* New York: SP Medical and Scientific Books.

Prieto, E., Hopson, L. Bradley, L., Byrne, M., Geisinger, K., Midax, D., &

Marchisello, P. (1980). The language of low-back pain: Factor structure of the McGill Pain Questionnaire. *Pain, 8*, 11–19.

Price, D. D., McGrath, P. A., Rafii, A., & Buckingham B. (1983). The validation of visual analogue scales as ratio scale measures for chronic and experimental pain. *Pain, 17*, 45–56.

Ransford, A. O., Cairns, D., & Mooney, V. (1976). The pain drawing as an aid to the physiologic evaluation of patients with low-back pain. *Spine, 1*, 127–134.

Reading, A. E. (1979). The internal structure of the McGill Pain Questionnaire in dysmenorrhea patients. *Pain, 7*, 353–358.

Reading, E., Everitt, B. S., & Sledmere, C. M. (1982). The McGill Pain Questionnaire: A replication of its construction. *British Journal of Clinical Psychology, 21*, 339–349.

Ready, L. B., Sarkis, E., & Turner, J. A. (1982). Self-reported vs. actual use of medications in chronic pain patients. *Pain, 12*, 285–294.

Richards, J. S., Nepomuceno, C., Riles, M., & Suer, Z. (1982). Assessing pain behavior: The UAB pain behavior scale. *Pain, 14*, 393–398.

Rosenbaum, J. F. (1982). Comments on "Chronic Pain as a Variant of Depressive Disease: The Pain-Prone Disorder." *Journal of Nervous and Mental Disease, 170*, 412–414.

Sanders, S. H. (1979). Behavioral assessment and treatment of clinical pain: Appraisal of current status. In M. Hersen, R. M. Eisler, & P. M. Miller (Eds.), *Progress in behavior modification* (Vol. 8). New York: Academic.

Sanders, S. H. (1980). Toward a practical instrument system for the automatic measurement of "up-time" in chronic pain patients. *Pain, 9*, 103–109.

Sanders, S. H. (1983). Automated versus self-monitoring of "up-time" in chronic low-back pain patients: A comparative study. *Pain, 15*, 399–405.

Sanders, S. H. (1985). Cross-validation of the Back Pain Classification Scale with chronic, intractable pain patients. *Pain, 22*, 271–277.

Saper, J. R. (1983). *Headache disorders: Current concepts and treatment strategies*. Littleton, MA: PSG Publishing.

Scott, J., & Huskisson, E. C. (1976). Graphic representation of pain. *Pain, 2*, 175–184.

Scott, J., & Huskisson, E. C. (1979). Vertical or horizontal visual analogue scales. *Annals of Rheumatic Disease, 38*, 560–561.

Shealy, C., & Shealy, M. (1976). Behavioral techniques in the control of pain: A case of health maintenance versus disease treatment. In M. Weisenberg & B. Tursky (Eds.), *Pain: New perspectives in therapy and research*. New York: Plenum.

Sriwatanakul, K., Kelvie, W., Lasagna, L., Calimlim, J. F., Weis, O. F., & Mehta, G. (1983). Studies with different types of visual analog scales for measurement of pain. *Clinical Pharmacological Therapy, 34*, 234–239.

Sternbach, R. A. (1974). *Pain patients: Traits and treatment*. New York: Academic.

Sternbach, R. A., Wolf, S. R., Murphy, R. W., & Akeson, W. H. (1973). Traits of pain patients: The low back "loser." *Psychosomatics, 14*, 226–229.

Strassberg, D. S., Reimherr, F., Ward, M., Russell, S., & Cole, A. (1981). The MMPI and chronic pain. *Journal of Consulting and Clinical Psychology, 49*, 220–226.

Sutton, E. P., & Belar, C. D. (1982). Tension headache patients versus controls: A study of EMG parameters. *Headache, 22*, 133–136.

Swanson, D., Swenson, W., Maruta, T., & McPhee, M. (1976). Program for managing chronic pain: Part I and II. *Mayo Clinic Proceedings, 51*, 401–411.

Thelen, M. H., & Frye, R. A. (1981). The effect of modeling and selective attention on pain tolerance. *Journal of Behavior Therapy and Experimental Psychiatry, 12*, 225–229.

Thompson, J. K., & Adams, H. E. (1984). Psychophysiological characteristics of headache patients. *Pain, 18*, 41–52.

Trief, P. M., & Yuan, H. A. (1983). The use of the MMPI in a chronic back pain rehabilitation program. *Journal of Clinical Psychology, 39*, 46–53.

Turk, D. C., & Flor, H. (1984). Etiological theories and treatments for chronic back pain. II. Psychological models and interventions. *Pain, 19*, 209–233.

Turk, D. C., Meichenbaum, D., & Genest, M. (1983). *Pain and behavioral medicine: A cognitive-behavioral perspective.* New York: Guilford.

Turk, D. C., Rudy, T. E., & Salovey, P. (1985). The McGill Pain questionnaire reconsidered: Confirming the factor structure and examining appropriate uses. *Pain, 21*, 385–397.

Turk, D. C., & Salovey, P. (1984). "Chronic Pain as a Variant of Depressive Disease": A critical reappraisal. *Journal of Nervous and Mental Disease, 172*, 398–404.

Tursky, B., & Sternbach, R. A. (1967). Further physiological correlates of ethnic differences in responses to shock. *Psychophysiology, 4*, 67–74.

Turner, J., & McCreary, C. (1978). Short forms of the MMPI with back pain patients. *Journal of Consulting and Clinical Psychology, 46*, 354–355.

Turner, J. A., Robinson, J., & McCreary, C. P. (1983). Chronic low back pain: Predicting response to nonsurgical treatment. *Archives of Physical Medicine and Rehabilitation, 64*, 560–563.

Violon, A., & Giurgen, D. (1984). Familial models for chronic pain. *Pain, 18*, 199–203.

von Baeyer, C. L., Bergstrom, K. J., Brodwin, M. G., & Brodwin, S. K. (1983). Invalid use of pain drawings in psychological screening of back pain patients. *Pain, 16*, 103–107.

Wallston, K. A., & Wallston, B. S. (1978). *Development of the Multidimensional Health Locus of Control (MHLC) Scales, 6*, 160–170.

Weisenberg, M. (1977). Pain and pain control. *Psychological Bulletin, 84*, 1008-1044.

White, B., & Sanders, S. H. (1985). Differential effects on pain and mood in chronic pain patients with time- versus pain-contingent medication delivery. *Behavior Therapy, 16*, 28–38.

Whitehead, W. E., Fedoravicius, A. S., Blackwell, B., & Wooley, S. (1979). A behavioral conceptualization of psychosomatic illness: Psychosomatic illness as learned responses. In J. R. MacNamara (Ed.), *Behavioral approaches to medicine: Application and analysis.* New York: Plenum.

Wolf, S. L., Nacht, M., & Kelly, J. L. (1982). EMG feedback training during dynamic movement for low back pain patients. *Behavior Therapy, 13*, 395–406.

Woodforde, J., & Merskey, H. (1972a). Personality traits of patients with chronic pain. *Journal of Psychosomatic Research, 16*, 167–172.

Woodforde, J. M., & Merskey, H. (1972). Some relationships between subjective measures of pain. *Journal of Psychosomatic Research, 16*, 173–178.

Zborowski, M. (1969). *People in pain.* San Francisco: Jossey-Bass.

9

Psychological Responses to Chronic Pain

Neil Spence

Dibden Research Unit
Glenside Hospital
Eastwood, Australia

INTRODUCTION

Marked changes in mood and manner, in attitude and activity, are often reported by patients with a range of chronic pain syndromes including headache, back pain, arthritis, cancer pain, neuralgia, phantom limb pain, dysmenorrhea, and temporomandibular joint dysfunction. This chapter examines the affective, behavioral, and cognitive sequelae of chronic pain and the factors that determine the nature and extent of individual reactions. It also alludes to the effects of chronic pain on the families of patients and on the clinicians who treat such disorders.

The literature on psychological responses to chronic pain is truly vast, and the present review is selective both in terms of findings and concepts. The basic framework utilized in this chapter is drawn from

Table 9.1.
The Conceptualization of Chronic Pain as a Stressor, Distinguishing between Sources, Mediations, and Manifestations of Stress (From Pearlin & Schooler, 1978; Pearlin et al., 1981).

Sources of Pain-Related Stress	Mediators of Pain-Related Stress	Manifestations of Pain-Related Stress
1. *Clinical characteristics of pain*	1. *Specific coping strategies*	1. *Affective changes*
a. sensory and affective qualities of the pain itself	Perceptions, thoughts, and actions that are systematically employed to	a. depression and grief
b. spatial distribution (e.g. site, lateralization)	a. directly avoid or eliminate the sources of pain-related stress	b. anger and irritability
c. temporal factors (e.g. duration, gradual vs. sudden onset, continuous vs. intermittent, predictable vs. unpredictable)	b. redefine, reinterpret, or rationalize the meaning or significance of pain-related stress	c. anxiety and apprehension
d. symptoms associated with the pain (e.g. numbness, pins and needles, nausea, photophobia)	c. control and regulate the psychological consequences of pain-related stress	d. apathy and indifference
e. irreversible physical changes associated with the pain (e.g. amputation, surgery, paralysis)		2. *Behavioral changes*
f. diagnostic issues (e.g. benign vs. life-threatening, organic vs. functional)	2. *Psychological resources*	a. verbal complaints
	Personality factors, attitudes, skills that aid in the formulation of coping strategies	b. increased intake of analgesic or psychotropic medication
		c. decrease in uptime and activity levels
		d. grimacing, moaning, gasping, etc.
		e. restricted posture, gait, or range of motion

2. *Disruption to daily living activities* a. sleep b. self-care c. mobility and transport d. sexual functioning e. eating f. smoking and drinking g. social activities h. recreation and hobbies i. domestic tasks j. paid work	a. high self-esteem b. internal locus of control c. cognitive ability and adequate educational development d. social competence e. delay of gratification and impulse control f. tendency to avoid sick role	f. greater utilization of medical and treatment services
3. *Involvement in complex treatment and service systems* a. medical and paramedical b. unemployment c. legal and compensation d. welfare and financial e. rehabilitation	3. *Social support* Networks of family and friends that reinforce the individual's own psychological resources and coping strategies by providing a. instrumental and practical assistance b. emotional and moral support c. appropriate contingencies for illness behavior	3. *Cognitive changes* a. retardation of thinking and information processing b. disruption of concentration, learning, and short-term memory processes c. restricted concept formation (e.g. concreteness of thinking, idiosyncratic reasoning) d. altered ideational content (e.g. fixed beliefs, rumination, preoccupation)

the literature on stress and coping, as exemplified by Pearlin and Schooler (1978), Andrews, Tennant, Hewson, and Vaillant (1978), Brown and Harris (1978), Folkman and Lazarus (1980), Pearlin, Menaghan, Lieberman, and Mullan (1981), Kanner, Coyne, Schaefer, and Lazarus (1981), Billings and Moos (1981), Viney and Westbrook (1982), and Monroe (1983). The work of such investigators covers three conceptual domains: the sources, mediators, and manifestations of stress. Their broad approach is valuable because it provides some insight into normal coping responses to life events and problems, including data on longitudinal changes. Moreover, their results emphasize the complex interaction that occurs between the stressor itself, the resources of the "stressee," and the ways in which distress may be experienced or shown. Particularly when the stressor is a chronic one, it becomes increasingly hard to distinguish between these three elements of the stress experience. Conceptually, however, such a division remains convenient as a framework for investigating how individuals cope with stress.

Anyone who has dealt with chronic pain patients knows the difficulty of trying to unravel the interplay that occurs between pain, personality, mood, outlook, work, family, and so on in their illness presentation. Table 9.1 provides a working model of the various factors that interact in the individual's experience of chronic pain, based on the conceptual approach used by Pearlin and associates in studying the sources, mediators, and manifestations of normal stress.

It should be emphasized that the allocation of variables to the different conceptual domains represented in Table 9.1 is somewhat arbitrary. While it is methodologically appealing to distinguish three major components of the stress process, there are some factors that might easily be thought of as more readily belonging to an earlier or later stage of the pain experience. For example, disruptions to daily living activities are treated in Table 9.1 as an additional source of stress for those who have chronic pain. However, these same activities could also be used to measure behavioral manifestations of pain or to assess coping strategies. Similarly, manifestations of chronic pain are not only dependent measures, but can additionally function as independent variables capable of generating new sources of stress or influencing the factors that mediate stress.

Such difficulties in categorizing classes of variables as belonging exclusively to one particular domain of the stress process serves to remind us that the evaluation of chronic pain and its psychological sequelae can never be approached naively. The model outlined in Table 9.1 is simply a means of providing a descriptive framework in which to examine relationships between different measures. It is a descriptive tool, a method of ordering observations, rather than a means of causal analysis. Accordingly, the structure of this chapter is organized with these limitations in mind. Psychological responses to chronic pain are discussed only in terms of affective, behavioral, and cognitive changes. The extent and nature of such changes are examined primarily in relation to clinical characteristics of pain, its impact on daily living, and the engagement in various treatment systems it often involves. Studies pertaining to these major sources of pain related stress are reviewed. The factors cited in Table 9.1 that appear to mediate this process—coping strategies, psychological resources, and social support—are not systematically examined in this review.

THE MEASUREMENT OF PSYCHOLOGICAL RESPONSES

Before discussing the research and clinical findings in these areas, it is important to briefly address some issues in the measurement of affective, behavioral, and cognitive changes occurring as manifestations of pain-related stress. Traditionally, affective responses to chronic pain have been most frequently studied. The measurement of depression, anxiety, anger, and so on has depended largely upon self-report instruments that would normally be used in psychiatric settings. These include the Minnesota Multiphasic Personality Inventory (Sullivan & Welsh, 1952), Hostility and Direction of Hostility Questionnaire (Foulds, Caine, & Creasy, 1960), Zung Depression Scale (Zung, 1965), Middlesex Hospital Questionnaire (Crown & Crisp, 1966), State-Trait Anxiety Inventory (Spielberger, Gorsuch, & Lushene, 1970), Wakefield Depression Scale (Snaith, Ahmed, Mehta, & Hamilton, 1971), Levine-Pilowsky Depression Questionnaire (Pilowsky & Spalding, 1972), Symptom Check List—90 (De Rogatis, Rickels, & Rock, 1976), Eysenck Personality Questionnaire (Eysenck & Eysenck, 1976) and General Health Questionnaire (Goldberg & Hillier, 1979).

The types of variables used to measure behavioral changes are, however, more specific to chronic pain patients. Since Fordyce (1976) introduced a range of operant techniques to pain management, there has been increasing interest in the assessment and modification of pain behavior. This has led to the development of observational methods to monitor the behavior of patients with back pain (Keefe & Block, 1982), headache (Philips & Hunter, 1982), rheumatoid arthritis (McDaniel et al., 1986), and chronic pain at other sites (Richards, Nepomuceno, Riles, & Suer, 1982; Cincirupini & Floreen, 1983). Methodological attention has also been paid to differences between observer-based and self-report measures of pain behavior in terms of medication use (Ready, Sarkis, & Turner, 1982), activity level (Sanders, 1983), and socialization (Kremer, Block, & Gaylor, 1981).

The evaluation of cognitive changes in chronic pain patients reflects a mixture of orthodox neuropsychological measures and content-oriented attitudinal scales. Sprock, Braff, Saccuzzo, and Atkinson (1983) assessed the cognitive functioning of pain patients using measures of abstraction, associative tightness, and speed of information processing. Patients studied by McNairy, Maruta, Ivnik, Swanson, and Ilstrup (1984) were administered selected tests from the Wechsler Adult Intelligence Scale, the modified Halstead-Reitan Battery, and Rey's Auditory-Verbal Learning Test. Other investigators have been more concerned with the attitudes, expectations, and attributions held by chronic pain patients. Lefebvre (1981) has constructed a questionnaire measuring cognitive distortion in patients with back pain, while Roberts et al. (1984) have developed a series of health belief scales, again for back pain patients. A measure of sociomedical orientation specifically for patients with facial pain has been used by Marbach and Lipton (1978). Instruments suitable for delineating the attitudes and assumptions of patients regardless of pain site include the Illness Behaviour Questionnaire (Pilowsky, Spence, Cobb, & Katsikitis, 1984), the Illness Behaviour Assessment Schedule (Pilowsky, Bassett, Barrett, Petrovic, & Minniti, 1983), and the Health Index (Sternbach, Wolf, Murphy, & Akeson, 1973a). The Hypochondriasis scale of the MMPI can also be used for this purpose, although its factorial structure appears to be somewhat complex (Comrey, 1957).

In reviewing the measurement of psychological responses to chronic pain, it should be emphasized that pain sequelae must be conceived as multidimensional changes. While not listed in Table 9.1, this would include physiological and biochemical responses to pain in a broader analysis. A second point is that none of the manifestations of pain-related stress should be considered more "real" than any other, although some may be more reliable or practical to measure. Third, none should be seen as intrinsically more desirable than any other as goals for treatment (Trief, 1983). Fourth, it is likely that affective, behavioral, and cognitive changes interact with each other in response to chronic pain. However, this does not always mean that there will be concordance between them (Philips, 1978), and it is not logically invalid to anticipate that in some patients affective improvement, for example, may be accompanied by behavioral deterioration. Bearing these points in mind, the following sections will examine the relation of psychological responses to the various sources of pain-related stress.

CLINICAL CHARACTERISTICS OF PAIN

This section examines how various aspects of the patient's pain relate to affective, behavioral, and cognitive variables. For most of their information about pain it is obvious that both clinicians and researchers have to rely on what the patient describes. This has traditionally been done by asking the patient to rate the severity of pain along a single dimension of intensity, a method formally known as magnitude estimation (Wolff, 1978). The most popular form of this technique is probably the visual analogue scale (Clarke & Spear, 1964). A different approach to pain measurement now widely applied in descriptive and intervention studies is the McGill Pain Questionnaire (MPQ) developed by Melzack (1975). The MPQ consists of a large number of pain adjectives, grouped in such a way that the patient's choice of descriptors can be analyzed to provide three separate scores representing the sensory, affective, and evaluative dimensions of pain perception.

In the following discussion, pain descriptions based on both analogue ratings and MPQ measures will be cited where they have been related to patterns of psychological response to chronic pain. While some studies of the internal structure of the MPQ find considerably more dimensions than expected (Leavitt, Garron, Whisler, & Sheinkop, 1978; Hunter, 1983; Burckhardt, 1984; Kremer & Atkinson, 1984), the utility of its three-dimensional scoring system has been generally supported (Reading, 1979; Prieto et al., 1980; McCreary, Turner, & Dawson, 1981; Byrne et al., 1982). It is interesting to note that the factor structure of the MPQ for acute pain does not appear to be as clearly differentiated along sensory, affective, and evaluative lines in comparison to chronic pain (Reading, 1982). Descriptions of acute pain reveal a normal distribution of sensory scores, but low affective and evaluative scores (Melzack, Wall, & Ty, 1982). Correspondingly, these latter dimensions are used more frequently by chronic pain patients, and in some factor analyses their content accounts for most of the variance (Leavitt et al., 1978; Kremer & Atkinson, 1984). Turk, Rudy, and Salovey (1985) have recently warned that it may not be possible to establish discriminative validity for the sensory, affective, and evaluative scores of the MPQ. These findings emphasize the difficulty of identifying in chronic pain patients the "pure" sensory aspects of their experience. This has led some observers to conceptualize chronic pain not so much as a primary perceptual process but rather as a need state (Wall, 1979) or an emotion in itself (Swanson, 1984).

Despite the strong role of affect in descriptions of chronic pain, qualities of the pain itself do not always correspond closely with the changes cited as manifestations of stress in Table 9.1. Fordyce, Brena, Holcombe, De Lateur, and Loeser (1978) compared the pain descriptions given by patients on 25 bipolar adjectives with their MMPI scores and activity levels. Twenty-six MMPI scales were used, but only seven significant correlations occurred from the total of 650 adjective-scale comparisons. Stronger relationships emerged between adjectives and the amount of "uptime" reported by patients, but the authors concluded that pain description seemed to have little practical bearing on psychological state or activity level. The severity of pain reported by patients was likewise found by Fordyce et al. (1984) to be only weakly related to measures of medication use, treatment frequency, and participation in daily living activities.

Patients with chronic pain were allocated to high and low affect groups, on the basis of their MPQ affective scale scores by Kremer and Atkinson (1981). Those using many affective terms to describe their pain showed more anxiety, depression, and somaticization, but not hostility. The same patients also reported significantly greater changes in their physical and psychosocial functioning. In a later study with a different sample of patients, Kremer, Atkinson, and Kremer (1983) found that global psychological impairment could be predicted from MPQ affective descriptors but not from sensory descriptors.

Patients with chronic low back pain were administered the MPQ and the MMPI by McCreary et al. (1981). The authors factor-analyzed patients' MPQ responses and derived four factor-based scales, similar but not identical to the sensory, affective, and evaluative dimensions normally scored. The relationship of their descriptive factor scores with MMPI results was modest in that only four significant associations occurred. These were confined, however, to those MMPI scales that are so often elevated in the clinical presentation of chronic pain patients (Sternbach, 1974). Both affective and evaluative descriptors were positively related to higher Hypochondriasis scores, while affective descriptors alone indicated higher Depression and Hysteria scores. The authors also found that a simple visual analogue rating of pain intensity correlated significantly with each of these three MMPI scales, and that this measure could in fact account for more variance in the prediction of Hypochondriasis, Depression, and Hysteria scores than either of their affective or evaluative factors.

Skevington (1983a) correlated intensity and MPQ measures with affective and cognitive variables in patients attending a rheumatology clinic for chronic pain. For patients with organic findings, no significant associations occurred. In patients without organic findings, however, pain intensity was positively correlated with feelings of sadness and skepticism. Pain rating was also associated with higher scores on Scales 1 (General hypochondriasis), 2 (Disease conviction), and 5 (Affective disturbance) of the Illness Behaviour Questionnaire (IBQ). These same three scales were each significantly related to the sensory, affective, and evaluative descriptors of the MPQ. Additionally, higher sensory scores were correlated with lower scores on Scale 6 (Denial of life problems) and higher scores on Scale 7 (Irritability) of the IBQ.

In a study of headache patients, Demjen and Bakal (1981) could identify only one IBQ scale that related to pain intensity. Higher pain ratings were negatively correlated with scores on Scale 3 (Psychological vs. sematic perception of illness), such that greater intensity was reported by patients with a less psychological view of their disorder. Hunter and Philips (1981) reported that pain intensity in patients with tension headache was positively associated with depression, but not with extraversion or neuroticism.

In a group of back pain patients having acupuncture treatment, Mendelson et al. (1983) found that pain intensity correlated with measures of state anxiety, trait anxiety, and depression. Like Skevington (1983a), the authors identified significant associations between intensity and Scales 1, 2, and 5 of the IBQ. No relationship was found between pain intensity and the degree of work disability reported by patients. Measures of illness behavior, depression and anhedonia were not related to pain ratings in back patients studied by Marbach, Richlin, and Lipton (1983). However, for a group of patients with facial pain, given the same assessments, a significant relationship emerged between pain and illness behavior. Lipton and Marbach (1983) used factor analysis to develop two scales reflecting the attitudes and behaviors of patients with facial pain. Both measures—labeled "emotional and expressive description of and response to pain" and "effect of severe pain on daily functioning" were positively related to pain intensity.

Keefe and Block (1982) measured five indices of pain behavior—guarding, bracing, rubbing, grimacing, and sighing—in a group of patients with low back pain. For all behaviors except grimacing there was a significant correlation with level of reported pain intensity. In a later study of back pain patients, Keefe and Hill (1985) found that gait patterns were not strongly related to self-reported pain severity. At admission to an inpatient treatment program, Richards et al. (1982) reported that neither pain intensity nor MPQ descriptors were associated with incidence of overt pain behavior. At discharge, however, there was a significant correlation between intensity and behavioral measures.

With regard to medication use, Turner, Calsyn, Fordyce, and Ready (1982) identified patients taking no addictive drugs, those taking narcotics, and those taking both narcotics and sedatives. No differences in pain rating distinguished the three groups. The same lack of association was reported by McNairy et al. (1984). These results can be contrasted with those reported by McCreary and Colman (1984) who found significant variation in both intensity and MPQ-derived measures for back pain patients according to drug use. Mendelson et al. (1983) noted that in their back pain group, intensity was positively correlated with psychotropic drug use, but not with analgesic intake.

Lefebvre (1981) attempted to measure distortion of thinking and attribution in back pain patients by means of a Cognitive Error Questionnaire. He found that pain per se was not associated with distortion, but that depression was a significant correlate of the latter. Neuropsychological aspects of cognition were investigated by Sprock et al. (1983). They found that pain rating was significantly associated with degree of depression, which in turn was related to deficits in information processing. There was no direct correlation, however, between cognitive performance and levels of either depression or drug use. McNairy et al. (1984) reported, on the other hand, that neuropsychological functioning was impaired in a group of pain patients who abused or depended upon narcotics and/or psychotropic medications.

It is clear from this brief survey of the literature that the relationships between the sensory and affective qualities of chronic pain and the psychological responses that accompany it are not straightforward. Severity of pain, whether it is defined in terms of pain intensity or MPQ measures, does not correlate consistently with changes in affective, behavioral, or cognitive variables. Linton (1985) has suggested that pain and activity levels may well be correlated when the latter are based on global reports, but that the association tends to disappear as the activity ratings become more specific and objective. The importance of sex differences in the relation between pain, activity, and depression has been noted by Haley, Turner, and Romano (1985), with females showing greater consistency between these measures. Philips and Jahanshahi (1985) have observed that the links between pain intensity and the affective and behavioral responses it elicits appear to become more closely related as symptoms endure over many years.

The next set of clinical variables cited in Table 9.1 involves the spatial distribution of pain. Merskey and Watson (1979) have hypothesized that when pain is exclusively lateralized on the left side of the body, there is a greater probability that psychological factors are involved in its etiology. The argument behind this is that the nondominant hemisphere (usually controlling the left side of the body) has a special role in regulating emotional experience. In response to these suggestions Hall, Hayward, and Chapman (1981) studied lateralization and its psychological concomitants in a large group of pain clinic patients. No relationship was found between degree of depression and the laterality of their pain site, nor were any of the scales of the IBQ and the MMPI substantially correlated with this variable. Schwartz and DeGood (1984) examined the distribution of symptoms drawn by chronic pain patients, and rated the degree to which they were anatomically appropriate. Patients with inappropriate patterns tended to be more somatically preoccupied, obsessive, hostile, and reported a higher level of general distress.

Site of pain was examined in a pain clinic population simply in terms of number of discrete locations by Toomey, Gower, and Jones (1983). It was predicted that extensive pain distribution would be associated with greater reported functional and health behavior deficits and with greater degree of psychological disturbance, including somatic preoccupation and less perceived personal control. Patients were classified according to distribution pattern into low, moderate, or high groups, but the authors also reported correlation analyses for the total population studied. From the latter data it was found that number of discrete pain sites was significantly associated with impairment of self-rated functional abilities in the areas of general activity, walking, work, socialization, and recreation. Site frequency correlated with number of recent physician visits, and with total number of health professionals consulted. Number of sites correlated with the number of different sedative-hypnotic drugs used, and with the number of different drugs taken overall. Greater distribution of pain was associated with higher scores on Scales 1 (General hypochondriasis), 2 (Disease conviction), 5 (Affective disturbance) and 7 (Irritability) of the IBQ, and with lower scores on Scale 3 (Psychological versus somatic perception of illness) of the IBQ. Although locus of control is conceptualized as a mediating factor in the present review rather than a manifestation of stress in its own right, it is interesting to note that Toomey et al. (1983) found that number of sites was negatively correlated with internality.

Other studies have examined the effect of spatial distribution simply in terms of whether certain locations seem to be more stressful than others. Again, bearing in mind that it is identified as a mediating variable in Table 9.1, Armentrout (1979) used self-concept as a means of assessing the impact of chronic pain on headache and back pain patients. Contrary to expectation, he found that patients with headache had a lower evaluation of who and what they were, and of their physical capacities. Demjen and Bakal (1981) recorded the topographical properties of pain in patients with chronic headache, but could find no relationship with IBQ profile. Patients with facial pain and back pain were compared by Marbach et al. (1983). The two groups did not differ with regard to depression and anhedonia, but back pain patients showed significantly higher levels of illness behavior.

Toomey, Gover, and Jones (1984) divided their heterogeneous pain clinic sample into patients whose pain was located in the head and/or neck ($N=60$), neck/head and low back ($N=18$), low back ($N=9$), and none of these sites ($N=5$). Differences between these groups were examined using the same measures of behavioral and psychological functioning applied in Toomey et al. (1983). It was hypothesized that, in view of the particular salience of the head and neck region to the self-concept, patients with facial pain would endorse greater levels of psychological distress. In contrast, patients with pain at other sites were expected to report more physical and functional impairment. These relationships were partially confirmed. Patients with head/neck pain reported less disability in terms of downtime, walking, social, work, and recreational behavior. Measures of treatment seeking and medication usage did not generally discriminate between the groups, although patients with head/neck pain had undergone significantly less surgery. The IBQ profiles of the groups differed on Scales 2 and 3, with head/neck patients reporting less conviction of disease and a more psychological view of their illness. It was not apparent, however, that patients with head/neck pain were in greater psychological distress. Their scores on Scales 5 (Affective disturbance) and 7 (Irritability) of the IBQ were no higher than those of the other groups.

It is obvious from the results discussed above that the effect of pain site on pattern of psychological response can be approached in several different ways. Perhaps the clearest findings at the moment are those indicating that the number of discrete sites at which pain is experienced does seem to consistently correlate with a range of affective, behavioral, and cognitive measures. The significance of the different anatomic regions in which pain occurs is, however, harder to generalize about. It would seem unlikely that site per se would help predict manner of psychological response, unless its meaning to the individual (in terms of body image, illness history, etc.) was somehow taken into account.

The third set of variables to be considered under the heading of clinical characteristics of pain are temporal factors. The best studied of these is duration; that is, the amount of time since the pain first began. Of course, the term "chronic" pain reflects this variable, and most clinicians and researchers define chronic pain as having a duration of six months or more. In practice, the mean duration of pain for patients attending a pain clinic or specialized treatment facility is usually in the order of several years. Implicitly, it would be expected that patients would display greater psychological distress with time. Sternbach, Wolf, Murphy, and Akeson (1973b) compared the MMPI profiles of patients with acute and chronic back pain, defining the latter as more than six months duration. Chronic patients showed significant elevations on the Hypochondriasis, Depression, and Hysteria scales. Perhaps surprisingly, they displayed lower scores than acute patients on the Paranoia and Hypomania scales.

No consistent relationship between duration of pain and illness behavior was identified by Pilowsky and Spence (1976b). They analyzed the IBQ profiles of a heterogeneous sample of pain clinic patients whose mean length of illness was 7.4 years. For male patients, scores on none of the seven IBQ scales correlated with duration. There was a significant negative correlation, however, between duration and Scale 7 (Irritability) for female patients. That is, the longer their symptoms had existed, the less likely these women were to report that they were hard to get along with, let illness interfere in their interpersonal relations, and that they got angry easily. To check whether clearer findings might emerge in patients with more serious medical conditions, correlations between duration and illness behavior were repeated only for patients (male and females combined) with substantial organic pathology. No significant associations were obtained, and it was concluded by the authors that illness behavior patterns in chronic pain cannot easily be ascribed to chronicity itself.

Cox, Chapman, and Black compared the MMPI profiles of pain clinic patients who had had their pain for several years with those of surgical patients whose operations had been performed less than a week beforehand. The chronic pain group had significantly higher scores on Hypochondriasis, Depression, and Hysteria. Two groups of patients with facial pain (mean duration 31 months) and back pain (mean duration 41 months) were studied by Marbach et al. (1983). The period of time since the pain had started was found not to be predictive of illness behavior, depression, or anhedonia in either group of patients. In a large sample of facial pain patients, two-thirds of whom had had their symptoms for at least 6 months, Marbach and Lipton (1983) derived two factor-based scales of emotionality and interference with functioning. Scores on these dimensions were unrelated, however, to pain duration. Negative results have also been reported by Mendelson et al. (1983). They assessed patients with back pain (mean duration 12.2 years) and a range of psychological tests, including measures of neuroticism, extraversion, hostility, state and trait anxiety, depression, and IBQ profile. No significant correlation was found between any of these variables and chronicity. Similar results were reported by Merskey et al. (1985) for headache patients assessed on a variety of psychological tests, and by Keefe, Wilkins, and Cook (1984) for back patients rated on overt pain behaviors during physical examination.

A comprehensive study of the relation between duration of pain and psychological disturbance was carried out by Garron and Leavitt (1983) in patients with back pain. Three groups of patients were identified on the basis of duration: pain less than 6 months ($N=39$), between 6–24 months ($N=35$), and more than 24 months ($N=74$). There were no differences between the groups on pain intensity or MPQ-derived measures. The authors found that their MMPI profiles varied significantly in levels of Hypochondriasis, Depression, Hysteria, Paranoia, Psychasthenia, and Mania. The chronic group consistently showed the highest scores on these scales. For patients with pain of less than 6 months duration, clinically significant elevations (T score >70) did not occur on any means scale score. The profiles of the two remaining groups, however, both showed mean Hypochondriasis and Hysteria scores that were raised two standard deviations. On other measures of psychological disturbance, Garron and Leavitt (1983) found that the three groups differed significantly in trait anxiety (chronic group highest) but did not vary in current levels of anxiety, depression, and hostility. Taking into account other findings as well as their own, Garron and Leavitt concluded that pain duration can be seen to adversely effect psychological functioning when the latter is measured in terms of heterogeneous and complex indicators, such as the MMPI. They further argued that measures that have been factorially derived (such as current mood scales or the IBQ) are unlikely to reflect disturbance because their content is too narrow. The most robust changes appear to occur on the MMPI scales of Hypochondriasis, Depression, and Hysteria.

There are other temporal aspects of chronic pain that merit attention apart from its duration. Whether the original onset of pain was sudden or gradual is a variable that some clinicians consider important to the patient's adjustment. Where painful symptoms build up slowly over several years, an individual may literally have more time to modify attitudes and activities and to minimize future disruption. In the case of sudden onset, however, a multitude of changes can be experienced without warning over a short time period. Another temporal variable that might influence the stressfulness of chronic pain is continuity. Some pain patterns are episodic in nature, while in others the pain seems unrelenting in its severity. Sternbach, Dalessio, Kunzel, and Bowman (1980) reported that patients with vascular headaches had less elevated scores on the MMPI compared to patient with headaches related to muscle contraction. This they attributed to the occurrence of longer and more frequent pain-free intervals in the vascular group. Continuity of headache was found by Demjen and Bakal (1981) to be related to Scale 3 (Psychological versus somatic perception of illness) of the IBQ. Patients with episodic pain were more likely to consider psychological factors as relevant to their headache symptoms. Finally, the last temporal aspect of chronic pain that should be mentioned is its degree of predictability. Where patients experience pain on an episodic basis, they will often be thinking about what contributes to its exacerbation (Wiener, 1975). This search for meaning may identify a variety of perceived causal agents (such as overactivity, diet, stress, noise, temperature, etc.). Whether or not these factors really contribute to the individual's pain is besides the point. If an attributional link is made, and the individual can exert some control over the factors perceived to be causal, then pain may be less aversive (Thompson, 1981).

The next group of variables listed in Table 9.1 that form part of the clinical makeup of pain are other physical symptoms that may accompany it. These changes, such as pins and needles or nausea, may be quite distressing, and sometimes even more debilitating than the pain itself. There has been little investigation of the effects of such symptoms, independent of the pain with which they are so closely associated. In Demjen and Bakal's (1981) study of chronic headache patients, reports of throbbing and nausea were related to scale 3 (Psychological vs. somatic perception of illness) of the IBQ. Patients with either of these symptoms were significantly more likely to view their disorder in somatic terms. Keefe et al. (1984) found that back pain patients with clear neurological signs exhibited more frequent pain behaviors than those without such findings. The same trend existed for mechanical signs, but was not quite significant.

Another set of clinical variables that may be important in influencing adjustment to chronic pain are irreversible physical changes that result from trauma, illness, or treatment. Examples of these sequelae might include epilepsy in conjunction with headache, disfigurement in conjunction with rheumatoid arthritis, amputation in conjunction with phantom limb pain, and spinal fusion in conjunction with back pain. Such changes are not symptoms in the sense discussed earlier, whereby physical sensations (e.g., nausea) could be seen as belonging to a familiar clinical picture. The sequelae identified in this section are more like "complications," and they have a greater permanence about them. However, like accompanying symptoms, their implications for the psychological adjustment of the chronic pain patient are largely unknown. Incidental data relevant to this area are sometimes reported. In their study of drug utilization patterns, Turner et al. (1982) found that pain clinic patients taking addictive medication were almost three times as likely to have undergone pain-related surgery than other patients. Number of lumbar surgeries was more likely to be associated with overt pain behaviors as assessed by Keefe et al. (1984) and Keefe and Hill (1985).

The last category of clinical variables cited in Table 9.1 is related to diagnostic issues. The question here is whether membership of diagnostic subgroups within the common syndromes (such as headache or backache) has different implications for psychological functioning. To some extent, this type of variable cuts across some of the others that have been previously discussed. For example, it has already been pointed out that continuity of pain—which has some bearing on psychological adjustment—is more likely where headaches are of muscular rather than vascular origin (Demjen & Bakal, 1981). No doubt there are other instances in which the different clinical characteristics of chronic pain listed in Table 9.1 are confounded with each other, but it is not the aim of this review to analyze such interrelationships. Diagnosis remains an important variable in its own right, and its association with psychological functioning will be examined in patients with headache, facial pain, back pain, and cancer. In many cases of chronic pain, however, no firm diagnosis is possible because of the absence of organic findings. Thus the most common diagnostic subgrouping across virtually all chronic pain syndromes is along an "organic vs. nonorganic" dimension. The relevance of this variable to affective, behavioral, and cognitive measures will be looked at first.

It should be recognized that the terms organic or nonorganic are used here purely in a descriptive (rather than an aetiological) sense. The absence of organic findings does not by itself mean that pain is "psychogenic" or "hysterical," although both clinicians and patients sometimes implicitly make this diagnostic leap. Conversely, the presence of psychological findings should not be interpreted to mean that the pain cannot have an organic basis (Rook, Pesch, & Keeler, 1981). Conceptually at least, the dimensions of "organic vs. nonorganic" and "psychological disturbance vs. nondisturbance" are independent. How patients are distributed in practice along these two continuums depends upon a number of factors including the thoroughness of the physical workup, the manner in which psychological functioning is assessed, the types of pain disorders referred, and the setting in which patients are seen. The importance of these factors can be illustrated by comparing two studies which evaluated patients for both physical and psychological findings, and reported these results in a two-by-two format. Brena, Chapman, Stegall, and Chyatte (1979) assessed 101 patients with pain at various sites, and measured psychological disturbance by means of MMPI scores, drug use, activity level, and MPQ-derived descriptors. Leavitt and Garron (1979) assessed 102 patients with back pain, and documented their psychological status by MMPI scores, current mood measures, projective testing, recent life events, and clinical interview. The ratio of patients in each category can be compared across studies. The ratio of patients with positive findings from both physical and psychological assessments is 25:23 (where the first number represents Brena et al.'s data) and the ratio for findings on neither dimension is 16:18. However, for patients with physical findings and no psychological findings the ratio is 0:35, while for patients with psychological findings and no physical findings the ratio is 60:26. The difference in distribution between these two populations of chronic pain patients is obvious, and demonstrates the need for methodological care in interpreting the following results.

Hanvik (1951) compared the MMPI profiles of male back pain patients with and without organic findings. Those without findings had higher scores on Hypochondriasis, Depression, Hysteria, Psychopathic deviancy, Psychasthenia, and Schizophrenia. Patients with back pain attending an orthopaedic clinic were divided by Sternbach et al. (1973b) into organic ($N = 81$) and nonorganic groups ($N = 36$). The MMPI results of each group were almost identical, although organic patients had a significantly higher Hypomania score. Freeman, Calsyn, and Louks (1976) studied three groups of male patients who had either sufficient physical findings, some findings, or no findings to account for their back pain. There was significant MMPI variation between the groups on the same scales identified by Hanvik (1951), with the exception of Psychopathic deviancy. The organic patients had no mean scores that were clinically significant ($T = 70$) on any MMPI scale, whereas patients with some findings had at least 3 such elevations, and patients with no findings had at least 4 elevated mean scores. Using contemporary MMPI norms, Ahles, Yunus, Gaulier, Riley, and Masi (1986) similarly found that no patients with documented rheumatoid arthritis ($N = 30$) had four raised scores, while 18 percent of nonorganic patients with comparable symptoms ($N = 45$) showed that degree of psychological disturbance. The authors demonstrated, moreover, that the use of the original MMPI norms tended to increase the profile discrepancy between organic and nonorganic patients in their study.

Organic patients ($N = 42$) and nonorganic patients ($N = 37$) with back pain were compared by McCreary, Turner, and Dawson (1977) using MMPI measures. Differences were significant on 6 of the 10 clinical scales, with organic patients having lower scores. As reported in earlier studies, patients without physical findings were higher on Hypochondriasis, Hysteria, Psychopathic deviancy, and Schizophrenia. The authors additionally found that their nonorganic patients were higher on Mania and Social introversion. Unlike earlier studies, no differences between the groups on Depression and Psychasthenia were obtained. Physicians in his study were also asked to rate severity of impairment and ability to return to normal activities for each patient. The presence or absence of physical findings did not relate to impairment, but nonorganic patients were rated as significantly more able to return to normal activities.

Marbach and Lund (1981) classified patients with facial pain into three diagnostic groups: trigeminal neuralgia, degenerative temporomandibular joint disease, and myofascial syndrome. Despite the fact that patients in the last category lacked organic findings, no differences between the groups in depression, anxiety, or anhedonia were identified. A modified diagnostic system was used by Lipton and Marbach (1983). Patients with facial pain were considered to have organic findings ($N = 61$) if they had degenerative joint disease or facial neuralgia, and to lack organic findings ($N = 68$) if they had myofascial pain. A third group ($N = 41$) had mixed symptoms that could be considered partly organic. The authors note that patients with psychogenic pain were excluded from the study. The scores of the three groups were not significantly different on measures of psychological distress, sociomedical orientation, and treatment history.

Fordyce et al. (1978) examined both MMPI and activity scores in a heterogeneous sample of pain clinic referrals. One hundred consecutive patients were assessed, but organic vs. nonorganic ratings were not predictive of their MMPI results or self-reported activity measures. Neurological patients with pain were given the Middlesex Hospital Questionnaire and the Eysenck Personality Inventory by Woodforde and Merskey (1972). Patients were divided into those with physical findings ($N = 27$) and those lacking evidence of organic disease ($N = 16$). No differences in personality scores was found between the groups. Pilowsky and Spence (1976c) administered the IBQ to 100 pain clinic patients. The mean profile of patients with little or no pathology ($N = 55$) did not vary from that for patients with major pathology ($N = 20$). From the above results, it can be seen that in patients unselected for site of pain, the presence or absence of physical findings bears no relationship to their psychological status. In patients with back pain, however, there is evidence to suggest that those with no identifiable pathology will consistently have higher scores on the Hypochondriasis, Hysteria, and Schizophrenia scale of the MMPI. For patients with facial pain, no relationship between lack of organic findings and psychological status is apparent.

Diagnostic subgroups other than those based on the organic vs. nonorganic distinction will now be examined. Sternbach et al. (1980) evaluated the MMPI profiles of 182 headache patients in the three most common diagnostic groups: vascular ($N=83$), muscle contraction ($N=41$), and mixed vascular and muscle contraction ($N=58$). Vascular patients obtained lower MMPI scores than patients with other diagnoses, a finding consistent with that reported by Kudrow and Sutkus (1979). The same diagnostic categories were used by Demjen and Bakal (1981) in analyzing headache patients' responses to the IBQ. There were 32 patients with muscle contraction headache, 25 patients with migraine, and 18 patients with mixed symptoms. No IBQ differences between the groups were evident.

Merskey et al. (1985) compared patients with classical or cluster headache ($N=19$), common migraine ($N=42$), tension headache ($N=22$), and mixed symptoms ($N=20$) on a wide range of psychological measures. Differences were minimal, with patients in the classical or cluster headache group reporting slightly less depression and social dysfunction than patients in other groups. A large sample of headache patients, consisting of classic migraine ($N=51$), common migraine ($N=235$), and tension headache ($N=74$), was studied by Philips and Jahanshahi (1985). Patients with classic migraine were found to report higher levels of overt pain behavior, but to acknowledge less depression, than their fellow sufferers.

Gordon and Hitchcock (1983) divided facial pain patients into trigeminal neuralgic ($N=32$) and nonneuralgic ($N=28$) groups. Patients with postherpetic pain were excluded from the study. Levels of neuroticism and extraversion were similar in the two groups, but there was some variation in IBQ measures. Patients with trigeminal neuralgia obtained higher scores on Scale 6 (Denial of life problems) and lower scores on Scale 7 (Irritability). A final diagnostic subgroup that should not be ignored is whether chronic pain is associated with a life-threatening medical condition or not. The most familiar example of the importance of this variable is probably in cancer, where the patient's psychological functioning is threatened both by pain and impending death. Kremer, Atkinson, and Ignelzi (1982) identified cancer patients who scored either very high or very low on the affective dimension of the MPQ. They found no differences between these patients, however, on measures of somaticisation, depression, anxiety, and hostility. This was in contrast to an earlier study (Kremer & Atkinson, 1981) in which patients with chronic benign pain had been divided in the same way, and corresponding differences on other psychological measures were demonstrated. The authors interpreted the apparent lack of consistency in cancer patients as stemming from the meaning of their pain, in contrast to the nonfatal symptoms of the patients with benign pain.

This concludes discussion of the clinical characteristics of chronic pain. Several groups of variables listed in Table 9.1 have been reviewed, some in more detail than others. There is a reasonable volume of literature on sensory and affective qualities of pain, and on spatial and temporal differences in how it is experienced. Little information is available on the effect of associated symptoms or irreversible physical changes. Many studies have been done on the organic vs. nonorganic distinction in chronic pain, but other diagnostic subgroups of patients with pain in the same body region have not been widely investigated. The implications of the clinical characteristics of chronic pain for patient adjustment are still not well understood.

DISRUPTION TO DAILY LIVING TASKS

There are various medical, social, and psychological factors that lead to disability in chronic pain patients. In some of the studies already cited in this review, mention has been made of the fact that limitations in activity are not simply a function of pain severity or the presence of physical findings (Fordyce et al., 1978; Brena et al., 1979). Environmental and learning influences are also at work which, when modified, can result in drastic improvement in performance (Fordyce, 1976). However, whatever the conditions under which disability arises or wanes, it is important to see such changes as more than dependent variables in the chronic pain equation. Disability-related measures provide some assessment of the individual's quality of life. Limitations and changes in activities are sources of stress in their own right, and have an impact on the chronic pain patient over and above that exerted by the pain itself.

The changes in function and performance that accompany chronic pain can vary from major life events to minor alterations of routine. It is assumed here that both types of change can be stressful. The effect of significant life events on physical and mental health has been widely documented (Rahe & Arthur, 1978). More recently, the role of minor life events ("hassles") in contributing to psychological disturbance has also been confirmed (Kanner et al., 1981). Table 9.1 lists 10 areas of daily living that often change in the context of chronic pain. Before attempting to examine the affective, behavioral, and cognitive consequences of such disruptions, we will look more closely at the known incidence of these changes.

Holmes and Rahe (1967) originally developed the Social Readjustment Rating Scale as a means of measuring life events before physical illness or psychological disorder. Few studies have used this instrument or its variants to assess the aftermath of ill health. Caplan, Gibson, and Weiss (1984) assessed recent life change in a group of 50 individuals who had undergone rehabilitation mainly for spinal cord injury or stroke. During the first six months of illness, changes in the following areas were most frequently experienced: recreation (reported by 92% of subjects), personal habits (84%), social activities (82%), financial status (72%), sleeping (72%), and eating habits (58%). Life events in the 6-month period preceding illness were also measured. It was found that subjects experienced an average of 3.3 events before illness compared to 11.8 events after illness. When these events were weighted and summed, subjects had a mean "life change unit" (LCU) score of 75 before illness compared to 259 after illness. One-third of the sample had LCU scores above 300, a level which was equivalent to the onset of major life crisis if accumulated within a 12-month period.

Levenson, Hirschfeld, and Hirschfeld (1980) undertook a similar assessment of life events in 164 patients who had been injured in industrial accidents. All subjects were being evaluated for complaints of pain combined with other physical symptoms, and 85 percent had injuries of the lower back. Two-thirds of the sample had had their accidents more than 12 months beforehand. Life events were measured four years preinjury and up to two years postinjury. In the first 12-month period after injury, patients in Levenson et al.'s study experienced a mean frequency of 12.5 life events and had an average LCU score of 249. In their second year post-injury, 9.6 life events occurred with a mean LCU score of 291. The nature of life event changes before and after each patient's accident was also analyzed. Changes in the following areas were reported significantly more often postinjury: eating, sleeping, personal habits, recreation, being fired or laid off work, social activities, decreased income, credit card difficulties, sexual difficulties, and arguments with spouse. Feuerstein, Sult, and Houle (1985) investigated environmental stressors in a small group of patients with chronic back pain who were currently employed. None were grossly disabled or psychologically disturbed. Their mean LCU score was found to be significantly higher than that demonstrated in a matched group of healthy controls. However, pain intensity was not related to the total number of life events reported in either group.

The results of these studies are important for several reasons. First, they demonstrate in a quantitative fashion the amount of change and readjustment that may be inherent in serious (or not-so-serious illness). A substantial proportion of subjects in these studies had LCU scores that were beyond the major life crisis threshold. The second point is that the changes most frequently reported were not always drastic events but involved relatively routine activities such as sleeping, eating, recreation, and socialization. Third, the incidence of reactive life events appears to be only loosely linked to pain severity itself. To what extent disruption of daily living occurs in traditional chronic pain populations—and with what consequences—is considered next.

Pelz and Merskey (1982) assessed 83 patients with chronic pain on a number of psychological measures. The average duration of pain for the group was just over three years, and a significant degree of disturbance was reported by patients in the areas of work, sleep, sport, exercise, leisure, social activities, and sexual relationships. A more detailed analysis of the effects of chronic pain on day-to-day functioning was carried out by Deyo, Inui, Leininger, and Overman (1982) with rheumatoid arthritis sufferers. Seventy-nine patients with a mean pain duration of 12 years completed the Sickness Impact Profile (SIP). This comprehensive instrument contains 136 items covering 12 different activities of living. It was found that nearly half or more patients in the sample recorded problems with walking, self-care, work, leisure, social activities, sexual behavior, and sleeping.

Pilowsky and Bassett (1982) compared patients attending a pain clinic with patients hospitalized for depression on a range of measures, including the SIP. About one-half of the pain sample considered that their general activity level was in need of improvement. The same need was affirmed in less than one-quarter of the depressed group. The SIP scores of the pain patients were significantly higher than those of the depressed patients in the areas of body care and ambulation. Scores on work disruption were not reported by the authors. The pain group was significantly less disabled, however, in the categories of home management, emotional behavior, social interaction, alertness, and communication. These results can be informally compared with the SIP profile obtained by Deyo et al. (1982) for rheumatoid arthritis patients. The highest mean dysfunction scores for pain clinic patients, followed by each corresponding score for the arthritis sample, are as follows: social interaction (27.3 vs 11.7), body care and movement (32.7 vs 12.7), home management (23.0 vs 26.3), alertness (21.2 vs 13.0), and emotional behavior (21.0 vs 13.2). It appears that the pain clinic patients studied by Pilowsky and Bassett experienced greater disruption in most areas. Follick, Smith, and Ahern (1985) also compared the SIP results of 107 patients with chronic low back pain to those obtained by Deyo et al. (1982) for rheumatoid arthritis sufferers. Back pain patients reported disruption scores of greater than 20 percent in almost all categories, with the exception of body care, communication, and eating. In contrast, arthritis patients acknowledged equivalent scores in only three areas, namely ambulation, work, and home management.

In a later study with a different group of pain clinic patients, Pilowsky, Crettenden, and Townley (1985) examined how good ($N = 28$) and poor sleepers ($N = 72$) varied on SIP, IBQ, physiological and psychological measures. Poor sleepers reported significantly greater difficulties in the areas of emotional behavior, body care, home management, social interaction, ambulation, and recreation. Additionally, on the IBQ they reported higher scores on Scales 1 (General hypochondriasis), 2 (Disease conviction), and 5 (Affective disturbance). No physiological differences were recorded, and other psychological measures confirmed the greater anxiety and depression of the poor sleep group. However, when sleep status was regressed on a range of SIP, IBQ, and affective scores, only pain intensity and degree of depression were significantly associated with sleep disturbance.

A large group of patients with back pain were evaluated by Main and Waddell (1982). Ratings of disability were found to be positively correlated with neuroticism, depression, and Scale 2 (Disease conviction) of the IBQ. Disability was negatively correlated with Scale 3 of the IBQ, such that greater dysfunction was associated with a more physical view of symptoms. Naliboff, Cohen, Swanson, Bonebakker, and McArthur (1982) investigated the MMPI profiles of back pain patients, migraine patients, and patients with diabetes or hypertension. Some differences were observed, but generally it was found that MMPI scores were more strongly related to self-rated functional limitation than to group membership, age, or pain duration. On the Hypochondriasis, Depression, and Hysteria scales, level of disability accounted for 31 percent, 20 percent, and 30 percent respectively of the variance for all patients. The authors concluded that MMPI elevations in chronic illness, regardless of whether pain occurs or not, are closely tied to the limitations in activity reported by patients.

In a later study, Naliboff et al. (1985) compared patients with chronic low back pain ($N = 68$) to a sample of age-matched, pain-free control subjects ($N = 35$) on a range of disability and psychological measures. They found that back pain patients reported significantly greater disruption in the areas of social activity, time spent at work, and time spent sleeping. Within the back pain group, it was found that psychological dysfunction was much more closely related to physical limitation than to pain severity. The authors noted that while pain intensity and duration were frequently used in clinical practice to quantify chronic pain disorder, these measures did not closely reflect its associated psychological and physical changes. In particular, they concluded that activity disturbance was an important and complex area of disability that required sensitive measurement on a number of dimensions.

Three groups of subjects with pain complaints were assessed by Skevington (1983a). The organic group had active rheumatoid disease for which they received regular outpatient treatment. The nonorganic group also attended for treatment for treatment but had no identifiable pathology. The nonpatient group had pain without detectable pathology but no longer sought regular outpatient treatment. Relative to a healthy control group, organic patients carried out less recreational activities, while both the nonorganic and the nonpatient subjects reported more passive activities. Sleep disturbance was significantly greater in nonorganic patients compared to organic patients. Limitation of activity was examined in relation to IBQ scores and mood disturbance for each group of subjects. In the organic sample, sleeping difficulties were significantly correlated with lower scores on Scale 2 (Disease conviction), 5 (Affective disturbance), and 7 (Irritability) of the IBQ, with less aggression, and with more skepticism. For this group, a high frequency of passive activities was also associated with lower levels of elation. Nonorganic patients reported that sleep disturbance was positively correlated with disease conviction and with sad mood. Passive activities were associated with higher levels of elation. For the nonpatient group, sleeping difficulties were indicative of more aggression, while infrequent reporting of recreational activities was related to greater surgery and social affection. In this study, the nature of the relationship between self-reported limitation and psychological measures seemed quite specific to each group of subjects.

Lipton and Marbach (1983) derived two factors of pain response—emotionality and interference—in facial pain patients. The second dimension accounted for 13 percent of the variance in their factor analysis and dealt with the effect of pain on work, socialization, and enjoyment. The authors found that scores on this factor were related to the severity of pain but not to its duration. Neither treatment history nor sociomedical orientation was associated with degree of interference, although some relationship with level of psychological distress was found. The strength of the relationship between interference and distress was dependent upon diagnostic factors. For patients with organic diagnosis there was no significant association, while for patients with nonorganic diagnosis there was a low but significant correlation. The highest correlation between degree of interference in daily functioning and level of psychological distress occurred in the mixed group where over 80 percent of the variance was shared. Again, these results suggest that the psychological effects of limitation in daily living activities are difficult to generalize across patient groups. Indeed, Carron, DeGood, and Tait (1985) have noted that even within the same diagnostic samples, there can be significant variation. They compared patients with chronic back pain from the United States and New Zealand, and found that patients from New Zealand reported less disruption to their daily routine and fewer dysphoric symptoms.

To conclude this section, it is worth repeating that the operant approach to chronic pain management focuses very much on modifying disability rather than pain. As Fordyce (1976) himself has stated: "When a patient is helped to do more while requiring less ongoing treatment and those effects seem destined to persist to the lasting benefit of the patient, it is for others to worry, if they so desire, about whether the patient has undergone any beneficial change in pain." While the efficacy of this type of treatment is well documented (Turner & Chapman, 1982), there are few studies that compare the relative effects of behavioral intervention in different activities of daily living. Catchlove and Cohen (1982) evaluated the treatment outcomes of worker's compensation patients who received multimodal therapy for chronic pain. For one group, returning to work was presented as a necessary part of treatment; for a second group, work was regarded as a result of the program. It was found that 60 percent of patients in the first group returned to work during treatment and that 90 percent of these were still working at follow-up. In contrast, only 25 percent of patients in the second group returned to work during treatment, and 75 percent of these remained at follow-up. The study demonstrates the importance of the active restoration of work activity, a finding consistent with Feuerstein et al.'s (1985) observation that among employed patients with back pain, work pressure negatively correlated with depression. The relative contribution to well-being of other discrete areas of living for chronic pain patients requires further investigation.

SYSTEMS INVOLVEMENT

Not all of the life-event changes that accompany chronic pain are minor. While many of the smaller changes are indeed disruptions to existing work and domestic routines that can be slowly readjusted to, there are other types of changes that are often entirely new and more threatening. These life events are tied to involvement in the treatment and service systems upon which patients with chronic pain can easily become dependent. Receiving conflicting diagnoses, waiting for appointments, not understanding treatment rationales, applying for unemployment or sickness benefits, requiring legal advice, going to court, having weekly compensation payments terminated, being unable to pay bills, mortgages or other debts, undergoing rehabilitation, trying to establish alternative work options—these are all examples of unfamiliar changes that can befall chronic pain patients. Thus not only do patients lose established activities, but they often become enmeshed in substitute routines which deplete them of time and energy and impinge negatively on their self-image and role performance. The effect of these changes, summarized in Table 9.1, must also be considered in understanding how patients react to chronic pain.

Most patients involved in medical, paramedical, or rehabilitation treatment have, of course, received previous therapy. Marbach and Lipton (1978) observed that almost half their sample of patients with facial pain had seen three or more doctors. Headache patients investigated by Packard (1979) had seen four doctors or more in about one-third of cases. Pain clinic patients using addictive medications were found by Turner et al. (1982) to have undergone an average of two pain-related surgeries and seven pain-related hospitalizations. Pelz and Merskey (1982) reported that their pain clinic population had a mean rate of 0.9 pain-related operations. Interestingly, some 18 percent of patients felt that previous surgery (not necessarily pain-related) had caused or increased their pain. The effects of inappropriate lumbar spine surgery for patients presenting with back pain have been studied by Fager and Freidberg (1980), who noted a high incidence of iatrogenic symptoms. In reviewing the management of facial pain patients, Marbach et al. (1983) pointed out that most medical consultations resulted in either no treatment or further referral. Where treatment was attempted it had a high failure rate. The authors considered that such experiences must contribute to the distress of the chronic pain patient and result in illness behavior that is more emotional and expressive. Rook et al. (1981) found no clear pattern between the number of surgeries reported by chronic pain patients and their MMPI profiles, but did observe some elevation in profiles corresponding to increases in number of hospitalizations and number of physicians seen.

Certainly there is evidence to suggest that the illness behavior of patients with chronic pain is often abnormal (Pilowsky, 1978). Whether this is the product of continuous treatment failure or, on the other hand, the very basis of intractibility can be hard to judge. Probably it is both. Dissatisfaction about previous treatment often occurs in the context of a personal belief system that sees illness as a purely somatic process in which complete pain relief should be possible. Such attitudes have many corollaries. Thomas and Lyttle (1980) found that back pain patients attending a hospital orthopaedic clinic initially had very high expectations for treatment efficacy. Approximately two-thirds of the patients with facial pain evaluated by Marbach and Lipton (1978) were demanding of doctors yet skeptical of their ability. They also were relatively ignorant about health matters, dependent when ill, and prepared to "shop around" for health care. Levenson et al. (1980) noted that most of their sample of industrially injured patients saw themselves as having only physical problems and were very sensitive to any implication that they had a psychological or stress-related disorder. Headache patients studied by Barnat and Lake (1983) were similarly reluctant to accept that emotional problems were the main cause of their condition. Finally, the MMPI profiles of chronic pain patients are frequently characterized by elevations in Hypochondriasis, Depression, and Hysteria in a manner consistent with somatization or conversion reaction (Sternbach, 1974). Against this background, it can be seen that many chronic pain patients find medical, paramedical, and rehabilitation treatments to be frustrating and confusing.

Fitzpatrick and Hopkins (1981) interviewed headache patients about their satisfaction with initial neurological consultation. About 8 percent of the sample were dissatisfied with the doctor's medical actions, for example, expressing critical views for not having received appropriate tests or physical examination. About 11 percent were dissatisfied with communication from the doctor, while a further 17 percent were dissatisfied with both medical actions and communication. Thus over a quarter of the sample were unhappy about the information outcome of the consultation, generally criticizing the lack of expansion upon the diagnosis offered or the absence of discussion about aetiology and prognosis. The authors found that two groups of patients were more likely to be dissatisfied with the doctor's communication: Those who had fixed ideas about how their symptoms should be diagnosed, and those who were worried about the possibility of serious illness. These attitudes are not unlike those described in pain clinic patients, some of whom have high levels of disease conviction or hypochondriasis (Pilowsky & Spence, 1976a).

The treatment expectations of patients with headache were compared by Packard (1979) with those of their physicians. About two-thirds of the physicians thought the patients were primarily seeking pain relief, but only one-third of patients endorsed pain relief as the prime reason for medical consultation. Patients were more interested in receiving an explanation of their symptoms, and receiving reassurance from the doctor. Marbach and Lipton (1978) have commented upon the importance of understanding the motives of patients with chronic facial pain who seek treatment, such that their somatic view of symptoms is not inadvertently reinforced by the provision of only physical therapies.

The difficulties that may be encountered by chronic pain patients in interacting with various treatment systems are not helped by the fact that many may feel uncomfortable in asserting themselves. Pilowsky and Spence (1976d) found that more than one-half of a sample of pain clinic patients reported that they characteristically bottled up angry feelings rather than expressing them. This tendency can be seen to have important implications for their medical management. As Sternbach (1978) has noted:

> In his patienthood, the person with pain is involved in a struggle for power which is primarily a vertical relationship. The middle-class patient can usually negotiate a treatment contract with the physician on a horizontal basis, as a social peer, for the physician is usually also of the middle class. The working class patient, however, is likely to perceive himself as having to deal with an authority-figure—and resents it.

This view may help to explain Rook et al.'s (1981) observation that the scores of chronic pain patients on the MMPI scales of Hypochondriasis, Depression, and Hysteria were negatively related to their years of schooling.

Such problems in the doctor–patient relationship are not, however, entirely attributable to social or educational factors (Larson & Marcer, 1984). Other difficulties may emerge from what Singh, Nunn, Martin, and Yates (1981) have referred to as "abnormal treatment behavior" on the part of the doctor. This may occur for a variety of reasons, both conscious and unconscious, and result in patterns of diagnosis, investigation, referral, and prescription that are inappropriate. The inherent difficulties of maintaining a flexible "biopsychosocial model" of medical practice have been identified by Beitman, Williamson, Featherstone and Katon (1982). Such problems apply to all clinicians involved in the management of chronic pain, where there is a particular need to integrate somatic, psychological, and sometimes family factors in treatment.

Skevington (1983c) has emphasized how professionals may readily embrace fixed beliefs about chronic pain and the patients who experience it. The influence of such assumptions on patient management was observed by Pilowsky and Bond (1969) in a hospital radiotherapy ward. Whether the provision of medication was initiated by staff or patients, and the strength of analgesia given, in part depended upon the age and sex of the patient. The general issue of under what conditions patients are seen by clinicians to "deserve" care and attention has been explored by Pilowsky (1977) in his discussion of altruistic behavior in doctors, with the recognition that the impulse to help others is often accompanied by some ambivalence towards the recipients of such help. In the case of chronic pain, there is a particular need for clinicians to acknowledge and monitor their own feelings of distress and frustration that patients may engender.

A note of caution is appropriate here. While it is true that for many patients with chronic pain, their treatment experiences can be negative and stressful for the reasons discussed above, it would be inaccurate to imply that this is inevitably the case. We know most about those patients who are referred for multidisciplinary pain clinic evaluation. But the characteristics of pain clinic patients, and their particular treatment histories, may well not be representative of the greater population of chronic pain sufferers. Chapman, Sola, and Bonica (1979) compared the IBQ profiles of pain clinic patients with those of patients with persistent pain who were managed in private practice. Pain clinic patients showed high disease conviction, low psychological view of illness, moderately high affective disturbance, and high denial—a familiar pattern reported by other pain clinics (Pilowsky, Murrell, & Gordon, 1979). However, the profile of patients managed privately was significantly different on several dimensions of illness behavior. Private patients displayed less disease conviction, a more psychological perception of illness, less depression, and also less hypochondriasis. The authors concluded that care must be taken not to stereotype patients with chronic pain, and that the setting in which they are seen must always be taken into account.

Perhaps the most difficult treatment context, for both patient and doctor is that set against the backdrop of compensation and litigation (Goldney, 1984). Mutual stereotyping can easily develop under such conditions, with distrust and anger prevailing on both sides (Rubinstein, 1982; Pilowsky, 1985). For patients with chronic pain, the inherent difficulties of the treatment process are often aggravated by their involvement in compensation or legal proceedings. More symptoms, increased complaints, unrealistic attitudes, and inflexible behaviors may be readily demonstrated by patients under these circumstances. To dismiss these reactions as manifestations of "compensation neurosis" would be grossly simplistic. It has already been suggested in this discussion that even without the prospect of legal involvement, the chronic pain patient may be ill-equipped to cope with orthodox treatment systems. Lloyd and Stagoll (1979) use the term "accident victim syndrome" to describe the physical and psychological symptoms of the industrially injured worker who fails to recover. They emphasize that while legal involvement can be seen to worsen the prospects of rehabilitation, the illness career of the patient is by this stage already under way due to previous medical management and family reactions.

Compensation and litigation are thus important variables in the responses of patients to chronic pain, but they are by no means the only sources of distress and abnormal illness behavior. Pelz and Merskey (1982) compared pain clinic patients receiving compensation with those who were not. The only difference between the groups in terms of psychological functioning was a significantly higher somatization score for the compensation patients. The authors concluded that the view that compensation patients are specifically different from others with pain must be qualified.

Similar findings were reported by Mendelson (1984) when he compared patients with compensable (workers compensation or motor vehicle accident) and noncompensable back pain. No differences in degree of psychological disturbance were evident in measures of anxiety, depression, hostility, and neuroticism. In a comparable study, Melzack, Katz, and Jeans (1985) found that compensation status did not influence the scores of pain clinic patients on the MMPI scales of Depression, Hypochondriasis, and Hysteria.

Some variation in patterns of overt pain behavior displayed by back pain patients receiving disability or compensation payments has been reported (Keefe et al., 1984), including aspects of gait (Keefe & Hill, 1985). However, the former study found that compensation status did not maintain its significance under regression analysis. Carron et al. (1985) examined differences in the presentation of back pain patients on the basis of both compensation and the country (United States and New Zealand) in which such payment occurred. Patients were compared on 20 posttreatment items. Some significant differences were found between patients receiving and not receiving compensation, but these were not consistent across countries, with the exception of activity level. In both countries, compensation patients were at least twice as likely than no-compensation patients to report resuming less than full activity. In the United States, but not in New Zealand, compensation patients were significantly less likely to return to employment.

This raises the longstanding issue of to what degree compensation patients eventually recover and return to work once their claims are finalized. Mendelson (1982) reviewed the research literature on the outcome of such patients with a range of injuries and found that their prognosis often remained poor, even after settlement. Dworkin, Handlin, Richlin, Brand, and Vanucci (1985) concluded that involvement in the process of compensation or litigation per se was not necessarily deleterious to treatment response and activity resumption in pain clinic patients, but that unemployment was associated with poor prognosis. This suggests that the harmful effects often attributed to compensation and litigation may be more productively examined in terms of their propensity to interfere with the routine of working. The notion that financial gain is the sole motive of patients involved in compensation or litigation fails to do justice to the complex interaction of physical, psychological, and social changes that so often accompany the experience of chronic pain.

OTHER ISSUES

Before concluding the present chapter, it is necessary to comment briefly on some general issues that are often implicit in studies of psychological responses to chronic pain. These include the question as to whether the effects of pain are really any different to those of any other chronic illness; the difficulty of assessing the patient's premorbid state in order to gauge the impact of pain and the degree of possible secondary gain; and finally, the important of differentiating psychological syndromes of chronic pain.

The MMPI profiles of a large sample of chronic pain patients were compared to those of general medical patients by Swanson, Maruta, and Swenson (1979). Significant differences were found on most clinical scales. These results were similar to those reported by Sternbach et al. (1980) using the same normative data to evaluate the MMPI profiles of patients with chronic headache. Naliboff, Cohen, and Yellen (1982) also found that patients with chronic low back pain showed a mean MMPI profile that was more disturbed than that of patients with hypertension and diabetes. However, using regression analysis the latter investigators demonstrated that a substantial amount of the variation in MMPI scores between back pain patients and those with other chronic illness could be predicted by the degree of functional limitation reported by patients. They concluded that pain patients do not show any unique type of emotional disturbance other than that related to disruption of daily living activities.

The second issue concerns the premorbid psychological characteristics of persons with chronic pain, and the role of such factors in the aetiology of pain symptoms. A number of studies report findings related to this area of enquiry. Merskey and Boyd (1978) assessed the current and premorbid status of pain patients both with and without organic diagnoses, and concluded that a significant proportion of the emotional disturbance associated with chronic pain was a secondary effect. A similar view was expressed by Watson (1982), following detailed item analyses of the MMPI profiles reported by patients from several pain treatment centres.

Contrary evidence occurs when formal DSM-III psychiatric criteria are used to assess chronic pain patients. Reich, Tupin, and Abramowitz (1983) found that 20 out of 43 pain clinic patients had an Axis II (personality disorder) diagnosis. A higher proportion was reported by Fishbain, Goldberg, Meagher, Steele, and Rosomoff (1986) using the same criteria, such that 166 out of 281 pain clinic patients showed personality disorder. In a similar vein, Levenson et al. (1980) and Levenson, Hirschfield, Hirschfield, and Dzubay (1983) investigated the frequency of life events in patients with pain associated with industrial accidents, and found that there had been above average levels of change in the two years preceding injury.

Another approach to the relationship between pain and distress has been to evaluate the psychological consequences of pain relief in patients undergoing successful surgical treatment. Bond (1973) reported no significant mean variation on measures of neuroticism and extraversion following cordotomy for women with advanced cancer of the cervix. On the other hand, neurosurgical procedures were observed by Sternbach and Timmermans (1975) to result in reductions in the MMPI scales of Hysteria and Hypomania that were significantly greater than those reported by pain patients who received rehabilitation treatment that did not include surgery.

It would seem most reasonable to accept that there are significant psychological consequences to chronic pain, but to also consider that in a marked proportion of patients seen in pain clinics, there would appear to be psychological causal factors. This leads on to the final issue of how best to differentiate between the major subgroups that apparently exist within the chronic pain population. Sternbach (1974) aroused interest in such a task by distinguishing patient "types" that seemed identifiable in terms of both their MMPI responses and their clinical presentation. The degree and consistency of heterogeneity in chronic pain populations was formally investigated by Bradley, Prokop, Margolis, and Gentry (1978). The MMPI profiles of several hundred patients with back pain were subjected to cluster analysis. Replicable subgroupings were found for three profiles across both sexes, with a fourth profile identified only for female patients. Notably only the latter subgroup corresponded to the well known "Conversion V" pattern on the MMPI.

These subgroupings appear to be relatively stable, and have been essentially replicated in other samples of back pain patients (McGill, Lawlis, Selby, Mooney, & McCoy, 1983; McCreary, 1985) and general pain clinic patients (Armentrout, Moore, Parker, Hewett, & Feltz,

1982; Hart, 1984; Atkinson, Ingram, Kremar, & Saccuzzo, 1986). Some of these studies have successfully linked subgroup membership to other patient characteristics, and to response to treatment.

CONCLUSIONS

This chapter constitutes a selective review of some of the most common psychological responses to chronic pain. Studies have been examined in terms of the conceptual framework represented in Table 9.1, distinguishing between sources, mediators, and manifestations of pain-related stress. Most attention has been focused on the various clinical characteristics of pain and their relationship to affective, behavioral, and cognitive measures. It is evident, however, that both investigators and clinicians interested in psychosocial aspects of chronic pain are increasingly broadening the scope of their assessments to include factors such as disruption to daily living activities and iatrogenic treatment and welfare effects.

This has been paralleled by commensurate attention to the role of mediating variables in the chronic pain experience. It has not been possible in the present chapter to examine the literature pertinent to this area, although examples of studies that might be potentially analyzed within the framework offered in Table 9.1 can be readily cited. Thus Rosenstiel and Keefe (1983) and Turner and Clancy (1986) have employed the Coping Strategy Questionnaire to measure the cognitive and behavioral methods reported by patients with low back pain, and have attempted to relate such strategies to affective and behavioral indices of longer term adjustment. While coping responses can be conceptualized as some of the things that people actually *do* in the face of stress, psychological resources represent some of the things that people *are* (Pearlin & Schooler, 1978). Locus of control is an example of such a variable included in Table 9.1 as mediating the response to chronic pain. Its role has been investigated in a number of studies, including those of McCreary, Turner, and Dawson (1980) and Skevington (1983b).

Social support is the final set of mediating factors referred to in Table 9.1. The influence of the patient's immediate family in promoting or inhibiting adaptation is being more frequently investigated. There is a growing body of literature that provides information about the marital satisfaction of pain patients and their spouses, the level of psychological distress reported by spouses, and the role of the spouse in eliciting pain behavior (Mohamed, Weisz, & Waring, 1978; Shanfield, Heiman, Cope, & Jones, 1979, Swanson & Maruta, 1980; Block, Kremer, & Gaylor, 1980; Moore, Berk, & Nypaver, 1984; Ahern, Adams, & Follick, 1985; Rowat & Knafl, 1985; Feuerstein et al., 1985). These findings suggest that individual differences between the families of pain clinic patients in their reactions to illness should not be overlooked.

It is hoped that consideration of the various sources and mediators of pain-related stress outlined in Table 9.1 will assist clinicians and investigators in the formulation of treatment and research strategies. In this way the psychological responses of the chronic pain sufferer can be more clearly identified, better understood, and more effectively managed.

REFERENCES

Ahern, D., Adams, A., & Follick, M. (1985). Emotional and marital disturbance in spouses of chronic low back pain patients. *Clinical Journal of Pain, 1,* 69–74.

Ahles, T., Yunus, M., Gaulier, B., Riley, S., & Masi, A. (1986). The use of contemporary MMPI norms in the study of chronic pain patients. *Pain, 24,* 159–163.

Andrews, G., Tennant, C., Hewson, D., & Vaillant, G. (1978). Life event stress, social support, coping style, and risk of psychological impairment. *Journal of Nervous and Mental Disease, 116,* 307–316.

Armentrout, D. (1979). The impact of chronic pain on the self-concept. *Journal of Clinical Psychology, 35,* 517–521.

Armentrout, D., Moore, J., Parker, J., Hewett, J., & Feltz, C. (1982). Pain patient MMPI subgroups: The psychological dimensions of pain. *Journal of Behavioural Medicine, 5,* 201–211.

Atkinson, J., Ingram, R., Kremer, E., & Saccuzzo, D. (1986). MMPI subgroups and affective disorder in chronic pain patients. *Journal of Nervous and Mental Disease, 174,* 408–413.

Barnat, M., & Lake, A. (1983). Patient attitudes about headache. *Headache, 23,* 229–237.

Beitman, B., Williamson, P., Featherstone, H., & Katon, W. (1982). Reluctance to physician use of the biopsychosocial model. *General Hospital Psychiatry, 4,* 81–83.

Billings, A., & Moos, R. (1981). The role of coping responses and social resources in attenuating the stress of life events. *Journal of Behavioural Medicine, 4,* 139–157.

Block, A., Kremer, E., & Gaylor, M. (1980). Behavioural treatment for chronic pain: The spouse as a discriminative cue for pain behaviour. *Pain, 9,* 243–252.

Bond, M. (1973). Personality studies in patients with pain secondary to organic disease. *Journal of Psychosomatic Research, 17,* 257–263.

Bradley, L., Prokop, C., Margolis, R., & Gentry, W. (1978). Multivariate analyses of the MMPI profiles of low back pain patients. *Journal of Behavioural Medicine, 1,* 253–272.

Brena, S., Chapman, S., Stegall, P., & Chyatte, S. (1979). Chronic pain states: Their relationship to impairment and disability. *Archives of Physical Medicine and Rehabilitation, 60,* 387–389.

Brown, G., & Harris, T. (1978). *Social origins of depression.* New York: The Free Press.

Burckhardt, C. (1984). The use of the McGill Pain Questionnaire in assessing arthritis pain. *Pain, 19,* 305–314.

Byrne, M., Troy, A., Bradley, L., Marchisello, P., Geisinger, K., Van der Heide, L., & Prieto, E. (1982). Cross validation of the factor structure of the McGill Pain Questionnaire. *Pain, 13,* 193–201.

Caplan, B., Gibson, C., & Weiss, R. (1984). Stressful sequelae of disabling illness. *International Rehabilitation Medicine, 6,* 58–62.

Carron, H., DeGood, D., & Tait, R. (1985). A comparison of low back pain patients in the United States and New Zealand: Psychosocial and economic factors affecting severity of disability. *Pain, 21,* 77–89.

Catchlove, R., & Cohen, K. (1982). Effects of a directive return to work approach in the treatment of workman's compensation patients with chronic pain. *Pain, 14,* 181–191.

Chapman, C., Sola, A., & Bonica, J. (1979). Illness behaviour and depression compared in pain centre and private practice patients. *Pain, 6,* 1–7.

Cinciripini, P., & Floreen, A. (1983). An assessment of chronic pain behaviour in a structured interview. *Journal of Psychosomatic Research, 27,* 117–123.

Clarke, P., & Spear, F. (1964). Reliability and sensitivity in the self-assessment of well-being. *Bulletin of the British Psychological Society, 17,* 55.

Comrey, A. (1957). A factor analysis of items on the MMPI hypochondriasis scale. *Educational and Psychological Measurement, 17,* 568–577.

Cox, G., Chapman, C., & Black, R. (1978). The MMPI and chronic pain: The diagnosis of psychogenic pain. *Journal of Behavioral Medicine, 1,* 437–443.

Crown, S., & Crisp, A. (1966). A short clinical diagnostic self-rating scale for psychoneurotic patients. *British Journal of Psychiatry, 112,* 917–923.

Demjen, S., & Bakal, D. (1981). Illness behaviour and chronic headache. *Pain, 10,* 221–230.

De Rogatis, L., Rickels, K., & Rock, A. (1976). The SCL-90 and the MMPI: A step in the validation of a new self-report scale. *British Journal of Psychiatry, 128,* 280–289.

Deyo, R., Inui, T., Leininger, J., & Overman, S. (1982). Physical and psychosocial function in rheumatoid arthritis. *Archives of Internal Medicine, 142,* 879–882.

Dworkin, R., Handlin, D., Richlin, D., Brand, L., & Vannucci, C. (1985). Unraveling the effects of compensation, litigation, and employment on treatment response in chronic pain. *Pain, 23,* 49–59.

Eysenck, H., & Eysenck, S. (1976). *Manual of the Eysenck Personality Questionnaire.* London: Hodder and Stoughton.
Fager, C., & Freidberg, S. (1980). Analysis of failures and poor results of lumbar spine surgery. *Spine, 5,* 87–94.
Feuerstein, M., Sult, S., & Houle, M. (1985). Environmental stressors and chronic low back pain: Life events, family and work environment. *Pain, 22,* 295–307.
Fishbain, D., Goldberg, M., Meagher, B., Steele, K., & Rosomoff, H. (1986). Male and female chronic pain patients categorized by DSM-III psychiatric diagnostic criteria. *Pain, 26,* 181–197.
Fitzpatrick, R., & Hopkins, A. (1981). Patients' satisfaction with communication in neurological outpatient clinics. *Journal of Psychosomatic Research, 25,* 329–334.
Folkman, S., & Lazarus, R. (1980). An analysis of coping in a middle-aged community sample. *Journal of Health and Social Behaviour, 21,* 219–239.
Follick, M., Smith, T., & Ahern, D. (1985). The Sickness Impact Profile: A global measure of disability in chronic low back pain. *Pain, 21,* 67–76.
Fordyce, W. (1976). *Behavioural methods for chronic pain and illness.* St. Louis, MO: C. V. Mosby.
Fordyce, W., Brena, S., Holcombe, R., De Lateur, B., & Loeser, J. (1978). Relationship of patient semantic pain descriptions to physician diagnostic judgements, activity level measures and MMPI. *Pain, 5,* 293–303.
Fordyce, W., Lansky, D., Calsyn, D., Shelton, J., Stolov, W., & Rock, D. (1984). Pain measurement and pain behaviour. *Pain, 18,* 53–69.
Foulds, G., Caine, T., & Creasy, M. (1960). Aspects of extra- and intro-punitive expression in mental illness. *Journal of Mental Science, 106,* 599–610.
Freeman, C., Calsyn, D., & Louks, J. (1976). The use of the Minnesota Multiphasic Personality Inventory with low back pain patients. *Journal of Clinical Psychology, 32,* 294–298.
Garron, D., & Leavitt, F. (1983). Chronic low back pain and depression. *Journal of Clinical Psychology, 39,* 486–493.
Goldberg, D., & Hillier, V. (1979). A scaled version of the General Health Questionnaire. *Psychological Medicine, 9,* 139–145.
Goldney, R. (1984). Elucidation of psychological factors in compensable injury. *Medical Journal of Australia, 141,* 433–436.
Gordon, A., & Hitchcock, E. (1983). Illness behaviour and personality in intractable facial pain syndromes. *Pain, 17,* 267–276.
Haley, W., Turner, J., & Romano, J. (1985). Depression in chronic pain patients: Relation to pain, activity, and sex differences. *Pain, 23,* 337–343.
Hall, W., Hayward, L., & Chapman, C. (1981). On "The lateralization of pain." *Pain, 10,* 337–351.
Hanvik, L. (1951). MMPI profiles in patients with low back pain. *Journal of Consulting Psychology, 15,* 350–353.
Hart, R. (1984). Chronic pain: Replicated multivariate clustering of personality profiles. *Journal of Clinical Psychology, 40,* 129–133.
Holmes, T., & Rahe, R. (1967). The social readjustment rating scale. *Journal of Psychosomatic Research, 11,* 213–218.

Hunter, M. (1983). The Headache Scale: A new approach to the assessment of headache pain based on pain descriptions. *Pain, 16,* 361–373.

Hunter, M., & Philips, C. (1981). The experience of headache: An assessment of the qualities of tension headache pain. *Pain, 10,* 209–219.

Kanner, A., Coyne, J., Schaefer, C., & Lazarus, R. (1981). Comparison of two modes of stress measurement: Daily hassles and uplifts versus major life events. *Journal of Behavioural Medicine, 4,* 1–39.

Keefe, F., & Block, F. (1982). Development of an observation method for assessing pain behaviour in chronic low back pain patients. *Behaviour Therapy, 13,* 363–375.

Keefe, F., & Hill, R. (1985). An objective approach to quantifying pain behaviour and gait patterns in low back pain patients. *Pain, 21,* 153–161.

Keefe, F., Wilkins, R., & Cook, W. (1984). Direct observation of pain behaviour in low back pain patients during physical examination. *Pain, 20,* 59–68.

Kremer, E., & Atkinson, J. (1981). Pain measurement: Construct validity of the affective dimension of the McGill Pain Questionnaire with chronic benign pain patients. *Pain, 11,* 93–100.

Kremer, E., & Atkinson, J. (1984). Pain language: Affect. *Journal of Psychosomatic Research, 28,* 125–132.

Kremer, E., Atkinson, J., & Ignelzi, R. (1982). Pain measurement: The affective dimensional measure of the McGill Pain Questionnaire with a cancer pain population. *Pain, 12,* 153–163.

Kremer, E., Atkinson, J., & Kremer, A. (1983). The language of pain: Affective descriptors of pain are a better predictor of psychological disturbance than pattern of sensory and affective descriptors. *Pain, 16,* 185–192.

Kremer, E., Block, A., & Gaylor, M. (1981). Behavioural approaches to treatment of chronic pain: The inaccuracy of patient self-report measures. *Archives of Physical Medicine and Rehabilitation, 62,* 188–191.

Kudrow, L., & Sutkus, B. (1979). MMPI pattern specificity in primary headache disorders. *Headache, 19,* 18–24.

Larson, A., & Marcer, D. (1984). The who and why of pain: Analysis by social class. *British Medical Journal, 288,* 883–886.

Leavitt, F., & Garron, D. (1979). Psychological disturbance and pain report differences in both organic and non-organic low back pain patients. *Pain, 7,* 187–195.

Leavitt, F., Garron, D., Whisler, W., & Sheinkop, M. (1978). Affective and sensory dimensions of back pain. *Pain, 4,* 273–281.

Lefebvre, M. (1981). Cognitive distortion and cognitive errors in depressed psychiatric and low back pain patients. *Journal of Consulting and Clinical Psychology, 49,* 517–525.

Levenson, H., Hirschfeld, M., & Hirschfeld, A. (1980). Industrial accidents and recent life events. *Journal of Occupational Medicine, 22,* 53–57.

Levenson, H., Hirschfeld, M., Hirschfeld, A., & Dzubay, B. (1983). Recent life events and accidents: The role of sex differences. *Journal of Human Stress, 9,* 4–11.

Linton, S. (1985). The relationship between activity and chronic back pain. *Pain, 21,* 289–294.

Lipton, J., & Marbach, J. (1983). Components of the response to pain and variables influencing the response in three groups of facial pain patients. *Pain, 16,* 343–359.

Lloyd, J., & Stagoll, B. (1979). The accident victim syndrome: "Compensation neurosis" or iatrogenesis? *New Doctor, 13,* 29–34.

Main, C., & Waddell, G. (1982). Chronic pain, distress and illness behaviour. In C. Main (Ed.), *Clinical psychology and medicine.* London: Plenum Press.

Marbach, J., & Lipton, J. (1978). Aspects of illness behaviour in patients with facial pain. *Journal of the American Dental Association, 96,* 630–638.

Marbach, J., & Lund, P. (1981). Depression, anhedonia and anxiety in temporomandibular joint and other facial pain syndromes. *Pain, 11,* 73–84.

Marbach, J., Richlin, D., & Lipton, J. (1983). Illness behaviour, depression and anhedonia in myofascial face and back pain patients. *Psychotherapy and Psychosomatics, 39,* 47–54.

McCreary, C. (1985). Empirically derived MMPI profile clusters and characteristics of low back pain patients. *Journal of Consulting and Clinical Psychology, 53,* 558–560.

McCreary, C., & Colman, A. (1984). Medication usage, emotional disturbance, and pain behaviour in chronic low back pain patients. *Journal of Clinical Psychology, 40,* 15–19.

McCreary, C., Turner, J., & Dawson, E. (1977). Differences between functional versus organic low back pain patients. *Pain, 4,* 73–78.

McCreary, C., Turner, J., & Dawson, E. (1980). Emotional disturbance and chronic low back pain. *Journal of Clinical Psychology, 36,* 709–715.

McCreary, C., Turner, J., & Dawson, E. (1981). Principal dimensions of the pain experience and psychological disturbance in chronic low back pain patients. *Pain, 11,* 85–92.

McDaniel, L., Anderson, K., Bradley, L., Young, L., Turner, R., Agudelo, C., & Keefe, F. (1986). Development of an observation method for assessing pain behaviour in rheumatoid arthritis patients. *Pain, 24,* 165–184.

McGill, J., Lawlis, G., Selby, D., Mooney, V., & McCoy, C. (1983). The relationship of MMPI profile clusters to pain behaviours. *Journal of Behavioural Medicine, 6,* 77–92.

McNairy, S., Maruta, T., Ivnik, R., Swanson, D., & Ilstrup, D. (1984). Prescription medication dependence and neuropsychologic function, *Pain, 18,* 169–177.

Melzack, R. (1975). The McGill Pain Questionnaire: Major properties and scoring methods. *Pain, 1,* 277–299.

Melzack, R., Katz, J., & Jeans, M. (1985). The role of compensation in chronic pain: Analysis using a new method of scoring the McGill Pain Questionnaire. *Pain, 23,* 101–112.

Melzack, R., Wall, P., & Ty, T. (1982). Acute pain in an emergency clinic: Latency of onset and descriptor patterns related to different injuries. *Pain, 14,* 33–43.

Mendelson, G. (1982). Not "cured by a verdict": Effect of legal settlement on compensation claimants. *Medical Journal of Australia, 2,* 132–134.

Mendelson, G. (1984). Compensation, pain complaints, and psychological disturbance. *Pain, 20,* 169–177.

Mendelson, G., Selwood, T., Kranz, H., Loh, T., Kidson, M., & Scott, D. (1983). Acupuncture treatment of chronic back pain. *American Journal of Medicine, 74,* 49–55.

Merskey, H., & Boyd, D. (1978). Emotional adjustment and chronic pain. *Pain, 5,* 173–178.

Merskey, H., Brown, J., Brown, A., Malhotra, L., Morrison, D., & Ripley, C. (1985). Psychological normality and abnormality in persistent headache patients. *Pain, 23,* 35–47.

Merskey, H., & Watson, G. (1979). The lateralization of pain. *Pain, 7,* 271–280.

Mohamed, S., Weisz, G., & Waring, E. (1978). The relationship of chronic pain to depression, marital adjustment, and family dynamics. *Pain, 5,* 285–292.

Monroe, S. (1983). Major and minor life events as predictors of psychological distress: Further issues and findings. *Journal of Behavioural Medicine, 6,* 189–205.

Moore, M., Berk, S., & Nypaver, A. (1984). Chronic pain: Inpatient treatment with small group effects. *Archives of Physical Medicine and Rehabilitation, 65,* 357–361.

Naliboff, B., Cohen, M., & Yellen, A. (1982). Does the MMPI differentiate chronic illness from chronic pain? *Pain, 13,* 333–341.

Naliboff, B., Cohen, M., Swanson, G., Bonebakker, A., & McArthur, D. (1985). Comprehensive assessment of chronic low back pain patients and controls: Physical abilities, level of activity, psychological adjustment and pain perception. *Pain, 23,* 121–134.

Packard, R. (1979). What does the headache patient want? *Headache, 19,* 370–374.

Pearlin, L., Menaghan, E., Leiberman, M., & Mullan, J. (1981). The stress process. *Journal of Health and Social Behaviour, 22,* 337–356.

Pearlin, L., & Schooler, C. (1978). The structure of coping. *Journal of Health and Social Behaviour, 19,* 2–21.

Pelz, M., & Merskey, H. (1982). A description of the psychological effects of chronic painful lesions. *Pain, 14,* 293–301.

Philips, C. (1978). Tension headache: Theoretical problems. *Behaviour Research and Therapy, 16,* 249–261.

Philips, C., & Hunter, M. (1982). A laboratory technique for the assessment of pain behaviour. *Journal of Behavioural Medicine, 5,* 283–294.

Philips, C., & Jahanshahi, M. (1985). The effects of persistent pain: The chronic headache sufferer. *Pain, 21,* 163–176.

Pilowsky, I. (1977). Altruism and the practice of medicine. *British Journal of Medical Psychology, 50,* 305–311.

Pilowsky, I. (1978). A general classification of abnormal illness behaviours. *British Journal of Medical Psychology, 51,* 131–137.

Pilowsky, I., & Bassett, D. (1982). Pain and depression. *British Journal of Psychiatry, 141,* 30–36.

Pilowsky, I., Bassett, D., Barrett, R., Petrovic, L., & Minniti, R. (1983). The Illness Behaviour Assessment Schedule: Reliability and validity. *International Journal of Psychiatry in Medicine, 13,* 11–28.

Pilowsky, I., & Bond, M. (1969). Pain and its management in malignant disease. *Psychosomatic Medicine, 31,* 400–404.

Pilowsky, I., Murrell, T., & Gordon, A. (1979). The development of a screening method for abnormal illness behaviour. *Journal of Psychosomatic Research, 23,* 203–207.

Pilowsky, I., & Spalding, D. (1972). A method for measuring depression: Validity studies on a depression questionnaire. *British Journal of Psychiatry, 121,* 411–416.

Pilowsky, I., & Spence, N. (1976a). Illness behaviour syndromes associated with intractable pain. *Pain, 2,* 67–71.

Pilowsky, I., & Spence, N. (1976b). Is illness behaviour related to chronicity in patients with intractable pain? *Pain, 2,* 167–173.

Pilowsky, I., & Spence, N. (1976c). Pain and illness behaviour: A comparative study. *Journal of Psychosomatic Research, 20,* 131–134.

Pilowsky, I., & Spence, N. (1976d). Pain, anger and illness behaviour. *Journal of Psychosomatic Research, 20,* 411–416.

Pilowsky, I., Spence, N., Cobb, J., & Katsikitis, M. (1984). The Illness Behaviour Questionnaire as an aid to clinical assessment. *General Hospital Psychiatry, 6,* 123–130.

Pilowsky, I. (1985). Malingeraphobia. *Medical Journal of Australia, 143,* 571–572.

Pilowsky, I., Crettenden, I., & Townley, M. (1985). Sleep disturbance in pain clinic patients. *Pain, 23,* 27–33.

Prieto, E., Hopson, L., Bradley, L., Byrne, M., Geisinger, K., Midax, D., & Marchisello, P. (1980). The language of low back pain: Factor structure of the McGill Pain Questionnaire. *Pain, 8,* 11–20.

Rahe, R., & Arthur, R. (1978). Life change and illness studies: Past history and future directions. *Journal of Human Stress, 4,* 3–15.

Reading, A. (1979). The internal structure of the McGill Pain Questionnaire. *Pain, 7,* 353–358.

Reading, A. (1982). A comparison of the McGill Pain Questionnaire in chronic and acute pain. *Pain, 13,* 185–192.

Ready, L., Sarkis, E., & Turner, J. (1982). Self-reported versus actual use of medications in chronic pain patients. *Pain, 12,* 285–294.

Reich, J., Tupin, J., & Abramowitz, S. (1983). Psychiatric diagnosis of chronic pain patients. *American Journal of Psychiatry, 140,* 1495–1498.

Richards, J., Nepomuceno, C., Riles, M., & Suer, Z. (1982). Assessing pain behaviour: The UAB Pain Behaviour Scale. *Pain, 14,* 393–398.

Roberts, N., Smith, R., Bennett, S., Cape, J., Norton, R., & Kilburn, P. (1984). Health beliefs and rehabilitation after lumbar disc surgery. *Journal of Psychosomatic Research, 28,* 139–144.

Rook, J., Pesch, R., & Keeler, E. (1981). Chronic pain and the questionable use of the Minnesota Multiphasic Personality Inventory. *Archives of Physical Medicine and Rehabilitation, 62,* 373–376.

Rosenstiel, A., & Keefe, F. (1983). The use of coping strategies in chronic low back pain patients: Relationship to pain characteristics and current adjustment. *Pain, 17,* 33–44.

Rowat, K., & Knafl, K. (1985). Living with pain: The spouse's perspective. *Pain, 23,* 259–271.

Rubinstein, A. (1982). Mediterranean back and other stereotypes: A review of the Australian literature dealing with industrial back injuries. *Australian Journal of Social Issues, 17,* 295–303.

Sanders, S. (1983). Automated versus self-monitoring of "up time" in chronic low back pain patients: A comparative study. *Pain, 15,* 399–405.

Schwartz, D., & DeGood, D. (1984). Global appropriateness of pain drawings: Blind ratings predict patterns of psychological distress and litigation status. *Pain, 19,* 383–388.

Shanfield, S., Heiman, E., Cope, D., & Jones, J. (1979). Pain and the marital relationship: Psychiatric distress. *Pain, 7,* 343–351.

Singh, B., Nunn, K., Martin, J., & Yates, J. (1981). Abnormal treatment behaviour. *British Journal of Psychology, 54,* 67–73.

Skevington, S. (1983a). Activities as indices of illness behaviour in chronic pain. *Pain, 15,* 295–307.

Skevington, S. (1983b). Chronic pain and depression: Universal or personal helplessness? *Pain, 15,* 309–317.

Skevington, S. (1983c). Social cognitions, personality and chronic pain. *Journal of Psychosomatic Research, 27,* 421–428.

Snaith, R., Ahmed, S., Mehta, S., & Hamilton, M. (1971). Assessment of severity of primary depressive illness. *Psychological Medicine, 1,* 143–149.

Spielberger, C., Gorsuch, R., & Lushene, R. (1970). *Manual for the State-Trait Anxiety Inventory.* Palo Alto: Consulting Psychologists Press.

Sprock, J., Braff, D., Saccuzzo, D., & Atkinson, J. (1983). The relationship of depression and thought disorder in pain patients. *British Journal of Medical Psychology, 56,* 351–360.

Sternbach, R. (1974). *Pain patients: Traits and treatment.* New York: Academic Press.

Sternbach, R., Wolf, S., Murphy, R., & Akeson, W. (1973a). Aspects of chronic low back pain. *Psychosomatics, 14,* 52–56.

Sternbach, R., Wolf, S., Murphy, R., & Akeson, W. (1973b). Traits of pain patients: The low back "loser." *Psychosomatics, 14,* 226–229.

Sternbach R. (1978). Clinical aspects of pain. In R. Sternbach (Ed.), *The psychology of pain.* New York: Raven Press.

Sternbach, R., Dalessio, D., Kunzel, M., & Bowman, G. (1980). MMPI patterns in common headache disorders. *Headache, 20,* 311-315.

Sternbach, R., & Timmermans, G. (1975). Personality changes associated with reduction of pain. *Pain, 1,* 177–181.

Sullivan, P., & Welsh, G. (1952). A technique for objective configural analysis of MMPI profiles. *Journal of Consulting Psychology, 16,* 383–388.

Swanson, D. (1984). Chronic pain as a third pathologic emotion. *American Journal of Psychiatry, 141,* 210–214.

Swanson, D., & Maruta, T. (1980). The family's viewpoint of chronic pain. *Pain, 8,* 163–166.

Swanson, D., Maruta, T., & Swenson, W. (1979). Results of behaviour modification in the treatment of chronic pain. *Psychosomatic Medicine, 41,* 55–61.

Thomas, M., & Lyttle, D. (1980). Patient expectations about success of treatment and reported relief from low back pain. *Journal of Psychosomatic Research, 24,* 297–301.

Thompson, S. (1981). Will it hurt less if I can control it? *Psychological Bulletin, 90,* 89–101.

Toomey, T., Gower, V., & Jones, B. (1983). Spatial distribution of pain: A descriptive characteristic of chronic pain. *Pain, 17,* 289–300.

Toomey, T., Gover, V., & Jones, B. (1984). Site of pain: Relationship to measures of pain description, behaviour and personality. *Pain, 19,* 389–397.

Trief, P. (1983). Chronic back pain: A tripartite model of outcome. *Archives of Physical Medicine and Rehabilitation, 64,* 53–56.

Turk, D., Rudy, T., & Salovey, P. (1985). The McGill Pain Questionnaire reconsidered: Confirming the factor structure and examining appropriate uses. *Pain, 21,* 385–397.

Turner, J., Calsyn, D., Fordyce, W., & Ready, L. (1982). Drug utilization patterns in chronic pain patients. *Pain, 12,* 357–363.

Turner, J., & Chapman, C. (1982). Psychological interventions for chronic pain: A critical review. II. Operant conditioning, hypnosis, and cognitive-behavioural therapy. *Pain, 12,* 23–46.

Turner, J., & Clancy, S. (1986). Strategies for coping with chronic low back pain: Relationship to pain and disability. *Pain, 24,* 355–364.

Viney, L., & Westbrook, M. (1982). Coping with chronic illness: The mediating role of biographic and illness-related factors. *Journal of Psychosomatic Research, 26,* 595–605.

Wall, P. (1979). On the relation of injury to pain. *Pain, 6,* 253–264.

Watson, D. (1982). Neurotic tendencies among chronic pain patients: An MMPI item analysis. *Pain, 14,* 365–385.

Wiener, C. (1975). The burden of rheumatoid arthritis: Tolerating the uncertainty. *Social Science and Medicine, 9,* 97–104.

Wolff, B. (1978). Behavioural measurement of human pain. In R. Sternbach (Ed.), *The psychology of pain.* New York: Raven Press.

Woodforde, J., & Merskey, H. (1972). Personality traits of patients with chronic pain. *Journal of Psychosomatic Research, 16,* 167–172.

Zung, W. (1965). A self-rating depression scale. *Archives of General Psychiatry, 12,* 63–70.

10

The Behavioral Management and Prevention of Chronic Pain

Steven J. Linton

Department of Occupational Medicine
Örebro Medical Centre, Sweden

The behavioral approach as espoused in behavioral medicine has provided a major breakthrough in the management and prevention of chronic pain. The problem of chronic pain has reached alarming proportions and may be considered a major medical problem. While conventional medical treatments have had difficulties in successfully managing chronic pain problems, a behavioral approach has provided new insights into the syndrome. This penetration of the malady has also resulted in new approaches to the management and prevention of chronic pain. This chapter will provide a brief background into the behavioral approach to pain and then will evaluate behavioral programs for the management and prevention of chronic pain. It will be shown that behavioral programs have made a major contribution to the management of pain problems. However, although the best remediation programs lead to significant and clinically substantial improvements, problems in the effective management of chronic pain demand its prevention.

Before examining the behavioral approach to pain and its management or prevention, it may be useful to review some basic information concerning chronic pain. First of all, chronic pain may be defined as pain that persists for at least three months or more. Pain as a result of malignant disease is often excluded (Bradley, 1983). It is also important to point out that the pain may be related to several kinds of pathologies and it may be classified, for example, as myofascial, rheumatic, neurologic, causalgic, or vascular (Fricton, 1982). Not withstanding, a very significant proportion of patients with chronic pain suffer from disorders in the musculoskeletal system and this paper focuses primarily on those types of disorders.

The extent of the chronic pain problem is rather enormous. As an illustration, in virtually every country in the Western world neck, shoulder, and back pain are prominent problems (e.g., Anderson, 1980; Andersson, 1981; Ergonomics, 1985; Nachemson, 1982).

In general, it may be said that approximately 85 percent of the working population will seek help for pain problems in the musculoskeletal system at some time during their working lives (Andersson, 1981). Of these, more than 50 percent will have recurrent troubles and many of these will become chronic sufferers. In Sweden, where reliable records are available through the National Health Insurance Office, statistics show that 12.5 percent of all sick days are related to back pain and that pain in the locomotive system is the number one consumer of sick pay, compensation pensions, and health care visits (Arbetarskyddsfonden, 1976). Similar statistics are available from other countries. In the Netherlands, problems in the locomotive system are a leading cause of sick absenteeism and account for 20 percent of days absent from work (Zuidema, 1985). Almost identical statistics are available from the Federal Republic of Germany where skeletal diseases account for nearly 22 percent of sick absenteeism (Hettinger, 1985). Moreover, the number of persons suffering from chronic pain problems seems to be on the rise. Between 1970 and 1979 there was a more than 200 percent increase in musculoskeletal disorders in Australia (McPhee, 1982) and a similar increase for back disorders has been recorded in Luxembourgh (Metzler, 1985). Clearly, chronic pain is a prevalent disorder which is consuming large amounts of resources and resulting in severe social, personal, and familial difficulties.

A BEHAVIORAL VIEW OF PAIN

A behavioral view of pain has been expounded upon elsewhere (e.g., Fordyce, 1976; Linton, Melin, & Götestam, 1984) and need not be dwelled upon here, but a review of the basic tenets is valuable since an understanding of the behavioral approach is a prerequisite to understanding programs designed to manage and prevent pain problems. Traditionally, pain has been viewed as a simple neurological state where pain experience is in direct proportion to tissue damage. However, it is now recognized that pain is a highly subjective experience and as such it is a class of behavior (Fordyce, 1976). To understand the implications of this one might consider that, according to behavioral theories, actions an organism takes are actions of the whole organism (as opposed to the action of an arm or the nervous system) (Rachlin, 1985). In other words, pain involves several parts of the organism including its physiology, cognitive functioning, and overt behavior. In fact, the physiological processes associated with pain experience are extremely complicated and several opportunities for modulation of the nerves' signals are built into the system (Melzack & Wall, 1965). Pain is a set of behaviors rather than a neurological state and like any other behavior it may be modified by learning processes. When pain persists over a long period of time, the potential to modify behavior is high (Fordyce, 1976).

A considerable proportion of the behaviors we engage in when we are sick are learned behaviors. Communicating that we are in pain, seeking medical help, lying down, and taking medicines are all examples of behaviors that may be learned. The behavioral view is that patients learn behavior patterns that help them reduce pain—at least in the short run—and that these behavior patterns may maintain the experience of pain under certain conditions in the long run. Since physiological processes, experience, and overt behaviors are all part of the set of pain behaviors in a whole organism view, one cannot view these factors in isolation from one another. The learning of pain behavior is discussed in detail in other articles (e.g., Fordyce, 1976; Linton et al., 1984; Rachlin, 1985). These publications illustrate how maladaptive behaviors associated with chronic pain, such as excessive reliance on medications, overutilization of health care services, low activity level, and psychological symptoms may be learned.

THE DEVELOPMENT OF CHRONIC PAIN

The development of a pain problem from the acute to the chronic stage may be described in several ways, such as in a statistical, descriptive, or theoretical approach. It is of interest to know how many persons suffering from pain problems will actually develop chronic problems. Ordinarily, the development may be classified into subacute and chronic stages. By looking at incidence and prevalence rates one may obtain a rough idea of the number of persons developing chronic problems. One of the most thorough studies has been conducted in Denmark by Biering-Sörensen (1984) in which a whole community was evaluated. The study is valuable also in that it is representative of the data obtained by other researchers. Table 10.1 illustrates decreasing numbers from lifetime prevalence to point prevalence to the incidence rate during the last year. The percentage of persons having recurrent or persistent pain over a one-year period is also indicated in the table. These data suggest that the number of persons suffering from chronic problems should be considerably less than those suffering from acute and subacute problems. However, the data obviously do not allow one to draw any conclusions concerning the development of chronic pain problems.

Another way of examining the development of chronic pain problems from a statistical approach is to look at the number of persons sick listed over time. If one defines chronic pain, as was done above, in terms of pain persisting beyond a certain time point, then one may obtain rates from such data. A study of this nature has been completed in Sweden (Chöler, Larsson, Nachemson, & Peterson, 1985). In this study, all of the patients applying for acute back pain were registered in a district in the Gotenburg area over a considerable period of time. Each patient was followed up to see when they were able to return to work. As may be seen in Figure 10.1 the percentage of patients getting better after an acute back problem increased rapidly so that more than 85 percent could return to work after a six-week period. (Patients received ordinary medical treatment for their problem as directed by a general practitioner). Note, however, that the shape of the curve changes drastically after approximately 6 to 12 weeks and that few persons get better after this point. In other words, according to these statistics there is a very good chance of getting better within approximately 3 months of the occurrence of the acute attack of back pain, but

Table 10.1.
Rates of the Occurrence of Low Back Pain in the General Public (Based on Data from Biering-Sörensen, 1984)

	Rate*	
Measure	Men (30–60 yrs)	Women (30–60 yrs)
Life Prevalence	62.6	61.4
One-Year Prevalence	44.8	45.0
Point Prevalence	12.0	15.2
One-Year Incidence	6.0	6.0
Recurrence/Persistence	61.6	63.1

*In percent

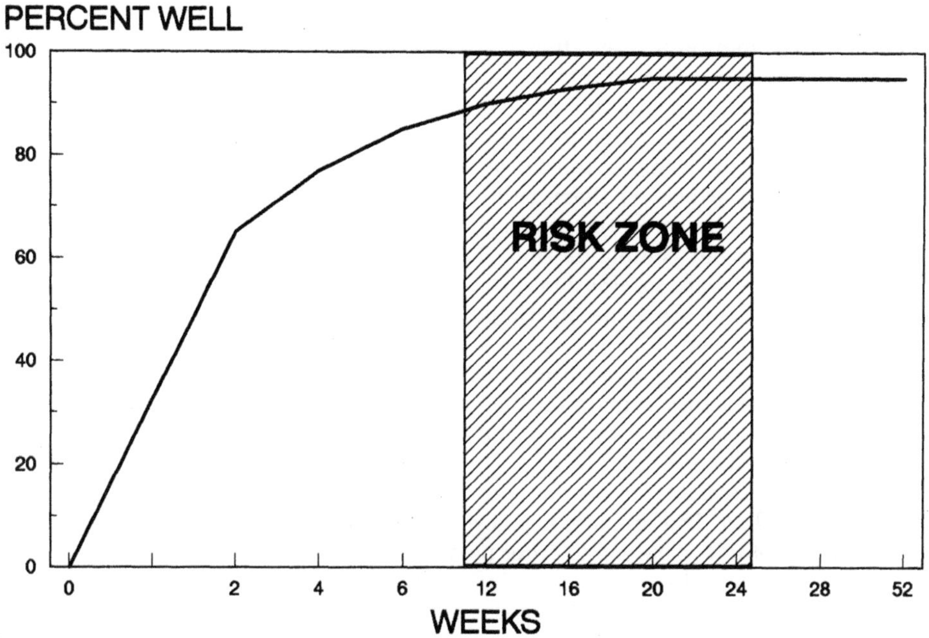

FIGURE 10.1. Percentage of patients over time that are well enough to return to work after suffering acute back pain. (Based on data from Chöler et al., 1985)

after 3 months the statistical chance of returning to work is very low indeed.

Another approach to the development of chronic pain is the descriptive one in which typical behaviors associated with each stage of development are described. An attempt at the representative description of the development of a case of chronic back pain has been made by Linton et al. (1984). A brief example is presented here to illustrate the process of lifestyle changes.

> The person is a female secretary who is healthy before the onset of the pain. Although some features of her background such as her family situation and work might be related to the development of pain problems, she is in most respects a fairly typical secretary. The acute phase of her pain problem is characterized by sharp pains in the low back region. Our secretary at this point is quite capable of taking command of the situation herself, obtaining medical care, and organizing her private life with regard to the problem. Upon medical examination the doctor finds positive organic signs and, as is quite usual in these cases, recommends that the patient rest for one to two weeks and prescribes a mild analgesic. For a good many patients, this regime would be successful and the

person would return to work. Yet, our secretary finds herself continuing to suffer from pain even after a few weeks rest.

She has now entered into the subacute phase of the development and we note that the symptoms have begun to change. The pain has spread from the low back region to include problems in the upper back region and neck. Furthermore, the character of the pain has begun to change; rather than attacks of sharp pain she is now also experiencing a deep-seated pain almost continuously. Other problems have begun to develop and the patient complains that she has problems getting to sleep at night. A medical examination reveals questionable positive organic findings, but there are some functional disturbances in the form of muscle tension. The continued pain poses a problem not only for the patient but for the presiding general practitioner and in this case he recommends that our secretary remain on the sick list (rest at home) and continue with analgesics. He also refers the patient to the X-ray department for an examination of the back.

Three months later our secretary returns again seeking help for back pain problem. The problem has now reached the chronic stage. We note that the pain has spread to other parts of the body such as referred pain in the legs and the character of the pain has changed to a diffuse ache. A number of other problems have also developed including sleep problems, anxiety, headache, and depression. A number of additional problems also seem to be developing in the form of economic troubles and strained family relationships. The X-ray and medical examinations show no clear positive findings, but instead some diffuse signs that might be related to the problem. Appropriate treatment measures are difficult to determine. Since the patient is complaining of more pain and sleep problems, and she maintains that she cannot return to work, our doctor continues to sick-list the patient and prescribes a stronger analgesic in addition to medication to help her relax so that she may sleep. The doctor recommends that she see a physical therapist and sends a referral to the rehabilitation department for possible rehabilitation treatment.

The above example illustrates the development of a chronic pain problem in terms of the associated problem behaviors as well as problems posed to the health care system.

A final method of examining the development of chronic pain is from a learning theory approach. We have seen statistically and descriptively that a small percentage of patients begin to deteriorate and that after approximately three months this deterioration translates into a chronic problem in which the patient has, statistically speaking, a very small chance of recovering. The question is: What happens during this time that results in such deterioration? One obvious answer is that the patient actually has a serious disease process which is irreversible and causes the deterioration. However, as the descriptive case illustrates and as other research shows, this is extremely rare indeed (Nachemson, 1983). Instead, one has begun to look at psychosocial factors which may influence the development of chronic pain. In particular, it is hypothesized that learning processes account for the development of problem behaviors as well as the experience of anxiety and depression (Linton et al., 1984).

In general, learning factors are thought to lead to a passive lifestyle which in the short run result in less pain but which in the long run helps create chronic problems.

It has been maintained that pain is as much a psychological phenomenon as it is a physical one. Although being exposed to noxious stimuli may or may not be related to learning, a person's reaction to noxious stimulation is. (Learning paradigms involving pain behavior have been outlined in detail by e.g., Fordyce, 1976; Linton et al., 1984.)

An important example is the learning of "sick behavior" in general. Here one notes that positive and negative reinforcement influence a person's verbal and overt behavior. In Western society, social practices provide for many potential reinforcers for sick behavior. Family members and friends ordinarily provide, for example, attention and relief from responsibilities on the basis of the number and intensity of sick behaviors (Kraft, 1975). Similarly, the medical profession administers drugs and attention on the basis of sick behavior: The greater the number and intensity of pain behaviors the more attention and drugs. Such outcomes may come to control sick behaviors and the person in question may come into the sick role. This may happen regardless of whether noxious stimuli are present. An illustration may help make this point. In an analogue laboratory situation pain reports have been controlled through the use of positive reinforcement and punishment (subtle verbal statements in both cases) so that subjects reported increasing amounts of pain, even when the noxious stimulus decreased (Linton & Götestam, 1985a).

A central process in the chronification of pain is the reinforcement of passive behaviors. Although positive and negative reinforcement of actual pain behavior and avoidance are often given a primary place in accounting for chronic pain behavior, such mechanisms probably account for only a relatively small part of the total behavior of a chronic pain patient (Linton et al., 1984).

While these processes are of vital importance, it appears that the development of behavior incompatible with "well" behavior also is of major importance. Over the course of time that a chronic pain problem develops, the patient may be selectively reinforced for engaging in passive behaviors and thereby learn a new "lifestyle." Compared with previous behavior levels and with norms for the same sex and age group, this new lifestyle is rather passive and tends not to include vigorous activities.

The key to understanding this process is that the patient with pain trouble will most likely be sick-listed over a substantial period of time and what happens during this period of time is crucial in the chronification of pain. If the patient's behavior results in as much or more reinforcement while being sick as compared to being well and if these reinforcers are similar in power, the probability for the occurrence of well behavior will decrease. In the acute and subacute phases, inactivity may be directly reinforced by reductions in pain, anxiety, and so on. After the development of a pain problem, the patient may spend considerable amounts of time resting, watching television, reading, or doing hobbies, and may in fact receive a good deal of reinforcement for this role in the home. Rather than buying "time out" from undesirable activities or rather than exhibiting pain behaviors throughout the day, the patient learns to take on a passive, inactive lifestyle. Consequently, the patient need not necessarily be described as engaging in either pain or avoidance behavior; rather, the patient may be said to be participating in behaviors that are of a passive nature in relation to the patient's prepain lifestyle.

There are also side effects of this development. One important development is that of depression, and another increased anxiety (Linton & Götestam, 1985b). Both depression and anxiety may have a tendency to change pain perception in such a way that the more depression and anxiety the less pain the patient tolerates. Furthermore, both depression and anxiety hinder the management of chronic pain problems since depression leads to a decrease in coping capacity and anxiety tends to limit the patient's activity.

Another distinction is important. The discussion above has featured learning processes after the onset of acute pain. For the purposes of prevention, however, one might also look at behavioral aspects of events leading up to the acute bout of pain. In other words, one may distinguish between processes involved in producing the first trauma and processes involved in the chronification of acute pain. An analysis might be made of the *behaviors that result in injury* since these behaviors may be quite different from those occurring after the appearance of acute problems. For example, the former may involve behaviors like sitting too much or lifting too often as well as behaviors associated with health promotion (e.g., exercise, weight control, smoking, alcohol consumption). A further examination of these factors is provided in the section on prevention.

In summary, one way of approaching the problem of chronic pain is to consider its development. After approximately 3–6 months the chances of fully recovering are quite small. The process of development, however, points to learned factors which alter the patient's lifestyle. Consequently, the problem of chronic pain might be tackled in at least two ways. First, one may attempt to analyze the existing problems of chronic pain patients to subsequently change these behaviors to more desirable ones. This involves the *management* of chronic pain. A second possibility also exists. If learning processes are important in the development of a chronic pain problem, then these processes could be influenced at an early stage in order to *prevent* the development of chronic pain problems. Let us now turn to an examination of management and prevention techniques.

BEHAVIORAL MANAGEMENT TECHNIQUES

There are a large variety of behavioral treatments for chronic pain, but they may be classified into three general categories: operant, relaxation, and cognitive approaches. In theory, these techniques are rather distinguishable, but in practice it is often difficult to classify a particular treatment regime into these categories. Operant programs involve contingency management techniques, but they may also include other kinds of treatments. The relaxation therapies vary considerably and are often mixed with cognitive techniques of the stress management type (Pearce, 1983). There are few programs which are "pure" regarding management techniques. Consequently, one must examine the studies with respect to the main management technique used.

Since several authors have already reviewed the effectiveness of behavioral treatments for chronic pain this section will concentrate on a summary of those results with particular emphasis on the most recent and best controlled studies (Aronoff, Evens, & Enders, 1983; Bradley, 1983; Follick, Zitter, & Ahern, 1983; Linton, 1982a, 1986; Tunks, 1988; Turk & Flor, 1984; Turner & Chapman, 1982). This review focuses on the effectiveness of the treatment techniques by considering what behaviors have been addressed, what results were obtained with these behaviors and whether treatment effects generalized to other behaviors.

OPERANT TECHNIQUES

Operant techniques or contingency management programs are aimed at identifying problem behaviors, functionally analyzing and modifying them, and finally maintaining improvements. Fordyce (1976) developed the classic operant program which included measures for decreasing medication intake, pain levels, and pain behaviors as well as increasing activity and other more constructive behaviors. Pain-related behaviors are seen as any other behaviors and may be modified by the appropriate contingency management. Details of these programs are available elsewhere (Fordyce, 1976).

The approximately 25 reports concerning effectiveness are nearly exclusively positive, but a number of methodological problems restrict the conclusions that can be made in many of these studies. As a result, the prospective controlled studies have been listed in Table 10.2. In any evaluation of the effectiveness of a treatment, well-designed and well-controlled studies must weigh more heavily than case studies or uncontrolled one-group outcome studies (cf. Rachman & Wilson 1980). In addition to being controlled studies the investigations in this group employed outcome measures covering a broad range of variables and the assessment methodology was generally admirable.

The earliest controlled studies dealt with the operant activity program (Cairns & Pasino, 1977; Doleys et al., 1982). The activity program developed by Fordyce includes activity training where one exercises to a quota. The quota level is determined in cooperation with the patient and based on the patient's pretreatment level of functioning. The goal quota is gradually increased in order to ascertain an overall increase in activity level. When the quota level is reached on any given trial the patient is provided with reinforcement in the form of graphic feedback, verbal reinforcement, and the chance to rest. Cairns and Pasino compared the usual physical therapy given to back pain patients with a group receiving verbal reinforcement only and a third group receiving verbal reinforcement plus graphic feedback. They found that the group receiving both verbal reinforcement and graphic feedback did about as well as the group receiving only verbal reinforcement and both of these groups were significantly better than the ordinary physical therapy group.

Another study of exercising to quotas was done by Doleys, Crocker, and Patton (1982). A single subject, multiple-baseline-across-responses design was used to evaluate the effects of exercising to quota with 26 chronic pain patients. Results for a representative patient clearly indicate that increases in exercising occurred only when the quota system was initiated. Substantial increases during the quota exercising were also noted for the entire group, even if some increases were also noted during the no-quota condition. Taken together these two studies provide considerable support for the contention that the operant activity training program leads to substantial and clinically significant increases in exercising levels.

Two additional studies employed single subject designs. Miller and Lelieuvre (1982) looked at pain problems in four geriatric patients living in a nursing home. They used an ABAB-reversal design and all outcome measures except for pain experience were observed. Activating the patients was the main emphasis of the treatment. In general, the program produced improvements for reported pain intensity, activity level, and medication intake. On the individual level, clear control was obtained for two of four patients for overt pain communication behaviors. However, there was some difficulty in increasing and maintaining ward activity and exercise levels. Apparently the patient's activity levels were already near their peak (ceiling effect) because they were participating in the nursing home's activity program. The need for a careful behavior analysis is indicated by this example.

A tightly controlled single-subject design was used to study four chronic low back pain patients provided with four different behavioral treatments (relaxation, activity program, assertiveness training, and a functional analysis of pain) in a multiple-baseline-across-subjects design (Sanders, 1983). It was found that relaxation training produced clinically meaningful changes in subjects' pain ratings, medication intake and up-time, while social reinforcement for activity also had consistent but somewhat less distinct effects on these variables. These data are particularly noteworthy since the study used relatively short periods of training (one week) for each of the four behavioral treatments.

One study combined single subject designs with a three group pre- and posttest design (Linton & Götestam, 1984). In this study applied relaxation used as a coping strategy was compared with a group receiving applied relaxation plus a complete operant program. Both of these active treatment groups were compared with a waiting-list control. The results on a wide range of variables indicated that both treatment groups—on the individual and group levels—had substantial and statistically significant improvements as compared to baseline and the waiting-list control. However, there were few statistically significant differences between the two treatment groups. The group including the operant procedures had quicker, and at posttest, somewhat larger improvements for the variables of medicine consumption and activity level than did the group receiving only applied relaxation. On the other hand, the subjects in the applied relaxation group had significantly less reported pain than the operant group at the nine month follow-up.

The utility of a behavioral program provided on an outpatient basis has been evaluated in a three group pre-post test study (Linton, Melin, & Stjernlöf, 1985). Twenty-eight chronic pain patients were randomly

Table 10.2.
Controlled Outcome Studies Using the Operant Approach

Study	N	Pain	Treatments	Design	Outcome
Cairns & Pasino (1977)	9	Back	In-patient activity training 1 = no special training, 2 = verbal reinforcement 3 = verbal reinforcement & graphic feedback	3 group pre/post	3 = 2 > 1 (S) for specified activities in physical therapy at post test. No follow-up.
Doleys et al. (1982)	26	Mainly back	Exercising to quota and reinforcement	Single-subject multiple-across-responses	Data from one S shows that substantial increases in activity occur only when quota program initiated. Data from entire group support this idea, but increases during nonquota periods blurs results.
Miller & Lelieuvre (1982)	4 (geriatric)	"Chronic"	a) Social reinforcement/extinction to increase activity, decrease pain behavior. b) Above plus quotas during physical therapy	Single-subject ABAB	Medication: 55% decrease and good control. Pain behaviors: Z of 4 pts decreased to 0 during treatment. Ward activity: 3/4 increased, but not maintained. Exercise: Only small increases. Pain Ratings: decreases in McGill intensity (37%) and word ranks (26%).

Sanders (1983)	4	Low back	1. Functional pain-behavior analysis 2. Progressive relaxation 3. Assertion training 4. Social reinforcement for activity increases	Nonconcurrent mult baseline across Ss with control for order	2 contributed most to overall improvement on up-time, medication intake and pain intensity followed by 4. 1 and 3 had minimal effect. No other effect observed.
Linton & Götestam (1984)	15	Low back	1. WLC 2. Applied relax as out-pat 3. Applied relax + operant dayward programme for meds, pain, activity	3 gr prepost + single-subject	Expectancy NS. Pain 2 > 1 (S). Exercise 3 > 1 (S). Act Daily Living 2,3 > 1 (S), down-time NS. Depression 2,3 > 1 (S). Anxiety & mood NS, goals 2 > 3 (S).
Linton et al. (1985)	28	Low back	1. WLC 2. Regular clinic treat 3. 2 as needed + behavior therapy: applied relax operant activity	3 gr prepost	Pain ratings 3 > 2, 1 (S). McGill NS. Act daily living 3 > 1 (S) improvement. Medications 3 > 2 + 1 (S). Sleep 3 > 2, 1 (S). Beck depression NS.
Heinrich et al. (1985)	51	Low back	1. Behavior therapy: goals, activity management, problem solving, assertiveness, exercise, pool, body mechanics 2. Physical therapy	2 gr pre-post	Dropouts = 5 for beh therapy, 13 for phy therapy. General improvements for both groups with few treatment specific differences.
White & Sanders (1985)	8	Mixed	1. Time-contingent medication delivery 2. Pain-contingent (as needed) medication delivery	2 gr repeated measures before, during, of the detoxification	Pain ratings 1 > 2 (S). Mood 1 > 2 (S).

assigned to a waiting-list control group, a regular rehabilitation treatment group or a behavior therapy group which received special training in applied relaxation as a coping strategy and an operant activities program to increase relevant activities at home. The behavioral group was shown to have significantly greater reductions in pain reports than the other two groups and furthermore, this group also had the greatest improvements for the variables of sleep, medication intake, and activity levels. A 20-month follow-up indicated that the improvements were generally maintained (Melin & Linton, 1988). This study provides considerable support for the usefulness of behavioral methods with outpatients.

A modified version of the operant approach was compared with physical therapy in a final study (Heinrich, Cohen, Naliboff, Collins, & Bonebakker, 1985). Since a routine method of treating chronic pain patients is physical therapy treatment, this study addressed the question of the comparative value of physical therapy and behavior therapy. The physical therapy program included instructions and training in the use of proper body mechanics, pain control strategies, relaxation training, and exercise. Each session included an educational component plus self-management and the training of activities. The behavioral program included education about pain perception, self-responsibility, personal effectiveness, pain control techniques such as relaxation, exercises and positive imagery, and goal setting for activity management. A large number of outcome variables covering both subjective ratings and staff ratings of physical abilities, current physical functioning, psychological functioning, and pain intensity were used. In general, subjects in both physical therapy and behavior therapy groups improved on all of the variables and there were only a few treatment-specific differences in outcome. Above all, the physical therapy group had significantly larger increases in low back control and back protection skills, while the behavior therapy group demonstrated an advantage in the reduction of psychological stress. Both groups were able to decrease reported pain levels. The results suggest that both physical and behavior therapy approaches might be useful, but some caution is warranted in drawing any such conclusions. Although the difference was not quite statistically significant, there was a considerable difference in the dropout rate between the groups. Forty-six percent of the 28 subjects that started the physical therapy treatment dropped out, whereas 21 percent of the subjects in the behavior therapy group dropped out. The number of dropouts is certainly an important factor in evaluating the effectiveness of any treatment program. In addition, the staff ratings on the various measures of functioning and abilities were apparently not blind. Another point has to do with compliance. Although the physical therapy group had greater increases in back protection skills these gains were not maintained at the 6-month follow-up evaluation. Furthermore, an additional two patients in the behavior therapy group and six patients in the physical therapy group did not complete the follow-up evaluations. Consequently, only 32 percent of the original patients are represented in the follow-up analysis for the physical therapy group and 70 percent for the behavior therapy group. If the missing data were counted as failures, this would surely affect the analyses of outcome.

An assumption central to the operant program is that reinforcement is usually provided on a "pain behavior" contingency. Medications, for instance, are given according to how much pain the patient has and when the patient is in pain. Consequently, the operant approach calls for providing medications (and some other reinforcers) on a time rather than pain contingency. A test of this proposition has been conducted during the detoxification of pain patients (White & Sanders, 1985). Two small groups of patients were intensely studied in a two-group design with continuous assessment. One group received time-contingent delivery of methadone with the amount per dose being gradually decreased over the course of five days. The pain-contingent group received their methadone doses on a pain-contingent "as-needed schedule." All other treatments and medications were held constant across groups. Although no differences were observed between the groups during baseline for the variables of recorded pain or mood, the time contingent group reported significantly lower pain intensity and significantly higher mood than did the pain contingent group at post-test. These data provide considerable support for the use of an operant drug optimization program. Indeed, the results for the group using operant methods actually demonstrated improvements in pain and mood levels at the same time that the analgesic level was being lowered.

The preceding review of the controlled studies demonstrates that operant techniques result in meaningful improvements and thereby provide support for the usefulness of the operant approach. There can no longer be any question as to whether the operant program is potent in increasing activity levels and decreasing medication use. Moreover, the operant approach is associated with moderate decreases in pain reports as well as on other variables such as depression, sleep quality and so on. Experiments are now needed to deal with specific components of the program and to answer the question of how well the program works, for whom, and why. At the current state-of-the-art, operant procedures are to be recommended for the objectives of increasing activity levels and decreasing medicine consumption and the opportunity for such treatment should probably be available in every rehabilitation program.

RELAXATION AND COGNITIVE–BEHAVIORAL THERAPIES

The title of this section is in the plural because there are many forms of such therapy and because there are many apparent inconsistencies in the literature that are resolved only when we distinguish among the various forms. Relaxation therapy is often assumed to mean progressive relaxation, but it also includes EMG biofeedback and more "muscle-directed" approaches used by physical therapists. Furthermore, there are various offspring within the progressive relaxation tradition such as the use of cognitive methods, autogenic training, hypnotic suggestion, meditation, and so forth. Cognitive-behavioral methods, moreover, have been included here since they almost always (when used in the pain context) involve the use of relaxation training.

Pearce (1983) has categorized cognitive behavioral approaches to chronic pain as being either "pain-directed" or "stress-directed." The former includes such things as restructuring or distraction but there is virtually only one study that has examined such a technique in a clinical setting. The latter named stress-directed strategies are usually coping strategies which combine relaxation with the modification of self-statements. Consequently, it is quite difficult to distinguish between relaxation and cognitive-behavioral programs. However, cognitive programs may be said to be interested in the patient's thoughts and feelings.

The goal of the relaxation therapies varies greatly with the program but generally entails two themes. The first has to do with respondent conditioning processes where a pain-muscle tension cycle is presumed to exist. Therapy is directed towards reducing tension levels which should affect a reduction in pain. The second theme is to disrupt the connection between anxiety, despair, and pain. Namely, therapy should result in an increase in ability to cope with pain problems, a decrease in anxiety levels, and consequently a decrease in pain ratings. The second conception is much broader than the first. A coping approach which results in decreases in anxiety should increase pain tolerance and perhaps affect the perception of pain by reducing muscle tension and changing pain perception. Furthermore, the coping approach should lead to more constructive behaviors in terms of, for example, activity levels, medication intake, and so on. In other words, the therapy is oriented towards teaching patients better ways of thinking about and dealing with their pain in everyday situations; patients learn to manage their pain and live with it in more appropriate ways.

BIOFEEDBACK

A summary of the biofeedback studies is provided in Table 10.3. Nine studies are included which have employed these methods. Ordinarily, biofeedback is trained during therapy sessions and there is limited practice at home or between training sessions. Criticism has been directed towards the biofeedback approach since it may be too simple of an approach to a very complex problem (Linton, 1982a; Turner & Chapman, 1982). Indeed, the results of the studies in Table 11.3 are mixed. As may be seen, several of the studies show decreases in EMG and pain reports but the significance, consistency, and maintenance of the improvements is not clear.

The earliest four studies (Dohrmann & Laskin, 1978; Nouwen & Solinger, 1979; Stenn, Mothersill, & Brooke, 1979; Casas, Beemsterboer, & Clark, 1982) show a questionable relationship between EMG and pain levels and in the two comparative studies the addition of biofeedback to other programs seems to have had little effect. Flor, Haag, Turk, and Koehler (1983) found that the group difference for EMG level was not significant in their study. An EMG decrease was reported by Keefe, Schapira, Brown, Williams, and Surwit (1981); however, pain reports were only modified during feedback sessions; not between sessions. Likewise, Nouwen (1983) produced significant decreases in EMG in the biofeedback group even though pain reports were not reduced significantly.

The data concerning biofeedback are not convincing and certainly do not provide clear evidence of its utility. Some of the variance might be accounted for by training schedules, type of chronic pain problem, and electrode placement. However, the relationship between EMG level and chronic pain problems is not lucid. Current research indicates that there is no consistent evidence that chronic pain patients of the low back type have elevated paraspinal EMG levels or that a reduction in EMG is likely to be an active ingredient in biofeedback therapy (Nouwen & Bush, 1984).

RELAXATION THERAPIES

Various other forms of relaxation training were used in the remaining studies. Three studies have employed ordinary progressive relaxation.

Table 10.3.
Controlled Outcome Studies Using Relaxation or Cognitive-behavioral Techniques

Study	N	Pain	Treatments	Design	Outcome
Dohrmann & Laskin (1978)	24	Temporomandibular joint	1. Masseter EMG biofeedback 2. Placebo control	2 gr pre-post	1 > 2 (S) in reducing EMG level. 11 of the 13 patients in gr 1 had remission as opposed to 4 of 8 in gr 2. At follow-up 75% of gr 1 had no further treatment compared to 28% in gr 2.
Nouwen & Solinger (1979)	26	Back	1. Back muscle EMG biofeedback 2. Waiting-list control	2 gr pre-post	1 > 2 (S) EMG and pain reductions. At follow-up EMG returned to pre-treatment levels for gr 1, but pain reductions were maintained.
Stenn et al (1979)	11	Temporomandibular joint	1. Progressive relaxation plus coping 2. Progressive relaxation, EMG biofeedback, and coping	2 gr pre-post	EMG levels decreased (S) 1 = 2, pain decrease (S) 2 > 1, and symptoms decreased (S) 1 = 2. Both groups maintained EMG decreases and symptom improvements at follow-up.
Keefe et al (1981)	18	Rheumatoid arthritis	1. EMG biofeedback progressive relax., transfer training with 30 one-minute repetitions/day	1 gr pre-post continuous measurement	EMG: decrease (S) within and between sessions, pain: decrease (S) within sessions, tension: decrease (S) within and between sessions. At 1 yr follow-up, pain NS, 56% of patients "improved."
Casas et al (1982)	16	Bruxism (temporomandibular joint)	1. Stress reduction counselling 2. Contingent nocturnal EMG feedback 3. 1 and 2 4. Waiting-list control	4 gr pre-post	At posttest 1 = 2 = 3 > 4 (S) improvement. At 2 mo follow-up symptoms (pain, grinding) were decreased for: 1. 3 of 4 pts 2. 3 of 4 pts 3. 2 of 4 pts 4. 1 of 4 pts

Turner (1982)	36	Low back	1. Waiting-list control 2. Progressive relaxation 1/day 3. Cognitive-behavioral: goals, relaxation, imagery, identifying cognitions, self-statements	3 gr pre-post	2 and 3 had improved pain (S), depression scores (S) and disability (S). 2, 3 > 1 (S) sickness impact profile, pain. Self-ratings abilities, goals 3 > 2 (S). At 1½ yr follow-up both 2 and 3 had reduced health-care use and 3 spent more time working.
Flor et al. (1983)	18	Rheumatoid arthritis	1. EMG BF (relevant muscles) + cognitive + home practice coupled to pain cues. 2. Pseudofeedback 3. WLC	3 gr pre-post	Pain: 1 > 2, 3 (S) intensity and duration. McGill sensory (NS), affective 1 > 2, 3 (S), cognition questionnaire: 1 > 2, 3 (S), medication: NS. Dr. Contact: 1 > 3 (S). EMG:?, 1 best reduction
Nouwen (1983)	20	Low back	1. EMG biofeedback 2. Waiting-list control	2 gr pre-post	EMG: 1 decrease (S), 2 NS pain: NS
Linton & Melin (1983)	17	Low back	1. Waiting list control 2. Rehabilitation treatment 3. 2 + applied relaxation	3 gr pre-post	Pain: 3 > 1 (S) (3 = 28% decrease), medication: 3 > 1 (S) (2 not applicable), activity test: 3 > 1, 2 (S), 3 > 1, 2 (S) social activities: 3 > 1, 2 (S), evaluation: 3 > 2 (S) satisfaction, activity.
McCauley et al. (1983)	17	Low back	1. Relaxation 2. Self-hypnosis	2 gr pre-post with placebo control	1 and 2 improved significantly compared to pretest and placebo on variables of pain, medicine intake, depression, sleep and quality of life. 1 > 2 (S) at follow-up for pain intensity.
Linton & Götestam (1984)		See Table II			
Linton et al. (1985)		See Table II			
Moore & Chaney (1985)	43	"Chronic" mainly back	1. Cognitive behavioral (relaxation, operant, goals, problem solving, cognitive strategies) in couples 2. Cognitive-behavioral (as above) individual 3. Waiting-list control	3 gr pre-post	1 = 2 > 3 (S) for pain intensity, pain beh., somatization and psychosocial adjustment. 2 > 3 (S) merital satisfaction and sickness impact profile. Pains maintained at 3 and 7 mos.

Sanders reported progressive relaxation to be the most important component in his comparative study, while Turner found progressive relaxation to be better than no treatment but not statistically better than a coping strategy based on relaxation and cognitive techniques. Intensive progressive relaxation training also has been compared with self-hypnosis (McCauley, Thelen, Frank, Willard, & Callen, 1983). However, in comparison to pre-test and placebo control conditions the only significant difference between the groups was that the relaxation group had significantly greater improvements on the variable of pain intensity reports than the hypnosis group at follow-up.

Applied relaxation has been used as a coping strategy in three studies. This type of relaxation training differs from progressive relaxation primarily in that patients are taught to relax very quickly and in a wide variety of situations so that they may *apply* the relaxation to control pain and anxiety in everyday situations (Linton, 1982b). In particular, patients are taught to identify bodily and environmental signals "warning" them that a pain problem is approaching. Next, patients are taught how to apply relaxation as soon as they discriminate a warning signal. Consequently, the technique is designed to prevent new attacks of pain or a worsening of the pain condition. Linton and Melin (1983) added applied relaxation to a dayward program and compared it to the ward's regular rehabilitation treatment and a waiting-list control. The group receiving applied relaxation in addition to the traditional rehabilitation program had the largest improvements on the variables of pain reports and medication intake and these improvements were significantly greater than the waiting list control. Furthermore, the applied relaxation group had significantly greater improvements than both the rehabilitation treatment control and the waiting list control on an activity test and for participation in social activities.

A continuation of this research examined the utility of applied relaxation as compared to a waiting-list control and a group receiving applied relaxation plus a concentrated operant (Fordyce, 1976) program (Linton & Götestam, 1984). Both of the treatment groups were found to have substantial and statistically significant improvements on a wide range of variables in comparison to the waiting-list control and baseline levels. Few specific differences between the two active treatment programs were noted; however, the applied relaxation (only) group tended to have better results on pain ratings while the group receiving applied relaxation and the operant program had quicker and at posttest larger improvements on the variables of medicine consumption and activity.

A third study attempted to combine the most potent aspects of the applied relaxation and operant approach (Linton et al., 1985). The experimental group received training in applied relaxation plus an operant activities program especially designed for outpatients. This behavior therapy group was compared to a waiting-list control and a group receiving the regular clinical treatment at the rehabilitation center. The results indicated that the behavior therapy group had superior results on the variables of pain reports, activities of daily living, medication consumption, and sleep and these differences were statistically significant.

In summary, these studies show that applied relaxation by itself or in combination with other treatment techniques was consistently associated with substantial treatment gains. Taken together these data support the proposition that applied relaxation can be useful in the remediation of chronic pain.

The remaining studies shown in Table 10.3 describe various other cognitive–behavioral methods for dealing with chronic pain. A couple of these studies deserve special mention. Turner (1982) conducted a well-controlled study comparing progressive relaxation with a coping strategy approach based on relaxation and cognitive strategies. A group waiting for treatment served as a control group. Few specific differences between the active treatment groups were found, although both resulted in significant improvements compared to the waiting list control. The evidence did suggest a tendency for the relaxation plus cognitive methods group to produce the best results. Moore and Chaney (1985) have looked at the effects of an outpatient cognitive behavioral program with respect to the involvement of the patient's spouse. They employed a multicomponent treatment program including education, progressive relaxation, a discussion of operant components, rational thinking, and cognitive methods such as distraction and reinterpretation. Although compliance may have been a problem in the study, it was found that the 16-hour cognitive-behavioral program produced reductions in pain, spasms, observed pain behavior, physical and psychosocial dysfunction, and utilization of health care. In particular, it was found that spouse involvement did not facilitate response to treatment on any of the variables.

Other recent studies of a controlled nature demonstrate the potential effectiveness of the combination of cognitive and behavioral methods (Kerns, Turk, Rudy, & Holzman, 1986; Philips, 1987). Moreover, Corey, Etlin, and Miller (1987) have demonstrated the possible importance for generalization of conducting the treatment in the patient's home environment.

RECAPITULATION OF THE TREATMENT RESULTS

The data reported over the past years provides clear evidence for the utility of some behavioral pain remediation techniques. The studies included in this review as well as in other reviews (e.g., Bradley, 1983; Linton, 1982a, 1986; Turk, Meichenbaum, & Genest, 1983; Turner & Chapman, 1982) have reported very positive outcomes. Nevertheless, earlier reviews have noted that methodological inadequacies limited the conclusions that could be drawn from the studies. The use of controlled studies with appropriate assessment methods has recently allowed us to draw more decisive conclusions. All of the studies included in this chapter are, for example, prospective, controlled studies. Based on these studies one may say that the operant package as developed by Fordyce has accumulated very strong evidence indicating that the main activity and medication techniques are indeed effective. While the operant approach has had a more difficult time showing that overt pain communication behaviors (such as pain talk, rubbing, grimacing) are reduced, there is currently some evidence showing this. Improvements in pain intensity ratings are usually moderate in size but consistently found. However, firm conclusion concerning pain ratings cannot yet confidently be made given the limited number of studies which reported pain rating decreases and which used proper pain intensity rating methods.

The relaxation and cognitive behavioral therapies continue to be widely used. Biofeedback studies reported mixed results and there are considerable questions regarding whether EMG tension levels are related to pain intensity ratings. Therefore limited support is found for biofeedback's efficacy. Relaxation training has accumulated a good deal more evidence supporting its usefulness. The controlled studies consistently showed meaningful and statistically significant reductions in pain reports and these improvements were accompanied by reasonable improvements in other areas such as activity level, mood, and medicine consumption. Using relaxation as a part of a coping strategy seems to be more effective than employing static training.

We find then that the operant and relaxation approaches are most effective in changing those behaviors towards which they are oriented. The operant program affects activity levels and medicine use mainly, while relaxation therapies work best with subjective pain ratings.

A number of comparative studies has been conducted and these are marked with an asterisk in Tables 10.2 and 10.3. In general, the comparative studies show that behavioral methods are superior to other types of rehabilitation techniques. Among the studies comparing various behavioral techniques there is some indication that the addition of various behavioral components does not result in significantly better results than relaxation therapy in itself. This is important since the complexity of treatment seems to be related to adherence.

Linton (1986) has reviewed the literature concerning how well patients adhere to training programs, for example, relaxing or physical exercises after the conclusion of treatment. Data were available from seven studies where one could determine the prescribed home practice and where follow-up results included measures of how often patients practiced these exercises. The method of evaluating the adherence results was generally rather global estimates or rating questionnaires. Nevertheless, the results indicate that patients do continue to practice exercises such as relaxation or activity training, but they do so at a substantially lower frequency than prescribed. For instance, Keefe et al. (1981) prescribed relaxation to be done two times per day with one minute repetitions 20–30 times per day, but they found at follow-up that patients on the average practiced their relaxation 1.37 times per day and did the one-minute repetitions only about four times per day.

With regard to treatment complexity Lutz, Silbert, and Ohlson (1983) found a clear relationship between the number of components (exercises) prescribed and the adherence rate. If, for instance, four exercises were prescribed (physical therapy exercises, relaxation, body mechanics, and a walk once per day) the adherence rate was only 7 percent whereas the highest adherence rate for an individual task was 50 percent. Consequently, questions of adherence are extremely important and there seems to be a clear relationship between the number of components prescribed and adherence. It is therefore necessary to investigate further the utility of broad-ranged programs which employ a large number of components. It may well be the case that while broad-based treatments are to be advocated, the use of unnecessary components should be strictly avoided. Furthermore, since a number of patients may not continue to practice their exercises (or practice them more infrequently than recommended) one needs to take this into consideration when designing, developing, and evaluating treatment programs.

PREVENTION

Although the above management techniques have been shown to result in meaningful and statistically significant improvements, patients seldom return to their prepain levels of pain experience, work, and activity. Apparently, remediation techniques help a patient to control the syndrome, but they do not rid the patient of the problem entirely. Even the best management programs do not result in all patients returning to a level of functioning matching their prepain levels. Many patients for example, are unable to hold a full-time job. Follow-up reports in the literature show that only 30–50 percent of such patients are gainfully employed one year after treatment (e.g., Cinciripini & Floreen, 1982; Gottlieb, Alperson, & Koller, 1982; Catchlove & Cohen, 1982). Another example of the limitations of rehabilitation is that reported pain levels are ordinarily decreased substantially but nevertheless far from a pain-free level. This state of affairs is not peculiar to chronic pain; there are many other types of chronic problems such as asthma and diabetes where a return to the preproblem state is virtually impossible. As a result, treatment should probably be oriented toward helping the patient live as normal and productive a life as possible. However, an alternative is to prevent the development of chronic pain. Given the difficulty of rehabilitating pain patients in addition to the high cost for society and the individual, prevention is indeed an attractive proposition.

The course of prevention is ordinarily the identification of risk factors and/or risk groups and a subsequent intervention to alter these factors. Primary preventive measures prevent the problem from occurring in the first place, while secondary ones prevent an acute problem from developing into a chronic one. Management techniques might even be considered to be tertiary prevention since they may prevent side effects and a worsening of the condition. In all cases prevention involves ways of interfering with or disrupting processes of disease or trauma (Kirscht, 1983).

Information about risk factors may be obtained in at least two ways. The first involves discovering relationships through epidemiological studies. For instance, a large group of subjects being exposed to a potential risk factor (e.g., heavy lifts, high levels of stress) may be followed in a prospective manner and compared to a control group which is not exposed to these factors. The incidence of back problems could then be determined for each group and the relative risk for developing back pain if exposed to the factor could be determined. As we shall see below, there have been considerable difficulties in producing clear results to date using these epidemiological methods. A second method, which is ordinarily used to generate ideas concerning potential risk factors that may subsequently be studied in epidemiological research, is to look at presumed relationships according to a particular theory. In the case of chronic pain, a behavioral view of the development of the problem provides many insights into potential risk factors. Let us briefly examine the literature concerning the isolation of risk factors for chronic pain. This discussion is restricted almost exclusively to back pain problems.

Risk Factors

Risk factors for the development of back problems involve three categories:

Individual factors. Considerable effort has been expended on identifying individual factors related to the onset or development of pain in the musculoskeletal system. However, most of these variables are extremely difficult or impossible to manipulate so they are therefore of minimal interest in prevention programs. Nevertheless, it is informative to review briefly the variables examined.

Anthropomorphic variables such as age, sex, height, weight, and posture have all been examined. Although age is related to degenerative processes and posture may be related to deformities, the evidence associating these factors to a higher frequency of back pain is inconsistent (e.g., Andersson, 1981). Any observed differences in relation to sex are colored by cultural aspects where men and women with the same degree of symptoms may be treated differently. For instance, men may be given surgical treatments more often than women, or men may be forced to apply for medical help more often than women since they may be engaged in work outside of the home and/or in work that is physically demanding more often than women. Nevertheless, the ratio of men to women undergoing rehabilitation programs for chronic pain is often reported to be two to three (Humphrey, 1980).

Muscle strength has been postulated to be an important variable in the development of back pain (e.g., Kraus, 1965). The proposition has been that decreased strength in the abdominal and back muscles makes one more susceptible to the development of pain. A review of the literature has shown that back pain patients generally have only very marginal reductions in muscle strength (Hansson, 1989). The evidence however, is contradictory. One line of research has compared groups of chronic suffers with healthy controls. The problem is knowing whether any observed differences are a result or a cause of the back pain. Furthermore, such studies have produced mixed results (Andersson, 1981; ASF, 1976). A recent prospective study found a *positive* correlation between back muscle strength and subsequent pain; that is, greater muscle strength increased the risk for back pain problems (Battié et al., in press). Other researchers have looked at activity levels and participation in sports as a measure of muscle strength. Here the results are more enlightening. Kelsey (1975a, 1975b) found insufficient physical exercise and participation in some sports to be associated with back pain. In a correlational study Cady, Bischoff, O'Connell, Thomas, and Allan (1979) examined strength and physical fitness and subsequent back injuries in firefighters. They found correlations that indicated a relationship between physical fitness and back injuries. This is also consistent with research indicating that exercise is related to the maintenance of health (Breslow, 1978).

However, it is not known whether exercise has an effect because it strengthens muscles or whether it has other effects. Exercising seems to release endorphines and serves as a buffer against depression, both of which can affect pain perception. Moreover, programs aimed at increasing muscle strength have had difficulty in demonstrating a decreased rate of back problems (e.g., Dehlin, Berg, Andersson, & Grimby, 1981; Schwartz, DeGood, Mohr, Bauerle, & Rowlingson, 1984). It appears that muscle strength in itself may not be as important as participation in moderate, regularly scheduled exercise.

Psychosocial factors have also been found to be related to the development of back problems. One serious problem in this area however, is the interdependence of the variables under study. It is difficult as a result, to isolate causal factors. An association between limited education, low income and low back pain has emerged from several studies (e.g., Beals & Hickman, 1972; Finneson & Freese, 1975; Gentry, Shows, & Thomas, 1974). Marital status, family problems, and social support have also been shown to be related to problems with musculoskeletal pain. There is a general consensus that pain patients have more marital disharmony, divorce, and family problems (Andersson, 1981; Biering-Sörensen, Bendix, & Vinterberg, 1980; Humphrey, 1980). The question remains as to whether these problems are a result or a cause of pain development. On the other hand, a relatively stable and cohesive social environment (social support) has consistently appeared as an important contribution to health in general (Winefield, 1984). Just as with exercising, social support may serve as a buffer and thereby protect persons from pain problems.

Another aspect of the family is the influence it may have on developing patterns of response to sickness. Family members might, for instance, serve as models for how one should react and may set the stage for "illness behavior." Craig (1978) has examined social modeling's influence on pain and concludes that it is substantial. Several authors, moreover, have noted that the prevalence of pain problems is higher among patients who have a family member with pain problems in comparison to patients who have not had such familial dynamics

(Crook, Rideout, & Browne, 1984; Mohamed, Weisz, & Waving, 1978; Violon & Guijea, 1984). Turkat and his associates (Turkat, 1982; Turkat & Noskin, 1983) reported that individuals who had a parental model who avoided work when ill reported more avoidance of responsibility when ill than did individuals without such parental models.

Personality characteristics have long been thought to be associated with pain problems. However, since pain of the back or extremities affects approximately 80 percent of the population it is exceedingly difficult to define a personality profile. On the other hand, many attempts have been made to isolate personality factors which may be associated with the development of chronic pain problems or which may serve as prognostic indicators. Detailed reviews of the area are available elsewhere (e.g., Humphrey, 1980; Sanders, 1979; Turk et al., 1983). The general conclusion from such reviews is that personality assessments may consistently find patterns such as high anxiety levels and depressive symptoms but that no personality profile can be isolated. The use of personality variables might be warranted in predicting response to medical or surgical treatment, but there is no evidence to date showing that it is useful in isolating risk groups.

Ergonomical work environment. Several articles have reviewed factors in the work place thought to be associated with the incidence of pain in the musculoskeletal system (Anderson, 1980; Andersson, 1981; Nachemson, 1982; Biering-Sörensen, 1983). A vast literature is reviewed in these articles and there is some agreement that six different factors are well-established risks for the development of acute pain. These are: heavy work, static work, bending or twisting, lifting, repetitive work, and exposure to vibrations. The interpretation of the data is complicated by the fact that there may be two processes which result in the development of acute pain. The first, and most often assumed process, is that work factors result in an acute trauma. This would be observed in the sudden onset of acute pain while working and may often be related to an accident, However, another possibility exists. This concerns long-term exposures which may result in pain and these may be referred to as "wear and tear" factors. Unlike major traumatic events, these factors may result in very minor but frequent trauma that, in the long run, can result in structural damage. As a result, the onset of the pain need not be sudden nor need to occur at the work place. Nevertheless, wear-and-tear factors might be related to pain which has an insidious onset or which has an onset outside of the work place.

The exact role the work environment plays in the onset of acute pain has not yet been established. Although the work environment may obviously be involved, it has also been found that the onset of more than half of the incidences of back pain occurred outside of the job situation (e.g., Buckle, Kember, Wood, & Wood, 1980; Stubbs, Rivers, Hudson, & Worringham, 1981). Another question is how often musculoskeletal pain is incurred via an accident at the work place. Statistics are available from several studies and they vary from 4 to 19 percent (ASF, 1976; Braitwaite, 1970). However, even if the onset of back pain does not occur at work, the pain still has considerable consequences for a person's ability to work. Among other things, substantial numbers of workers must adjust their work routines because of the pain (Biering-Sörensen, 1984; Gannik & Jespersen, 1980).

Despite the air of agreement, there are difficulties in untangling the relationship between work factors and the development of musculoskeletal pain problems. In particular, one seldom has the chance to examine a single factor since most variables are related to and confounded by other factors. Wood and Badley (1980) have pointed out difficulties in the research concerning occupational effects on the development of back pain and have consequently questioned the conclusions drawn. Their main criticism is that much of the published work seems to have sought evidence consistent with the authors' preconceived notions. In other words, the authors, according to Wood and Badley, were trying to verify certain relationships and this could well lead to distortions and oversimplifications. The most important is selection of the data where inconsistencies are glossed over and data which are consistent with the hypotheses highlighted. One example of this may be the reporting and interpretation of differences in morbidity rates between occupational groups. While the difference in absences due to back disorders between heavy and light industry is a striking and often cited statistic, Wood and Badley underscore a number of inconsistencies which they maintain are equally impressive. Most research in this area has been based on classification of patients by occupation rather than on representative samples of the population at large. This can lead to false impressions since, in addition to different levels of physical exposure, each occupation has its own distinct culture which may confound results. Furthermore, Wood and Badley point out that while supposed factors in the work environment causing back pain have been improved, we have witnessed a great increase in the number of persons suffering from back problems.

It is not an easy task to pinpoint which factors cause pain. As an illustration, Damkot and associates (Damkot, Pope, Lord, & Frymorer, 1984) used multivariate analysis to assess combinations of risk factors for the development of low back pain in men. Data were obtained for 150 variables including work history and work environment. The regression analysis which best discriminated between groups of men with or without pain problems explained only 27 percent of the variance. Although this is a significant amount of the variance representing factors that should be taken into account in prevention programs, more than 70 percent of the variance was attributable to factors other than those 150 used in the study. Finally, it should be remembered that the relationships found in such epidemiological studies are correlational rather than causal.

Psychosocial work environment. The identification of work-related psychosocial risk factors is even more difficult than identifying ergonomical ones, since an additional problem, subjective measurements, is encountered. Nevertheless, there is an increasing awareness that the problem of musculoskeletal pain may be better understood when such variables are considered. Indeed, it might be postulated that such factors are necessary if the onset and development of pain problems are to be understood.

There are several studies where the relationship between pain problems and the psychosocial work environment have been investigated. Usually, questionnaires have been used which ask participants about possible pain problems as well as their experienced work environment. These studies have almost always been of a correlational nature. Consequently, causal interpretations may not be made. Rather than psychosocial factors causing pain problems, pain might, in fact, color perceptions of the work environment.

Despite the above-mentioned methodological problems, research has generated several risk factors. The most important are:

- *job satisfaction*
- *work content*
- *social support*
- *work load*
- *overall combination of above*

With regard to satisfaction, Vällfors (1985), for example, has found that patients without back pain are more satisfied with their work than those with back pain. Interestingly, in a study of 21 people never having suffered back pain, one of the most striking results was their having very high levels of job satisfaction (Hultman, 1987).

A study of 23,000 workers illustrates the possible importance of the psychosocial work environment (Linton, 1990). Routine questionnaire data collected at occupational health-care centers were used to examine the relationship between experienced psychosocial and ergonomical variables, and musculoskeletal pain. Results demonstrated that an overall "poor" psychosocial work environment increased the risk for pain as much as three times. The most important aspects were work content and social support. Moreover, when a "poor" psychosocial environment was combined with ergonomical risk factors, such as heavy lifts, uncomfortable postures, or monotonous work, the effect was additive producing the highest relative risks.

The psychosocial work environment appears then to be important. In particular, social aspects of work, content, and satisfaction seem to be critical possibly to both the onset and development of pain problems. A good deal more information is needed, however, since the current investigations are hampered by methodological shortcomings.

A BEHAVIORAL MODEL

A short review of risk factors has been provided above. Although the work to date has isolated some factors, the puzzle of the development of pain problems is far from solved. In this section another approach will be looked at, namely, a behavioral perspective. By scrutinizing the development as explained by a behavioral model, it should be possible to generate ideas concerning prevention. In point of fact, a number of ideas about secondary prevention have already been put forward in the literature. A distinction also will be made between factors which can *result in an acute trauma* and in factors which can contribute to the *development of sick behavior*. There is no exact boundary discriminating primary from secondary prevention and in the literature there is considerable confusion concerning this. It is not possible, for example, to classify techniques since many of them are used as both primary and secondary preventive measures.

Consequently, the division below is not a strict one, but it does reflect the way in which the various methods are most often used currently. It also provides some needed structure in an area often marked by confusion. Since the literature has dealt exclusively with secondary prevention, let us examine it first.

Secondary Prevention

As pointed out above, the classification of secondary preventive measures is somewhat arbitrary. The timing of the intervention is often the variable discriminating between secondary and primary prevention rather than the actual content of the intervention.

The essential element of a behavioral view of secondary prevention is an understanding that the chronification of pain involves a developmental learning process whereby sick behaviors and a passive lifestyle are systematically reinforced. The process is rather circular and tends to produce negative side effects that complicate rehabilitation, for example, anxiety, depression, economic, and family problems. Prevention is consequently based on reinforcing well rather than sick behaviors and in trying to maintain "normal" sources of reinforcement in addition to providing various methods for controlling experienced pain. This should stop the gradual isolation and pacification of the patient which earmarks the chronification process, as well as prohibiting the development of negative side effects.

Prevention Programs

In this section a number of programs already in use will be described.

Low back schools. Developed by physical therapists as an information program, low back schools are designed as primary prevention. However, in practice the program is most often used as a secondary measure for sufferers. The program ordinarily involves information concerning the physiology of the musculoskeletal system, pain, and body mechanics. In addition, it contains information about applying this knowledge in everyday situations such as when lifting or doing household work. A recent review shows, however, that low back schools seem to have little or no effect on variables such as sick leave, treatment contacts, work status, pain intensity, activity levels, or medicine consumption (Linton & Kamwendo, 1987). On the other hand, the schools might result in changes in information level as well as in self-care behavior, but these variables have not been adequately tested. As a result, low back schools or some form of them might be considered in prevention programs in order to start important changes concerning information and self-care behaviors. However, it is important to point out that these programs need to be evaluated and that further measures are most likely needed to insure that changes in target behaviours actually occur.

Activation—return to work. A key concept in preventing the development of a pain problem from the acute to the chronic stage is activation. This involves limiting sick absences to prevent the development of a passive lifestyle. If the patient's condition should require that he or she be off from work for more than a week or two, then organized activity might be prescribed by the doctor. Furthermore, such programs could be based on "return-to-work" goal setting. There is some evidence to suggest that activation and direct job re-entry are more effective, at least for chronic pain patients, than more passive methods aimed at traditional rehabilitation (e.g., Catchlove & Cohen, 1982). Activation then involves physical training and above all the systematic application of health care so that active rather than "pain" behaviors are reinforced. This would also prevent the development of phobic-like avoidance of certain activities.

A recent development is the so-called "work hardening" programs which aim to restore work function. Those patients suffering recent onset of back pain are offered extensive physical and psychological treatments within the first 4 to 24 months of injury. A model program has been developed by Mayer and his associates (Mayer et al., 1985). They provided a comprehensive early rehabilitation program (more than 4 months since injury) 57 hours/week for 3 weeks. Functional restoration consisted of specific exercises where every effort was made to simulate a job experience. In addition, cognitive-behavioral techniques such as relaxation, coping, assertiveness, and family management were used. A two-year follow-up has shown impressive results (Mayer, Gatchel, Mayer, Kishino, Keeley, & Mooney, 1987). Of 116 patients undergoing treatment, 87% were actively working at follow-up compared to 41% in the reference group. Moreover, the reference group had more surgeries, health-care visits, and reinjuries than the treatment group. These results were striking, but need to be interpreted with some caution since the design employed is limited by the fact that subjects were not randomly assigned to the groups.

A somewhat different approach is to prevent back pain problems before they result in long absences from work. Linton, Bradley, Jensen, Spangfort, and Sundell (1989) conducted a controlled study which compared a physical and behavioral secondary prevention program with a waiting-list control group. Subjects were LPNs or nursing aides having a history of back trouble, but who were currently working. In a 40 hour/week, 5-week program, subjects participated in physical therapy aimed at improving physical condition and body mechanics as well as behavior therapy oriented towards coping and maintaining healthy behaviors. Results indicated that the treatment group had significantly greater improvements than the control group on pain intensity, anxiety, sleep quality and fatigue ratings, observed pain behavior, activities, mood, and helplessness. These differences were maintained at a 6-month follow-up. The treatment group, furthermore, broke a trend for increasing amounts of pain-related absenteeism. The authors conclude that a secondary prevention program which alters lifestyle factors may be an effective method for dealing with musculoskeletal pain problems.

A fairly simple, behavioral prevention program which tests some of the theoretical underpinnings of the behavioral approach has been evaluated by Fordyce, Brockway, Bergman, and Spengler (1986). Patients with acute back pain onset within the preceeding 10 days were studied. Traditional management methods (interventions based on pain) were compared with the behavioral approach where interventions were based on a time contingency. According to behavioral theory, a time contingency arrangement would reduce reinforcement of pain behaviors and thereby the frequency of such behaviors. In the behavioral group, any analgesics given were to be taken on a fixed time basis and the prescription was not renewable. Similarly, activity limits were "time-specified" and exercises were often prescribed on a fixed-time, fixed-number basis. In comparison, patients in the traditional group received analgesics as needed and participated in activities according to their pain experience. Patients in both groups were followed over the course of one year. Results showed that the behaviorally treated group tended to return to prepain onset levels of functioning, while the group treated traditionally showed significant increases in pain and claimed impairment. This study provides solid evidence that behavioral secondary prevention can be effective and it also provides support for the behavioral view of the development of chronic pain.

Another attempt at a comprehensive prevention program for patients with low back pain has been conducted in Gothenburg, Sweden (Chöler et al., 1985). Patients being sick-listed for back pain in Gothenburg were first studied in order to obtain control data concerning the length of sick absenteeism. Then, the traditional or regular treatment available from a general practitioner was compared to a special back pain clinic. The back clinic was organized so that general practitioners could refer patients with back problems of a duration greater than two weeks. After the referral, the patient was seen very quickly and given a thorough examination by an orthopedic surgeon. The patient was given specific information about his or her back problem and concrete advice concerning the treatment and prognosis. Treatment techniques included the low back school, traction, corsettes, technical aid, medicines, physical therapy, muscle strength training, TNS, relaxation, work place visits, and so on. The basic idea was to provide patients, at an early point in time, with a good back examination, and thorough and realistic information about the course of the problem. The information underscored the importance of self-care and back hygiene. Activation of the patient was also an important aspect and a return to work was discussed and planned for already at the first visit.

Ninety percent of the patients receiving care at the back pain clinic had positive opinions concerning their experience. Moreover, the patients receiving care at the back pain clinic had substantially shorter periods of being sick-listed as compared to a group receiving regular outpatient care. After 15 weeks all of the patients receiving care at the back clinic were back at work whereas nearly 20 percent of the general practitioners' patients remained on the sick list. In the preliminary report now available, however, these differences have not been tested for statistical significance. Another point is that since sick-listing certificates are made out by doctors, a bias in filling out the certificates might have occurred in the back pain clinic. Nevertheless, these data provide promise for the secondary prevention of chronic pain.

Primary Prevention

Problems in identifying risk factors have hindered the development of behavioral primary prevention programs. Nonetheless, there is reason to believe that behavior is important in the development of an acute injury. If one studies the six work place factors related to back injuries described earlier, it will be seen that all six are related to behavior and that at least three are behaviors. As an illustration, lifting, bending, twisting, and repetitive tasks are all believed to result in muscle loading on certain muscles in the back. Correct posture and work technique might reduce some of this loading, but changes in work routines to counteract this loading seem most relevant. This could involve learning new routines and/or the taking of short pauses where one might relax. Health promotion in the form of increased physical activity would also be relevant as an "insulation" factor. The combination of exercising, increased mobility at work, and engaging in frequent relaxation pauses could well result in a substantial lowering of physical muscle loading as well as in stress which also may contribute to muscle tension.

Health promotion may also be important in influencing the perception of pain. For instance, at a very early stage in the development of pain problems some people will be "complainers" while others will cope in more appropriate ways. Health promotion initiatives might teach people how to recognize and cope with such problems while they are still minor. Complaining—as opposed to engaging in alternate coping strategies—is also probably influenced by such things as work organization and job satisfaction which might also be dealt with in health promotion programs.

In short, acute trauma often seems to be related to long-term work patterns which place heavy loads on certain muscles. These muscles are tense and may easily be injured. By changing work routines one might prevent such tension and the consequent risk for injury. In addition, by providing for stress management one might reduce further muscle tension and also influence the perception of pain and the likelihood of complaint.

Pauses. An approach to primary prevention based on work physiology and relaxation is the use of pauses. These pauses may vary considerably but ordinarily they are short (micro = 2 seconds or less) rest periods where the participant may engage in exercises, or simply rest (Hagberg, ASF, 1982). The idea was generated from laboratory studies where it has been shown that a muscle's ability to do work, as seen in tolerance times, increases significantly if small pauses are interspersed with work (Hagberg, 1981). It is therefore believed that pauses could interrupt the muscle-tension-pain cycle and reduce overall muscle tension loads caused by work.

However, only a few studies have been conducted concerning pauses in the work place. Laporte (1966) looked at the influence of a gymnastic pause on post office workers. It was shown that those engaging in a single gymnastic pause had better scores on hand steadiness, general fatigue, and fatigue of the eyes and muscle strength after the pause in comparison to before. The study obviously suffers from a number of problems including the lack of a control condition, specification of rest content, and physiological measures.

Since relaxation training should result directly in reduced muscle tension as well as indirectly via stress reduction, the effects of relaxation gymnastics on neck and shoulder discomfort have been evaluated (Linton & Kamwendo, 1986). In this study, an ABAB design was used where one component involved working without relaxation gymnastics and the other involved working *with* relaxation gymnastics. Results were evaluated in terms of subjective ratings of discomfort, fatigue, functional impairment at work, and experienced stress. Seventeen subjects made these ratings five times per day so that the development of a problem during the course of the day could be evaluated. Indeed, the results showed no difference between the conditions during the early morning. However, small but statistically significant improvements in subjective discomfort and fatigue were recorded during the afternoons demonstrating the utility of relaxation gymnastics. One problem was the negative effect of disrupting work routines in order to participate which caused difficulties in maintaining adherence.

Although, at least in the Scandinavian countries, the use of pauses is widespread, there are too few studies with too poor designs and measurement techniques to draw any firm conclusions. Nevertheless, the use of pauses and relaxation gymnastics points to a simple method which may be worthwhile in the prevention of musculoskeletal pain problems.

CONCLUSIONS CONCERNING PREVENTION

In a word, a number of meritorious proposals for the prevention of chronic pain have been put forth. To date, these proposals have not been adequately tested. This is, in part, due to the fact that prevention is a relatively new area of interest and in part to the great practical and methodological problems in conducting research in this area. Just to illustrate this point, it may be observed that to evaluate primary prevention programs very large groups of subjects will be required (since only a few persons would be expected to develop *acute* musculoskeletal problems during, say, a one-year period). And, these subjects would have to be followed for a considerable period of time. Despite the problems, several attempts have been made to evaluate, above all, secondary prevention programs and as noted above some of these attempts were admirable in terms of the methodology used. Taken together, the product of these studies is certainly encouraging even if it is entirely too early to determine the utility of any of these programs. The data certainly warrant continued use and exploration of these techniques.

OVERALL RECAPITULATION

There is no doubt that chronic pain is a problem of major proportions. Although chronic pain has been refractory to traditional medical treatments, there is considerable evidence that behavioral methods are useful in the management of these problems. Operant and relaxation methods have been shown in several controlled studies to be effective in increasing activity levels, decreasing medication consumption, and pain intensity ratings. A number of other benefits also have been noted such as decreased depression, improved sleep, decreased anxiety, and so on.

On the other hand, the management of chronic pain problems seldom results in returning the patient to prepain levels of functioning. Management methods are, moreover, time-consuming and expensive. Consequently, the prevention of chronic pain is not only extremely important for humanitarian reasons, it is also quite attractive in socioeconomic terms.

Our knowledge about prevention programs is quite limited. However, behavior theory points to several avenues of prevention and the first studies appearing demonstrate great potential. Since behavior and lifestyle are key elements in the chronification of pain, behavioral methods appear to be applicable and probably necessary for the development of successful interventions. Despite the complexities of developing and testing preventive measures, it is concluded that the potential benefits are well worth the endeavor.

REFERENCES

Andersson, G. B. J. (1981). Epidemiological aspects on low-back pain in industry. *Spine, 6,* 53–60.

Anderson, J. A. D. (1980). Back pain and occupation. In M. I. V. Jayson (Ed.), *The Lumbar Spine* (pp. 57–82). Kent (England): Pitman Medical.

Arbetarskyddsfonden (ASF). (1976). *Ryggskador i arbetslivet: Kartläggning och analys av forskningsbehov (Back injuries at work).* Stockholm: Liber Tryck.

Aronoff, G. M., Evans, W. O., & Enders, P. L. (1983). A review of follow-up studies of multidisciplinary pain units. *Pain, 16,* 1–11.

Battié, M. C., Bigos, S. J., Fisher, L., Hansson, T. H., Jones, M. E. & Wortley, M. D. (in press). Isometric lifting strength as a predictor of industrial back pain complaints. *Spine.*

Beals, R., Hickman, N. (1972). Industrial injuries of the back and extremities. *The Journal of Bone and Joint Surgery, 54-A,* 1593–1611.

Biering-Sörensen, F. (1984). *A one-year prospective study of low back trouble in a general population.* Copenhagen: Laegeforeningens Forlag.

Biering-Sörensen, F., Bendix, T., & Vinterberg, H. (1980). Rygbesvaer—ikke arbejdsrelaterade risikofaktorer og profylakse. *Nordisk Medicin, 95,* 236–238.

Bradley, L. A. (1983). Coping with chronic pain. In T. G. Burish & L. A. Bradley (Eds.), *Coping with chronic disease: Research and application* (pp. 334–379). New York: Academic Press.

Braithwaite, G. H. (1970). *The pattern and cost of back injuries: I. Back injuries at work.* Auckland: The New Zealand Institute of Industrial Safety.

Breslow, L. (1978). Risk factor intervention for health maintenance. *Science, 200,* 908–912.

Buckle, P. W., Kember, P. A., Wood, A. B., & Wood, S. N. (1980). Factors influencing occupational back pain in Bedfordshire. *Spine, 5,* 254–258.

Cady, L. D., Bischoff, D. P., O'Connell, E. R., Thomas, P. C., & Allan, J. H. (1979). Strength and fitness and subsequent back injuries in firefighters. *Journal of Occupational Medicine, 21,* 269–272.

Cairns, D., & Pasino, J. (1977). Comparison of verbal reinforcement and feedback in the operant treatment of disability due to chronic low back pain. *Behavior Therapy, 8,* 621–630.

Casas, J., Beemsterboer, P., & Clark, G. (1982). A comparison of stress-reduction behavioural counseling and contingent nocturnal EMG feedback for the treatment of bruxism. *Behaviour Research and Therapy, 20,* 9–15.

Catchlove, R., & Cohen, K. (1982). Effects of a directive return to work approach in the treatment of workman's compensation patients with chronic pain. *Pain, 14,* 181–191.

Chöler, V., Larsson, R., Nachemson, A., & Peterson, L. E. (1985). *Ont i ryggen: försök med vårdprogram för patienter med lumbala smärttillståd* [Back Pain: An attempt at early intervention with low back pain patients]. Stockholm: Sjukvårdens och socialvårdens planerings—och rationaliseringsinstitut (SPRI).

Cinciripini, P. M., & Floreen, A. (1982). An evaluation of a behavioral program for chronic pain. *Journal of Behavioral Medicine, 5,* 375–389.

Cory, D. T., Etlin, D., & Miller, P. C. (1987). A home-based pain management and rehabilitation program: An evaluation. *Pain, 29,* 219–230.

Craig, K. D. (1978). Social modeling influences on pain. In R. A. Sternbach (Ed.), *The psychology of pain* (pp. 67–96). New York: Raven Press.

Crook, J., Rideout, E., & Browne, G. (1984). The prevalence of pain complaints in a general population. *Pain, 18,* 299–314.

Damkot, D. K., Pope, M. H., Lord, J., & Frymoyer, J. W. (1984). The relationship between work history, work environment and low back pain in men. *Spine, 9,* 395–399.

Dehlin, O., Berg, S., Andersson, G. B. J., & Grimby, G. (1981). Effects of physical training and ergonomic counselling on the psychological perception of work. *Scandinavian Journal of Rehabilitation Medicine, 13,* 1–9.

Dohrmann, R., & Laskin, D. (1978). An evaluation of electromyographic biofeedback in the treatment of myofascial pain-dysfunction syndrome. *Journal of the American Dental Association, 96,* 656–662.

Doleys, D. M., Crocker, M., & Patton, D. (1982). Response of patients with chronic pain to exercise quotas. *Physical Therapy, 62,* 1111–1114.

Ergonomics. (1985, January). [Special issue: Industrial back pain in Europe]. *28.*

Finneson, B., & Freese, A. (1975). *The new approach to low back pain.* New York. Berkley.

Flor, H., Haag, G., Turk, D. C., & Koehler, H. (1983). Efficacy of EMG biofeedback, pseudotherapy, and conventional medical treatment for chronic rheumatic back pain. *Pain, 17,* 21–31.

Follick, M. J., Zitter, R. E., & Ahern, D. K. (1983). Failures in the operant treatment of chronic pain. In E. B. Foa & P. M. G. Emmelkamp (Eds.), *Failures in behavior therapy* (pp. 311–334). New York: Wiley.

Fordyce, W. E. (1976). *Behavioral methods for chronic pain and illness*. St. Louis: C. V. Mosby.

Fordyce, W. E., Brockway, J., Bergman, J. A., & Spengler, D. (1986). Acute back pain: A control group comparison of behavioral vs. traditional management methods. *Journal of Behavioral Medicine, 9,* 127–140.

Fricton, J. R. (1982). Medical evaluation of patients with chronic pain. In J. Barber & C. Adrian (Eds.), *Psychological approaches to the management of pain*. New York: Brunner/Mazel.

Gannik, D., & Jespersen, M. (1980). Rygbesvaer og sygdoms adfaerd (Back trouble and illness behavior). *Nordisk Medicin, 95,* 247–250.

Gentry, W., Shows, W., & Thomas, M. (1974). Chronic low back pain: A psychological profile. *Psychosomatics, 15,* 174–177.

Gottlieb, H. J., Alperson, B. L., & Koller, R. (1982). Low back pain comprehensive rehabilitation proramme: A follow-up study. *Archives of Physical Medicine and Rehabilitation, 63,* 458–561.

Hagberg, M. (1981). Muscular endurance and surface electromyogram in isometric and dynamic exercise. *Journal of Applied Physiology, 5,* 1–7.

Hagberg, M. (1982). *Arbetsrelaterade besvär i halsrygg och skuldra: En kunskapsöversikt* [work related pain in the neck and shoulders]. Stockholm: Arbetarskyddsfonden (rapport 2).

Hansson, T. (1989). *Ländryggsbesvär och arbete* [Low back pain and work: A review]. Stockholm: Work Environment Fund.

Heinrich, R. L., Cohen, M. S., Naliboff, B. D., Collins, G. A., & Bonebakker, A. D. (1985). Comparing physical and behavior therapy for chronic low back pain in physical abilities, psychological distress, and patients perceptions. *Journal of Behavioral Medicine, 8,* 61–78.

Hettinger, T. (1985). Statistics on diseases in the Federal Republic of Germany with particular references to diseases of the skeletal system. *Ergonomics, 28,* 17–20.

Hultman, G. (1987). The healthy back, its environment and characteristics. *Ergonomics, 30,* 295–298.

Humphrey, M. (1980). The problem of low back pain. In S. Rachman (Ed.), *Contributions to medical psychology* (Vol. 2, pp. 131–152). London: Pergamon Press.

Keefe, F. J., Schapira, B., Brown, C., Williams, R. B., & Surwit, R. S. (1981). EMG-assisted relaxation training in the management of chronic low back pain. *American Journal of Clinical Biofeedback, 4,* 93–103.

Kelsey, J. L. (1975a). An epidemiological study of acute herniated lumbar intervertebral discs. *Rheumatology and Rehabilitation, 14,* 144–159.

Kelsey, J. L. (1975b). An epidemiological study of the relationship between occupations and acute herniated lumbar intervertebral discs. *International Journal of Epidemiology, 4,* 197–205.

Kerns, R. D., Turk, D. C., Rudy, T. E., & Holzman, A. D. (1986). Efficacy of cognitive-behavioral group approach for the treatment of chronic pain. *Clinical Journal of Pain, 4,* 195–203.

Kirscht, J. P. (1983). Preventive health behavior: A review of research and issues. *Health Psychology, 2,* 277–301.

Kraft, G. H. (1975). Treatment strategies of operant conditioning in rehabilitation. *Journal of Occupational Medicine, 17,* 658–662.

Kraus, H. (1965). *Backache, stress and tension.* New York: Simon and Schuster.

Laporte, W. (1966). The influence of a gymnastic pause upon recovery following post office work. *Ergonomics, 9,* 501–506.

Linton, S. J. (1982a). A critical review of behavioral treatments for chronic benign pain other than headache. *British Journal of Clinical Psychology, 21,* 321–337.

Linton, S. J. (1982b). Applied relaxation as a method of coping with chronic pain: A therapist's guide. *Scandinavian Journal of Behaviour Therapy, 11,* 161–174.

Linton, S. J. (1986). Behavioral remediation of chronic pain: A status report. *Pain, 24,* 125–141.

Linton, S. J. (1990). Risk factors for neck and back pain in a working population in Sweden. *Work and Stress, 4,* 41–49.

Linton, S. J., Bradley, L. A., Jensen, I., Spangfort, E., & Sundell, L. (1989). The secondary prevention of low back pain: A controlled study with follow-up. *Pain, 36,* 197–207.

Linton, S. J., & Götestam, K. G. (1984). A controlled study of the effects of applied relaxation and applied relaxation plus operant procedures on the regulation of chronic pain. *British Journal of Clinical Psychology, 23,* 291–299.

Linton, S. J., & Götestam, K. G. (1985a). Controlling pain reports through operant conditioning: A laboratory demonstration. *Perceptual and Motor Skills, 60,* 427–437.

Linton, S. J., & Götestam, K. G. (1985b). Relations between pain, anxiety, mood and muscle tension in chronic pain patients. *Psychotherapy and Psychosomatics, 43,* 90–95.

Linton, S. J., & Kamwendo, K. (1987). Low back schools: A critical review. *Physical Therapy, 67,* 1375–1383.

Linton, S. J., & Kamwendo, K. (1986). Relaxation gymnastics as preventive control for neck and shoulder pain: A case study. *Scandinavian Journal of Behavior Therapy, 15,* 39–44.

Linton, S. J., & Melin, L. (1983). Applied relaxation in the management of chronic pain. *Behavioral Psychotherapy, 11,* 337–350.

Linton, S. J., Melin, L., & Götestam, K. G. (1984). Behavioral analysis of chronic pain and its management. In M. Hersen, R. Eisler, & P. Miller (Eds.), *Progress in behavior modification* (Vol. 18, pp. 1–42). New York: Academic Press.

Linton, S. J., Melin, L., & Stjernlöf, K. (1985). The effects of applied relaxation and operant activity training on chronic pain. *Behavioral Psychotherapy, 13,* 87–100.

Lutz, R. W., Silbert, M., & Ohlson, N. (1983). Treatment outcome and compliance with therapeutic regiments: Long-term follow-up of a multidisciplinary pain program. *Pain, 17,* 301–308.

Mayer, T. G., Gatchel, R. J., Kishino, N., Keeley, J., Capra, P., Mayer, H., Barnett, J., & Mooney, V. (1985). Objective assessment of spine function following industrial injury. *Spine, 10,* 482–493.

Mayer, T. G., Gatchel, R. J., Mayer, H., Kishino, N. D., Keeley, J., & Mooney, V. (1987). A prospective two-year study of functional restoration in industrial low back pain. *Journal of the American Medical Association, 258,* 1763–1767.

McCauley, J. P., Thelen, M. H., Frank, R. G., Willard, R. R., & Callen, K. E. (1983). Hypnosis compared to relaxation in the outpatient management of chronic low back pain. *Archives of Physical Medicine and Rehabilitation, 64,* 548–552.

McPhee, B. (1982). Deficiencies in the ergonomic design of keyboard work and upper limb and neck disorders in operators. *Journal of Human Ergology, 11,* 31–36.

Melin, L., & Linton, S. J. (1988). A follow-up study of a comprehensive behavioural treatment programme for chronic pain patients. *Behavioural Psychotherapy, 16,* 313–322.

Melzack, R., & Wall, P. (1965). Pain Mechanisms: A new theory. *Science, 150,* 971–979.

Metzler, F. (1985). Epidemiology and statistics in Luxembourg. *Ergonomics, 28,* 21–24.

Miller, C., & Lelieuvre, R. B. (1982). A method to reduce chronic pain in elderly nursing home residents. *Gerontologist, 22,* 314–317.

Moore, J. E., & Chaney, E. F. (1985). Outpatient group treatment of chronic pain: Effects of spouse involvement. *Journal of Consulting and Clinical Psychology, 53,* 326–334.

Mohamed, S. N., Weisz, G. M., & Waving, E. M. (1978). The relationship of chronic pain to depression, marital adjustment, and family dynamics. *Pain, 5,* 285–292.

Nachemson, A. L. (1983). Work for all: For all those with low back pain as well. *Clinical Orthopedics and Related Research, 179,* 77–85.

Nouwen, A. (1983). EMG biofeedback used to reduce standing levels of paraspinal muscle tension in chronic low back pain. *Pain, 17,* 353–360.

Nouwen, A., & Bush, C. (1984). The relationship between paraspinal EMG and chronic low back pain. *Pain, 20,* 109–123.

Nouwen, A., & Solinger, J. (1979). The effectiveness of EMG biofeedback training in low back pain. *Biofeedback and Self-Regulation, 4,* 103–111.

Pearce, S. (1983). A review of cognitive-behavioral methods for the treatment of chronic pain. *Journal of Psychosomatic Research, 27,* 431–440.

Philips, H. C. (1987). The effects of behavioural treatment on chronic pain. *Behavioural Research and Therapy, 25,* 365–377.

Rachlin, H. (1985). Pain and behavior. *The Behavioral and Brain Sciences, 8,* 43–83.

Rachman, S. J., & Wilson, G. T. (1980). *The effects of psychotherapy* (2nd ed.). New York: Pergamon Press.

Sanders, S. H. (1979). Behavioral assessment and treatment of clinical pain: Appraisal of current status. In M. Hersen, R. Eisler, & P. Miller (Eds.), *Progress in behavior modification* (Vol. 8, pp. 249–291). New York: Academic Press.

Sanders, S. H. (1983). Component analysis of a behavioral treatment program for chronic low-back pain. *Behavior Therapy, 14,* 697–705.

Schwartz, D. P., DeGood, D. E., Mohr, E. M., Bauerle, J. A., & Rowlingson, J. C. (1984). *Can back pain be prevented in hospital employees?* Poster presented at the 4th World Congress on Pain, Seattle, WA. (Abstract p. 262, *Pain,* Suppl. 2, 1984.)

Stenn, P. G., Mothersill, K., & Brooke, R. (1979). Biofeedback and a cognitive behavioral approach to treatment of myofascial pain dysfunction syndrome. *Behavior Therapy, 10,* 29–36.

Stubbs, D. A., Rivers, P. M., Hudson, M. P., & Worringham, C. J. (1981). Back pain research. *Nursing Times, 77,* 857–858.

Tunks, E. (1988). Behavioral interventions and their efficacy. In R. Dobner, G. F. Gebhart, & M. R. Bond (Eds.), *Proceedings of the Vth World congress on Pain.* Amsterdam: Elsevier Science Publications.

Turk, D. C., & Flor, H. (1984). Etiological theories and treatments for chronic back pain. II. Psychological models and interventions. *Pain, 19,* 209–233.

Turk, D. C., Meichenbaum, D., & Genest, M. (1983). *Pain and behavioral medicine: A cognitive-behavioral perspective.* New York: Guilford Press.

Turkat, I. D. (1982). An investigation of parental modeling in the etiology of diabetic illness behavior. *Behavior Research and Therapy, 20,* 547–52.

Turkat, I. D., & Noskin, D. E. (1983). Vicarious and operant experiences in the etiology of illness behavior: A replication with healthy individuals. *Behavior Research and Therapy, 21,* 169–172.

Turner, J. A. (1982). Comparison of group progressive-relaxation training and cognitive behavioral group therapy for chronic low back pain. *Journal of Consulting and Clinical Psychology, 50,* 757–765.

Turner, J. A., & Chapman, C. R. (1982). Psychological interventions for chronic pain: A critical review. I, II. *Pain, 12,* 1–46.

Vällfors, B. (1985). Acute, subacute and chronic low back pain. *Scandinavian Journal of Rehabilitation Medicine,* Suppl. 11.

Violon, A., & Giurgea, D. (1984). Familial models for chronic pain. *Pain, 18,* 199–203.

White, B., & Sanders, S. H. (1985). Differential effects on pain and mood on chronic pain patients with time-versus pain contingent medication delivery. *Behavior Therapy, 16,* 28–38.

Winefield, H. R. (1984). The nature and elicitation of social support. *Behavioral Psychotherapy, 12,* 318–330.

Wood, P. H. N., & Badley, E. M. (1980). Epidemiology of back pain. In M. I. V. Jayson (Ed.), *The lumbar spine and back pain* (pp. 29–55). Kent, England, Pitman.

Zuidema, H. (1985). National statistics in the Netherlands. *Ergonomics, 28,* 3–7.

IV

BEHAVIORAL NEUROLOGY

11

Behavioral Causes and Management of Tension Headaches

Paul R. Martin

Department of Psychology
University of Western Australia

NATURE OF TENSION HEADACHES

A major obstacle to writing a chapter on tension headaches is the confusion surrounding the concept of the disorder. The classic headache classification system (Ad Hoc Committee, 1962) was developed over two decades ago and has been criticized on conceptual and empirical grounds (Martin, 1985). It is still in widespread use today but does not include a category called "tension headache." One category is labeled "muscle contraction headache," however, and the statement is made that "the ambiguous and unsatisfactory terms 'tension,' 'psychogenic' and 'nervous' headache refer largely to this group" (Ad Hoc Committee, 1962, p. 717). Muscle contraction headaches are defined as "ache or sensations of tightness, pressure or constriction widely varied in intensity, frequency, and duration, sometimes long-lasting and commonly suboccipital. It is associated with sustained contraction of skeletal muscles in the absence of permanent structural change, usually as part of the individual's reaction during life stress" (p. 717).

Reflecting modern approaches to taxonomy, a subcommittee of the International Association for the Study of Pain has developed, in draft form, a multiaxial system for classifying all chronic pain syndromes. This system defines two types of tension headaches "acute tension headaches" and "tension headaches: chronic form (scalp muscle contraction headache)," and includes much more information about each type of disorder than the Ad Hoc Committee's system. Consistent with the older system, tension headaches are considered to be musculoskeletal in origin although it is noted that the cardiovascular system or central nervous system are involved "according to some opinions."

In contrast to the two classification systems which have emerged from the headache/pain literature, the International Classification of Diseases (revision 9) lists tension headaches along with "psychogenic backache" under the heading "psychalgia" defined as "cases in which there are pains of *mental origin*, for example, headache or backache, when a more precise medical or psychiatric diagnosis cannot be made." In turn, psychalgia is classified under "Neurotic disorders, personality disorders and other non psychotic mental disorders" in the section on "Mental Disorders."

To those who are empirically oriented, the classificatory confusion can only be resolved via appropriate research investigations. Can a tension headache syndrome be identified; that is, are there a set of symptoms which covary and are distinct from related syndromes? And, what is the etiology of the syndrome? Unfortunately, these questions are less easy to answer than may first appear to be the case because they necessitate an unambiguous description of possible symptoms. Inspection of the various definitions of tension headaches (such as the ones above) indicates that symptoms are invariably described in nebulous terms. For this reason, both clinicians and researchers often diagnose tension headaches largely by exclusion; that is, no organic pathology and relative absence of migrainous features (which have been described much more precisely).

An early study by Ziegler, Hassanein, and Hassanein (1972) investigated headache syndromes by factor analyzing 27 "symptom" variables in a headache-prone population. This resulted in seven factors (accounting for about 47 percent of the total variation) which appeared to contain patterns of variables familiar to physicians in terms of clinical headache syndromes. "Factor 2" was characterized by "headaches of long duration" and "headaches lasting all the time," which might suggest the clinical entity of tension headaches. As the authors point out, however, it is curious that the symptom variables "brought on by stress" and "pain in the neck during headache" did not significantly load on Factor 2 despite the frequency of these phenomena in the entire headache population (44 and 36 percent, respectively). They go on to argue that the absence of these variables in Factor 2 headaches suggests the need for scrutinizing more carefully this large group of patients with headaches of long duration without preconceptions that their headaches must all be due to contraction of neck muscles as a manifestation of psychic "tension."

A number of studies have focused more on the issue of whether tension headaches and the other major group of "functional" headaches, namely, migraine, are readily differentiable, rather than on the integrity of the individual syndromes. A series of studies by Bakal and his colleagues (e.g., Bakal & Kaganov, 1977; Kaganov, Bakal, & Dunn, 1981) in which they have found migraine and tension headache patients to have similar symptoms, has led them to propose a psychobiological or severity model of headaches in which they argue that headache patients differ from occasional sufferers as well as from each other, primarily in terms of the frequency with which the various symptoms are experienced, and not in terms of the types of symptoms experienced. Similar findings leading to similar conceptualizations have been reported by others (the results of Arena, Blanchard, Andrasik, & Dudek, 1982, are an exception). Drummond and Lance (1984), for example, failed to obtain a clear distinction between migraine and tension headache, and found that patients described a broad spectrum of symptoms progressively declining from severe episodic headaches associated with many migraine features to constant headache with few or no migraine features. The results of such papers have led to the suggestion that the differences between tension headache and migraine are quantitative not qualitative, and that the two types of headaches should be viewed as lying at opposite ends of a spectrum or continuum rather than as discrete entities (e.g., Waters, 1973; Featherstone, 1985).

As a consequence of the difficulties associated with prescribing clear guidelines for diagnosing tension headaches, some studies have not even attempted to differentially diagnose headache sufferers (or done the job partially, such as categorizing into migraine vs. nonmigraine). This is particularly common in the epidemiological literature where subject samples are usually large (1,000–10,000) and data collected by questionnaire. Even when diagnoses are provided, the criteria on which they are based are often not specified. In this chapter, data on headache sufferers generally will be presented when sound data are not available on subjects specifically diagnosed as tension headache cases. This is considered justified as the evidence presented in this section and subsequent sections is generally consistent with the position that tension headaches are not fundamentally different from other types of functional headaches, namely, migraine and combined tension headache and migraine.

PREVALENCE OF TENSION HEADACHES

Data on headache prevalence have been reported from samples of children of varying ages (e.g., Sillanpaa, 1976), adolescents (e.g., Sillanpaa, 1983), University students (e.g., Ogunyemi, 1984), the elderly (e.g., Serratrice, Serbanesco, & Sambuc, 1985), and psychiatric patients (e.g., Philips & Hunter, 1982), in addition to various urban and rural communities (e.g., Nikiforow & Hokkanen, 1978). The samples have been drawn from many countries including Finland (e.g., Sillanpaa, 1983), Zimbabwe (e.g., Levy, 1983), Nigeria (e.g., Ogunyemi, 1984), Wales (e.g., Waters, 1973), Sweden (e.g., Ekbom, Ahlborg, & Schele, 1978), the United States (e.g., Schnarch & Hunter, 1979), Ecuador (e.g., Sachs, Sevilla, Barberis, Bolis, Schoenberg, & Cruz, 1985), and New Zealand (e.g., Paulin, Waal-Manning, Simpson, & Knight, 1985). Most of these studies have not attempted to diagnose tension headache cases so that the available data are on the prevalence of headaches generally (and factors that affect prevalence rates) rather than tension headaches specifically.

One of the most methodologically rigorous epidemiological studies was carried out by Nikiforow and Hokkanen (1978), in which questionnaires were sent to every inhabitant over 15 years of age in a defined area of Northern Finland. Analysis of the 3,067 questionnaires returned (response rate 77%) indicated the prevalence of headache in the year preceding the survey was 73.1% in women and 57.6% in men, a difference which was significant (and has been replicated in all comparable studies). The frequencies of severe (and mild) headache in 2,018 persons with a headache in the previous year were: approximately once a year 30% (10%), approximately once a month 40% (47%), approximately once a week 8% (20%), several times a week 7% (17%) and not stated 15% (6%).

Headache prevalence was slightly higher in the urban than the rural area, and declined sharply after 65 years of age. Education, social class, and mode of employment did not influence the prevalence of headache once pensioners were excluded. Headaches were significantly more common in married men and women.

There is considerable controversy over the frequency of tension headaches in children with some researchers suggesting that it is a commonly experienced type of headache and others reporting that it occurs infrequently (Werder & Sargent, 1984). Several researchers have found an increase in the prevalence of headache with age in the pediatric population (e.g., Bille, 1962).

One problem with interpreting the epidemiological data is that it is unclear the degree to which results can be generalized from one country to another. This point is well illustrated by comparison of the results of two studies (Andrasik, Holroyd, & Abell, 1979; Martin & Nathan, 1987) from different countries which asked the same questions of ostensibly similar populations (first-year undergraduate psychology students). These studies indicated the following cumulative frequencies of headaches in their samples (University of Western Australia vs. Ohio University) once per day (0.5% vs 3.2%), 3–4 per week (4.7% vs 20.0%), and 1–2 per week (20.0% vs 52.7%). These striking differences in headache frequency were paralleled in measures of headache intensity and duration.

PERSONALITY OF TENSION HEADACHE SUFFERERS

For many years it has been argued that headache sufferers tend to have a particular personality profile (Harrison, 1975). This is viewed as significant because the personality structure is argued to result in the individuals experiencing more stress which in turn precipitates headaches. Descriptions of the personality traits that characterize migraine have been remarkably consistent. Henryk-Gutt and Rees (1973), for example, suggested the prevalent view of a migraine sufferer as "tense, driving, obsessional perfectionist with an inflexible personality, who maintains a store of bottled-up resentments which can neither be expressed nor resolved. These characteristics would make him (or more often her) unable to adapt easily to circumstances, but liable to react excessively to environmental and interpersonal stresses sometimes with a migraine attack" (p. 142). Fewer descriptions of the personality traits associated with tension headaches have appeared in the literature, but those that have share much in common with the migraine profile. Martin (1966), for example, described tension headache patients as "sensitive, perfectionistic, worrisome, chronically tense and apprehensive" (p. 49).

While descriptions of headache personality in the literature have shown consistency, they have often been based on studies with major methodological limitations. Hence, assessment of personality has sometimes relied on clinical impressions or nonobjective instruments, samples of headache sufferers have not been representative of headache sufferers generally, and appropriate control groups have not been included. The dangers associated with ignoring these factors were well illustrated by the results of a study by Philips (1976). She found that in a "clinical" sample of tension headache cases (selected on the basis of the severity of their headaches and their desire for treatment), the female cases had significantly elevated neuroticism scores on the Personality Questionnaire (PQ) (Eysenck & Eysenck, 1976). However, when headache cases were selected from a community sample without reference to headache complaint made to their doctors, no significant differences were found on the psychoticism, neuroticism, or extraversion/introversion scales between this group and the appropriate mean age norms of the questionnaire.

Philips (1976) also reported no significant differences between migraine, tension headache, and mixed cases on any of the personality dimensions measured by the PQ. Since this study a number of other papers have appeared in the literature, and although the results have not been entirely consistent, they generally support the findings of Philips. Comparisons between migraineurs and tension headache or "nonmigrainous" cases have led to few significant findings. Schnarch and Hunter (1979), for example, only found differences on 2 of 26 scales used to measure personality variables. A number of recent studies (Andrasik et al., 1982; Kudrow & Sutkus, 1979; Sternbach, Dalessio, Kunzel, & Bowman, 1980) have reported that tension headache sufferers are more neurotic or psychologically disturbed than other headache groups, but Andrasik et al. (1982) have pointed out that their data suggest none of the headache groups were characterized by marked elevation in any of the very extensive battery of psychological tests used in their study.

Passchier, van der Helm-Hylkema, and Orlebeke (1984) recruited headache sufferers and nonheadache controls via advertisements in a local paper and reported tension headache and migraine cases had elevated achievement motivation, and tension headache cases showed greater rigidity. They found no evidence of higher neuroticism, or obsessive-compulsive behavior. In contrast, Blaszczynski (1984) reported higher levels of neuroticism and repressed hostility in female migraine and tension headache sufferers not attending clinics than with no pain controls, but equally elevated levels were present in a "pain" control group (chronic or recurring pain but no complaint of headache). Unfortunately, Blaszczynski does not specify how subjects were recruited. In summary, the evidence pertaining to the existence of a particular personality profile which predisposes individuals to developing headaches is not very convincing. Some studies have produced findings consistent with this hypothesis but others have not. The likelihood of obtaining significant results would appear to depend on the method of recruiting subjects with the probability decreasing from selecting from those attending a clinic, to selecting via advertising, to selecting from a community sample. If personality differences do exist they are likely to be small and may not be specific to chronic headaches but to chronic pain, chronic illness, complaining behavior, or some other factor. It is also possible that associations between personality profiles and headaches reflect causation in the opposite direction to the one usually hypothesized. Sternbach and Timmermans (1975) and Merskey (1972), for example, have presented evidence that chronic pain may lead to increases in neuroticism. In the former study, it was demonstrated that neurotic features decreased following a reduction of pain.

FUNCTIONAL ASPECTS OF TENSION HEADACHES

While medical practitioners assess headaches by eliciting signs and symptoms leading to formulation of a diagnosis, psychologists have argued for the advantages of adopting a functional perspective in which assessment seeks to elucidate the controlling variables of the problem behavior (Lake, 1981; Norton & Neilson, 1977; Scott, 1979). The two major classes of controlling variables are the antecedents and consequences of the problem behavior. The medical and psychological approaches to headache assessment have been contrasted in a recent chapter by Boudewyns (1982), and a review by Thompson and Figueroa (1983) considers some of the important issues involved in headache assessment such as the reliability of the assessment procedures.

A small study by Martin, Nathan, and van Keppel (1985) investigated the antecedents and consequences of headache sufferers. It was found that certain classes of antecedent stimuli such as negative affect ("stress," "anxiety," "anger"), visual disturbance ("flicker," "glare," "eyestrain"), and noise, were consistently reported across all types of headaches (tension, migraine, undifferentiated). Other antecedents did seem to be more associated with some types of headaches than others in the direction that the anecdotal headache literature would suggest. Hence, consumatory stimuli ("food," "hunger," "alcohol") seemed to be mainly associated with migraine, and muscle activity stimuli ("exercise," "fatigue," "neck movements") with tension headaches. Overall, however, the antecedent stimuli of the three types of headache did not differ significantly.

A recent investigation by Drummond (1985) found that menstruation, glare, and alcohol were more common antecedents for migraine than tension headaches. Other studies reporting data on the "precipitators" of headaches have usually been epidemiological ones and, hence, have had the advantage of large subject numbers but the disadvantage of no differential diagnosis. These studies usually list "stress" as the major precipitating factor, with heat, menstruation, and alcohol commonly reported. Other antecedents which are often listed include hunger, certain foods (particularly those rich in tyramine such as chocolate and aged cheeses), and exercise (Levy, 1983; Nikiforow & Hokkanen, 1978; Ogunyemi, 1984).

The results of all the above studies need to be treated with considerable caution as they are based on patient self-report, and are correlational in nature. Hence, whether the antecedents or "precipitators" are in any sense causal in inducing headaches remains a very open question. The results of a study by Moffett, Swash, and Scott (1974) underline the problem. While many studies have reported that migraine sufferers list chocolate as a precipitator of migraine attacks, these researchers demonstrated in two separate studies that eating chocolate under double-blind placebo conditions rarely led to headaches even in a group of subjects who had observed that their headaches regularly occurred after ingestion of small amounts of cocoa products.

With respect to the consequences of tension headaches, Martin et al. (1985) found that the most commonly reported reactions of tension headache sufferers to their headaches were to engage in the coping strategies of distraction and relaxation. Other common responses were to take medication and have something to eat or drink. The reactions of others to tension headaches were generally positive and supportive as the most commonly listed were "offer sympathy," "encourage stopping," "get a drink," "encourage sitting,"and "get medication", while tension headache sufferers reported that it was rare for others to ignore them, complain, or even to encourage them to keep going. These responses are obviously consistent with the suggestion that reinforcement of pain behavior might be an important maintaining factor in at least some cases of chronic tension headache.

PHYSIOLOGICAL MECHANISMS OF TENSION HEADACHES

The original research on headaches carried out by psychologists in the early 1970s was treatment-oriented and assumed that the prevailing medical view of tension headache etiology was correct. A number of researchers became skeptical of the beliefs, however, and began publishing psychophysiological studies of headache mechanisms from the mid-1970s (Martin, 1983). This literature is now quite extensive (over 30 papers to date) so that only a selective review will be possible here. More detailed reviews are provided by Martin (1980), Haynes, Cuevas, and Gannon (1982), and Pikoff (1984).

Skeletal Muscle Activity

A number of different methodologies have been employed to investigate the relationship between skeletal muscle activity and tension headaches. This has resulted partly from the advantages of exploring problems from a variety of perspectives, and partly because the proposed relationship might take any of several forms. One approach has been to compare the resting EMG levels (frontalis, neck, temporalis) of tension headache sufferers with no-headache or other control groups. This strategy is enquiring into whether tension headache sufferers have generally elevated EMG levels (as implied by the Ad Hoc Committee, 1962). The majority of studies investigating resting EMG levels have failed to find significant differences between tension headache and control subjects (e.g., Martin & Mathews, 1978; Andrasik, Blanchard, Arena, Saunders, & Barron, 1982; Gannon, Haynes, Safranek, & Hamilton, 1981). Many studies have found trends, however, and in some cases differences have reached statistical significance (e.g., Cohen et al., 1983).

Other studies have looked at differences in response to, and recovery from, stress on the grounds that those who suffer from frequent headaches might differ from those who do not, in terms of excessive increases in tension as a reaction to stress, or delayed return to baseline following stress. A large variety of different stressors have been used including mental arithmetic, noise stimuli, intellectual problems, cold pressor, and stressful imagery. In these studies, the majority have found no significant differences between tension headache and control subjects (e.g., Martin & Mathews, 1978; Andrasik et al., 1982; Feuerstein, Bush, & Corbisiero, 1982), but others have (e.g., Thompson & Adams, 1984; Cohen et al., 1983; Pritchard & Wood, 1983).

While some studies investigating EMG levels at rest and in response to stress have not reported whether headache subjects were experiencing headaches at the time of physiological recording, others have. The findings have been conflicting, however. Martin and Mathews (1978) found no significant differences between tension headache sufferers and controls whether all sufferers were included in the analysis or only those experiencing headaches at the time of recording. Hursey, Holroyd, Penzien, and Holm (1985) also found no significant differences between headache sufferers and controls when all the former group were included in the analysis (a trend was present), but differences in frontalis EMG attained significance when sufferers who were headache-free were withdrawn from the analysis.

Some researchers have reported within subject comparisons between headache and EMG activity. Again, the results have been very inconsistent. Haynes, Griffin, Mooney, and Parise (1975) found significantly higher frontalis EMG levels during headache periods; Martin and Mathews (1978) reported the reverse (significantly lower frontalis EMG during headaches), and no significant difference in neck EMG; and Philips (1977a) found no significant differences in frontalis, neck, trapezium, or temporalis EMG levels. Others have reported within subject correlations between EMG levels and headache intensity ratings recorded concurrently. Harper and Steger (1978) found a correlation of 0.12 between frontalis EMG and headache intensity ratings; and Martin and Mathews (1978) reported a correlation of −0.10 between frontalis EMG and headache intensity rating, and 0.02 between neck EMG and headache intensity rating.

Some researchers have responded to the negative findings by attempting to look for subgroups for whom the hypothesized relationships between tension headaches and excessive muscle tension holds. Martin and Mathews (1978) selected out the most diagnostically unambiguous cases of tension headaches for analysis on the grounds that results may have been distorted by including essentially incorrectly diagnosed patients. This approach did not affect the negative findings of the study. Haber, Kuczmierczyk, and Adams (1985) split headache sufferers into high and low EMG groups following a screening session carried out while sufferers were experiencing headaches. The authors were then able to show that the frontalis EMG levels of the high EMG group did differ from a control group, and that systematic changes in EMG levels from headache to headache-free conditions occurred for the high EMG group. While the results of this study warrant further investigation, there is obviously a danger of circularity in selecting out a high EMG subgroup and then demonstrating it differs from an unselected control group.

Some researchers have reasoned that the difference between tension headache sufferers and controls may not be so much in the level of muscle tension but the sensitivity to tension. This has led to a number of studies comparing pain thresholds and pain tolerances of headache and nonheadache subjects. Studies using standard procedures for measuring pain threshold and tolerance such as the Hardy-Wolff radiant heat method (Martin & Mathews, 1978) and Forgione-Barber pressure pain stimulator (Feuerstein et al., 1982) have not found significant differences between tension headache and control subjects. A recent paper by Borgeat, Hade, Elie, and Larouche (1984) evaluated the threshold hypothesis by asking subjects to tense their muscles and this more direct approach to assessing sensitivity to muscle tension resulted in a significant difference between tension headache sufferers and controls with the former group displaying lower thresholds.

Given the large number of negative findings and alternative explanations of positive findings (e.g., pain causing muscle tension rather than vice versa), few headache researchers now believe that one can symptomatically define a large group of headache sufferers the mechanism of which is "sustained contraction of skeletal muscles." Opinion varies as to how much of a departure from the original concept is necessary. Does the model need to be abandoned completely, reserved for a proportion of cases, or resurrected in some modified form?

Alternative Mechanisms

If tension headaches are not caused by excessive muscle tension, then what is the mechanism? Unfortunately, this question has not been widely investigated and no clear answer has emerged. Several studies have recorded a wide range of psychophysiological variables (e.g., forearm EMG, temporal artery blood flow, hand surface temperature, heart rate, systolic and diastolic blood pressure, skin resistance level), and failed to distinguish between tension headache sufferers and controls on any of them (e.g., Anderson & Franks, 1981; Andrasik et al., 1982; Feuerstein et al., 1982). Some studies have found significant differences on vascular measures (e.g., Bakal & Kaganov, 1977; Haynes et al., 1982) and this has led to the suggestion that the mechanism of tension headaches is vascular and similar to that of migraines. Martin and Mathews (1978) reported that tension headache sufferers rated increased headache intensity following inhalation of a vasodilating agent implying that the headache was associated with vasodilation, and these data also are consistent with the two types of headaches having fundamentally the same mechanism.

The available data linking vascular mechanisms to tension headaches are very tentative, however. Also, hypothesizing that similar mechanisms are responsible for tension headaches and migraines does not entirely clarify the issue as the basis for migraine attacks is not fully understood. The classic concept of migraines—that they result from a rebound phenomenon whereby cranial and cerebral vasoconstriction occurs in the preheadache phase (O'Brien, 1971; Ostfeld & Wolff, 1958) and cranial and cerebral vasodilation in the headache phase (Dalessio, 1972; Tunis & Wolff, 1953)—has been criticized by a number of writers. Feuerstein et al. (1982), for example, have cogently argued for the testing of a more complex 4-stage model of migraine pathology in which the temporal artery proceeds through a series of changes starting 36–72 hours prior to an attack including vasodilation with no associated pain, heightened lability, vasoconstriction, and finally, vasodilation with concomitant pain.

BEHAVIORAL TREATMENT OF TENSION HEADACHES

The initial and continuing focus of most psychologists carrying out research in the headache area has been on treatment. Publications on therapy outcome account for approximately 75 percent of the behavioral headache research literature (Martin, 1983), and by the author's estimate, papers have appeared at the fairly steady rate of 8 to 13 per year (mean 11) over the last decade. Obviously, the discussion of this large literature here will need to be selective, and more detailed reviews are available by Martin (1980), Holmes and Burish (1983), and Williamson (1981).

EMG Feedback Training

One form of treatment for tension headaches that has been investigated extensively is EMG feedback training. The rationale of this approach is that by giving headache sufferers information with respect to how tense are their head and neck muscles they can be trained to relax away the tension, and hence, prevent headaches from occurring. Feedback has usually been given from the frontalis muscle but some studies have given feedback from the neck muscles (e.g., Martin & Mathews, 1978), and others from the muscle showing the highest resting EMG levels (e.g., Peck & Kraft, 1977). The laboratory training has generally been accompanied by instructions to practice relaxing at home each day, but again there have been exceptions (e.g., Epstein, Hersen, & Hemphill, 1974).

Many studies have reported decreases in headache activity following EMG feedback training, improvement being maintained at least until the 12-month follow-up. Bruhn, Olesen, and Melgaard (1979) showed EMG feedback training to be superior to the "most suitable alternative" (drugs and/or physical therapy), and a series of early studies showed EMG feedback training to be superior to various control procedures such as "pseudofeedback" (e.g., Budzynski, Stoyva,

Adler, & Mullaney, 1973; Philips, 1977b) and "medication placebo" (Cox, Freundlich, & Meyer, 1975). It was argued that the control conditions ruled out the possibility that subjects were merely responding to a placebo effect, and the positive correlations between reduction in EMG activity and improvement found in some studies (e.g., Budzynski et al., 1973; Cox et al., 1975; Hutchings & Reinking, 1976) were cited as evidence for a causal link between these two variables. The control conditions looked less than satisfactory, however, as procedures such as "pseudofeedback" (recording of successful EMG feedback sessions played to patients who were told it was a monotonous tone that would help them relax) and "medication placebo" (patients given a glucose tablet which they were told would help them relax), seem unlikely to raise expectations of success to the same level as EMG feedback training, which has considerable face validity. The significance of the correlational data was also debateable both because it is not possible to argue from correlation to cause, and because many other studies failed to find significant correlations (e.g., Epstein & Abel, 1977; Haynes et al., 1975; Martin & Mathews, 1978).

Hence, the early literature on EMG feedback training was convincing with respect to the efficacy of the approach but not the mechanism of change. A recent series of studies by Holroyd and his colleagues has gone some way towards clarifying the treatment process. Holroyd, Andrasik, and Noble (1980) demonstrated that EMG feedback training was significantly superior in terms of headache reduction to a pseudotherapy condition ("meditation") which had been rated by subjects as equally credible to the EMG feedback training. This study seemed to rule out interpretations purely in terms of placebo effects. To clarify the relationship between changes in EMG and headache activity, Andrasik and Holroyd (1980) directly manipulated the former in three biofeedback conditions. While all biofeedback groups were instructed similarly and were led to believe that they were learning to reduce frontalis EMG, in fact training focused on teaching subjects to decrease, increase, or hold stable frontalis EMG. Results indicated that while EMG levels shifted in the intended directions, the headaches of the three biofeedback groups all improved significantly and equally. These findings have been interpreted by the authors as indicating outcomes obtained with biofeedback do not result merely from exposure to a credible treatment procedure, but are not mediated by learned control of physiological activity. They suggest that biofeedback works because subjects are implicitly encouraged to alter the cognitive and behavioral responses to headache-eliciting situations.

Holroyd et al. (1984) extended this model via an ingenious experiment in which subjects were assigned to one of four conditions: increase or decrease EMG (as in their earlier study), and high-success feedback or low-success feedback (achieved via bogus video displays). The authors reported that regardless of actual changes in EMG activity, subjects receiving high-success feedback showed substantially greater improvement in headache activity (53%) than subjects receiving moderate-success feedback (26%). Performance feedback was also found to be related to changes in locus of control and self-efficacy, and changes in these two cognitive variables during biofeedback training were also correlated with reduction in headache activity following treatment. These results have led to the authors devising a new model of therapeutic change in EMG feedback training in which it is hypothesized that "if patients perceive biofeedback training as a credible treatment and perceive themselves as succeeding at the biofeedback task through their own efforts, they will view (a) their headaches as having an internal locus of control, and (b) themselves as self-efficacious (i.e., as capable of influencing their headaches). These cognitive changes are expected to lead to new and more persistent efforts to cope with headache-related stresses that, in turn, alter psychological and physiological stress-responses triggering headaches" (p. 1040). The old and new models are presented in Figure 11.1 as paths A and B, respectively.

Parenthetically, one can point out that the research of Holroyd and his colleagues provides some of the strongest evidence against a simple muscular model of tension headaches, as they have demonstrated in two studies that training patients to increase muscle tension is as effective a treatment for tension headaches as training them to decrease muscle tension.

Relaxation Training

Another treatment for tension headaches that has been evaluated widely is relaxation training (usually progressive relaxation or autogenic training). Sometimes relaxation training and EMG feedback training have been given consecutively or concurrently. Like EMG feedback training, relaxation training has usually been accompanied by instructions to practice at home. The rationale of relaxation is obvious given the hypothesized mechanism of tension headaches.

Comparisons between EMG feedback and relaxation training have usually shown them to be equally effective (e.g., Cox et al., 1975; Haynes et al., 1975; Martin & Mathews, 1978). Hutchings and Reinking (1976), however, found EMG feedback and the combination of EMG feedback and relaxation training to be equally superior to relaxation training alone, and Chesney and Shelton (1976) found relaxation training and the combination of EMG feedback and relaxation training to be equally more effective than EMG feedback alone.

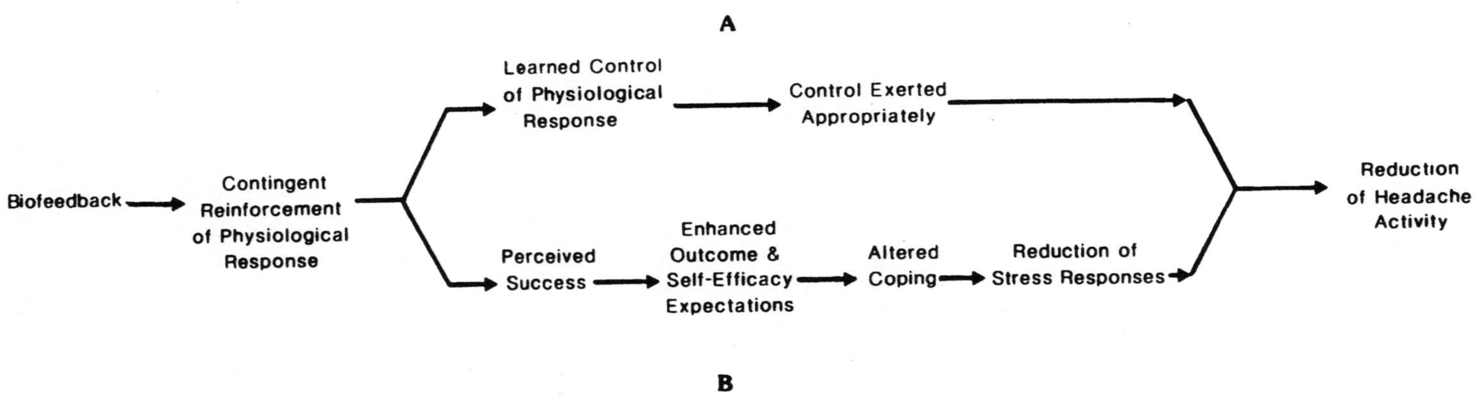

FIGURE 11.1. Two models of therapeutic change in EMG biofeedback training (From Holroyd et al., 1984).

Other Individual, Clinic-based Treatment Approaches

While the headache literature (tension and migraine) is generally replete with studies showing alternative treatment conditions to be equally effective, Holroyd, Andrasik, and Westbrook (1977) demonstrated that a cognitively oriented stress-coping training program was significantly more effective than EMG feedback training for alleviating headaches. Holroyd and Andrasik (1982) followed up this study, and reported that the very impressive results obtained by their stress-coping training group, persisted two years later. A number of other researchers have used a similar cognitive-behavioral approach, usually based on the work of Meichenbaum (1974), and reported very positive results (e.g., Anderson, Scott, & Olson, 1981; Bakal, Demjen, & Kaganov, 1981; Kremsdorf, Kochanowicz, & Costell, 1981).

Other treatments have been compared with EMG feedback and relaxation training and in almost all cases they have been shown to be equally effective: transcendental meditation (Winkler, 1978); hypnotic analgesia (Schlutter, Golden, & Blume, 1980); and digital temperature feedback (Daly, Donn, Galliher, & Zimmerman, 1983). Turkat and Adams (1982) found little support for the efficacy of covert positive reinforcement in treating tension headaches.

Home-based and Group Treatment

While most studies have reported on individual therapist-administered treatment, a literature is now emerging on lower cost approaches to therapy via utilizing group formats or minimal therapist-contact treatments. Figueroa (1982) compared a behavioral package (problem-solving techniques, relaxation training, anxiety management, stress inoculation, and pain management techniques) with traditional psychotherapy and self-monitoring, the two treatment conditions being administered in a group format. The authors reported that significant improvement occurred across all measures (frequency, severity, and duration of headache, type and amount of medication taken, etc.) in the behavioral group but not the other two groups. Williamson et al. (1984) compared two group relaxation programmes, one of which was called a self-help condition (four hours of group meetings encouraging patients to use a self-help manual or relaxation) and the other a therapist-administered condition (twelve hours of relaxation training with instructions to practice at home), with a waiting-list control group (four hours of discussion on basis of headaches). Results indicated that both treatment conditions were superior to the waiting-list control group at one-month follow-up.

Steger and Harper (1980) contrasted the efficacy of a comprehensive, clinic-based biofeedback and stress management strategy with a self-monitored, no therapist-contact, home relaxation program, and found the former to be significantly more effective. However, Teders et al. (1984) demonstrated that a minimal-therapist-contact home-based approach to relaxation training was highly effective and nearly equivalent for reducing headache complaints to a standard therapist-delivered relaxation treatment. The minimal contact, home-based treatment was shown to be more cost-effective when relating total amount of therapist contact to headache improvement. Similar results were reported by Blanchard et al. (1985).

Sherman (1982) reported on an even more abbreviated treatment approach in which the tension headache sufferers were merely lent 12-minute progressive muscle relaxation tapes and told to practice twice per day for one month. All but one subject showed sustained decreases in headache activity at 6-month follow-up.

Treatment of Tension Headaches in Children

Few studies have reported on the results of behavioral treatment with childhood headache sufferers. Most of the available studies focus on childhood migraine (these have been reviewed by Hoelscher and Lichstein, 1984), and all reports the author is aware of are on single cases or retrospective series. The data that are available, however, suggest that the techniques that have been developed with adults may also be efficacious with children. Werder and Sargent (1984), for example, report on the results of treating 31 children between the ages of 7 and 17 years (10 were diagnosed as "tension headache") with "biofeedback assisted self-regulating techniques." This apparently included progressive relaxation, autogenic phrases, self-awareness, and guided imagery. They reported that 28 children were able to control 51 percent or more headaches after the 2-month training period and that reduction in headache continued over the 1–3 year follow-up period. However, there was only a 39 percent reduction in mean headache hours for the tension headache subjects compared to a 71 percent reduction for migraine and combined headache subjects.

Waranch and Keenan (1985) described the treatment of 15 children aged 10–17 years (only one was diagnosed "tension headache") by a combination of relaxation, biofeedback (EMG and peripheral skin temperature), and behavioral counseling. At the end of treatment, eight of the children were headache-free and five others exhibited a marked reduction in headache frequency and severity. Improvements were maintained at follow-up periods of 6–22 months. Andrasik, Blanchard,

Edlund, and Attanasio (1983) reported the case of an 11-year-old girl suffering from tension headaches who was treated with EMG feedback training. Marked improvement was recorded on all measures of headache activity.

PROGNOSTIC INDICATORS OF TREATMENT RESPONSE

Blanchard et al. (1983a) investigated the capacity of a vast number of pretreatment measures to predict the response of tension headache patients to relaxation training. These variables were classified into four sets, the first of which was labeled "headache history" (21 variables). Using canonical discriminant function analysis these variables were found to correctly classify as improved or unimproved 89 percent of the patients. Two variables which stood out were the migrainous symptoms of "throbbing pain" and "pain is sometimes one-sided," both of which were strongly associated with positive outcome. The second set of variables was derived from headache diaries patients completed over a 4-week period prior to treatment (pain ratings recorded four times per day). The utility of these variables for predicting outcome was found to be low (70 percent correctly classified) implying that the initial level of headache activity is not relevant to treatment outcome. The third set of variables was derived from six psychological tests (Minnesota Multiphasic Personality Inventory, Psychosomatic Symptom Checklist, Rathus Assertiveness Scale, etc.). This resulted in 76 percent correct classifications. The fourth set of variables was psychophysiological measures (forehead EMG, heart rate, skin resistance level, and fingertip temperature), taken under the following conditions: baseline, three self-control, three responses to stress, and six reactivity measures. These variables led to 78 percent correct classification. When all four predictive sets were used the correct classification only came to 90 percent virtually the same figure as for headache history variables alone (89%).

A number of studies have found that younger patients tend to respond better to biofeedback and relaxation training than older patients (e.g., Blanchard et al., 1985; Diamond, Medina, Diamond-Falk, & De Veno, 1979). Diamond et al. (1979) reported that women improved more with biofeedback than men. Several investigators have found no significant relationship between diagnosis and treatment response (e.g., Diamond et al., 1979; Bakal et al., 1981). Researchers have reported that presence of depressive symptoms is associated with poor prognosis for relaxation training (Jacob, Turner, Szekely, & Eidelman, 1983), EMG feedback training (Levine, 1984), and their combination (Diamond et al., 1979); and Bakal et al. (1981) found that headache patients who experienced continuous or near-continuous pain during their waking hours were not responsive to cognitive-behavior therapy. Blanchard, Andrasik, Neff, Saunders, Arena, Pallmeyer, Teders, Jurish, and Rodichok (1983b) reported that therapist variables such as level of experience, warmth, competence, or helpfulness were not significant predictors of response to relaxation training and biofeedback. Several investigators have found regularity of home relaxation practice to be a significant predictor of treatment success (e.g., Blanchard et al., 1983b; Reinking & Hutchings, 1981).

METHODOLOGICAL ISSUES IN HEADACHE RESEARCH

While fairly consistent results have been obtained in some areas of headache research, inconsistencies and conflict have characterized other areas (investigation of physiological mechanisms is perhaps the most extreme example). Resolving the discrepancies is usually impossible due to methodological differences between studies or insufficient information in the published reports to compare results in any depth. The majority of studies are open to numerous criticisms as demonstrated by the results of various reviews. Thompson and Adams (1984), for example, reported that between 43 percent and 93 percent of studies (mean 69%) did not control for the 13 subject and procedural variables they perceived as seminal, while Andrasik et al. (1982) found that between 53 percent and 87 percent of studies (mean 67%) failed to meet the six methodological criteria they considered important. Listed below are a series of guidelines for behavioral headache research drawn from the above papers, Raczynski and Thompson (1983), and the author's own experience. While some may seem painfully obvious and elementary, the list has been compiled on the basis of errors commonly made.

1. *Selection of experimental sample*
   (i) There is a need for clear specification of the diagnostic criteria which define eligibility for the study. While the headache classification systems currently available do not give unambiguous guidelines as to what the criteria should be (see first section), it is incumbent on researchers at least to explicitly state what they have used.

   (ii) Researchers should demonstrate that the diagnostic criteria can be applied reliably.
   (iii) Headache sufferers should be screened by appropriate medical specialists.
2. *Selection of control sample*
   (i) Control samples should be recruited from similar sources and using similar procedures to the experimental sample. Gross deviations from this ideal have been a problem in the headache literature as many researchers have recruited headache sufferers via doctors or advertising, and control groups from colleagues and students in their own department.
   (ii) Control groups should be matched with experimental groups on age and sex, as Basmajian (1978) has reviewed data suggesting that muscular changes occur during aging, and Schwartz, Brown, and Ahern (1980) have reported that sex differences exist in facial muscle activity.
3. *Reporting of subject characteristics:* There is a need for providing detailed information about the subject sample such as age, sex, chronicity, symptomatology, treatment history, and so on so that the results of different studies can be meaningfully compared.
4. *Control of extraneous variables:* There is a need to control for factors that might affect the dependent variables under study. Many medications, for example, influence muscular and vascular activity. Even nicotine (Stephens, 1977) has been demonstrated to have vasoactive effects and effects upon skeletal muscle tone (Domino, 1973). Behavioral treatments might also affect psychophysiological functioning during or after treatment.
5. *Technical factors:* There is a need for researchers to employ the correct electrodes/transducers and amplifiers and use them most appropriately (e.g., placing electrodes accurately, attaching electrodes with low impedence, using appropriate band-pass filters, eliminating noise and movement artifact). Perhaps the most problematic area for headache research has been measuring the vasoconstriction/dilation alleged to underlie migraine and perhaps tension headaches. Some notion of the lack of technical consensus in this area can be gained by the plethora of transducers that have been used in recent years and include ultrasonic, reflectance photoelectric, pressure-transducing plethysmographs, and photoelectric back scatter techniques. Few researchers would claim they know exactly what they are measuring even if they can measure it reliably.

6. *Methodological factors*
   (i) Experimental sessions should be structured such that there are adequate habituation periods (for subjects to adapt to the laboratory environment), and baseline periods (for recording resting levels of activity).
   (ii) Instructions to subjects with respect to variables such as eyes open/closed and posture should be precise and reported in publications.
   (iii) Recording should take place during headache-free and headache periods.
7. *Laboratory stressors:* Stressors used in laboratory studies have usually been discrete, brief (few minutes) physical or cognitive stimuli whereas headache sufferers report the stresses that precipitate their headaches tend to be of long duration and socioenvironmental in nature, such as job, school, family, or interpersonal problems (Haynes et al., 1982). Hence, there is a need for researchers to use longer duration stressors that more closely approximate naturalistic ones (e.g., imagining aversive, interpersonal situations).
8. *Nonspecific demand factors:* Differences in outcome between studies may be expected as a function of whether subjects were or were not aware of the hypotheses under investigation, the manner in which experimenters communicated experimental procedures to the subjects, and whether experimenters were aware of the diagnostic classification of a subject (Haynes et al., 1982). Hence, there is a need for experimenters to reduce these potential sources of bias to a minimum (e.g., use automated procedures, "blind" experimenters) and report procedures used in detail.
9. *Data analytic techniques:* Perhaps the most common data analytic error in recent headache research is using numerous univariate analyses to analyse multivariate data without any form of adjustment to compensate for the increased probability of type I errors that this approach engenders.
10. *Interpretation of results*
    (i) While all researchers are presumably aware that it is inappropriate to argue from correlation to cause, such an inferential leap is at least implied in many papers in the headache literature. Correlations from treatment studies between decreases in EMG and headache improvement are frequently cited as evidence for a muscular pain mechanism despite the obvious alternative explanations. It is rarely pointed out that an association between elevated muscle

tension and headache might be the result of pain causing tension rather than the reverse.

(ii) Most samples of headache sufferers have been recruited from student populations, the community, or patient populations, via advertisements or requests for referrals. Arguing that results gained with one group (e.g., student volunteers) apply to another group (e.g., referred patients) is, of course, unjustified. A recent paper by Belar, Sutton, and Wilson (1983) emphasized this point by reporting differences in headache activity, personality profiles, and muscle tension between a recruited subject sample and a clinic-based subject sample.

HEADACHE MANAGEMENT: BEYOND THE RESEARCH LITERATURE

Unfortunately, the research literature on headaches is of limited value to clinicians at the present time, for three main reasons. First, much of the literature casts doubt on traditional assumptions without providing clearly superior alternatives. Secondly, the treatment literature focuses on evaluating standardized, usually unimodal approaches, while clinicians tend to favor individualized, multimodal approaches for problems as complex as headaches. And, third, treatment studies usually do not include enough procedural details for clinicians to replicate the techniques. With respect to this last point, the final chapter in Don Bakal's book (1982) consists of his manual for the cognitive behavioral treatment of chronic headaches, and this contains a wealth of information on therapy techniques.

The literature does contain some clear messages for clinicians, however. There is little point, for example, in attempting differentially to diagnose tension headaches and migraines as such a decision would be somewhat arbitary and would not provide useful information with respect to the pain mechanism, how the problem should be treated, or the likely prognosis. As most treatments are equally effective, clinicians may feel free to choose between them on grounds other than efficacy. Treatments that are relatively cheap in terms of therapist time should probably be considered as a first step. A cognitive behavioral approach focusing on stress-coping training may be the best treatment currently available. It appears to be important to strongly encourage patients to practice relaxation at home.

The author's own approach to headache management based on the headache research literature, broader theoretical and empirical considerations, and clinical experience is summarized in Figure 11.2 and

PRE-ASSESSMENT

Medical screening

↓

ASSESSMENT

A. Personal and social history

B. Headache history

C. Functional analysis of headaches

- 1. Antecedents
  - 1.1. Predisposing factors
  - 1.2. Onset factors
  - 1.3. Setting factors
  - 1.4. Immediate factors
- 2. Consequences
  - 2.1. Positive reinforcement
  - 2.2. Negative reinforcement
- 3. Exacerbating factors
  - 3.1. Reactions to antecedents
  - 3.2. Reactions to headaches

↓

TREATMENT

A. Modification of antecedent factors

B. Coping with antecedent factors and headaches

C. Contingency management of headache consequences

FIGURE 11.2. An individualized approach to headache management.

outlined below. This material is included due to the limited practical guidelines provided by the headache research literature in isolation.

All headache cases need thorough medical investigation to ensure that the headaches are not the result of organic pathology such as infections or tumors (these are rare but must be excluded). Therapists who are not medically qualified are well advised to only treat cases for whom a medical practitioner has confirmed in writing that behavioral management would be appropriate.

Assessment takes account of a wide range of variables to provide a context or framework within which to understand the headache problem. The assessment particularly concentrates on clarification of the controlling variables of the problem. The assessment techniques that seem most useful are interviewing and self-monitoring. With respect to the latter, both time sampling (e.g., regular recordings of rated headache intensity) and event sampling (e.g., recording activities thoughts and feelings before and after headaches begin, end, or change in severity) (Martin, 1983), can be useful.

The aim of assessment is for the therapist and patient to develop an understanding of the variance in the patient's problem (why their headaches occur or get worse at one time rather than another). The main focus of the assessment is on the three areas shown in the figure, namely the antecedents and consequences of headaches, and exacerbating factors. With respect to antecedents, four subcategories have been listed according to their temporal relationship with the headaches. The more remote factors (onset and predisposing) are more difficult to identify and of less importance to management. Predisposing factors include personality traits that might make an individual more vulnerable to headaches (e.g., high-trait anxiety leading to frequent tension states). Onset factors refer to events or situations that resulted in the headache problem developing (e.g., psychological or physical trauma, menopause). Setting factors are the life situations or lifestyles that are conducive to headaches by virtue of frequently leading to the specific conditions under which headaches occur (e.g., marital discord or child management problems resulting in stress). Immediate factors are the stimuli which precipitate or aggravate headaches (e.g., stress, noise, flicker, etc.).

Assessment should take into account the immediate and long-term consequences of the headaches both for the patient and those with whom they interact regularly. Obviously the key issue is whether headaches regularly lead to positive reinforcement (e.g., rest, medication, sympathy, attention, massage) or negative reinforcement (avoidance or escape from undesirable activities or situations) as this might account for the maintenance of the problem.

An area that seems very important clinically but that has received virtually no attention in the research literature is reactions of headache sufferers to the antecedents of headaches and the headaches themselves. Often the reactions are likely to increase the likelihood of a headache developing or getting worse so that a negative feedback loop is established. One example of such a reaction is rushing to complete aversive tasks on the grounds that if a headache develops or gets worse then it will not be possible to carry out the tasks. This, of course, virtually guarantees the prophesized problem occurring. Another example is responding by becoming irritable and snapping at those in the immediate vicinity. This often provokes negative reactions, and hence, increases stress levels.

Assessment of the controlling variables of the headache problem can be used to guide treatment planning by considering strategies under three headings (see Figure 11.2). One approach is to try and reduce or eliminate the stimuli, situations, or events that give rise to headaches (i.e., modify the setting or immediate factors). Possibilities range from simply avoiding situations that precipitate headaches (e.g., loud, noisy parties), to relatively complex and time-consuming approaches such as marital therapy or child management training. If headaches are associated with anxiety or depression then focusing treatment on these negative emotions might be desirable.

A second approach is to train patients to cope more adequately with the antecedent factors or the headaches themselves. Techniques such as relaxation training, self-instructional training, attention-diversion training, and imagery training (Bakal, 1982) come under this heading and are appropriate for virtually all sufferers from chronic headaches. Procedures for training patients to react to the antecedents of headaches and the headache themselves in more appropriate ways also fit into this category.

A final approach which is only appropriate in some cases is contingency management of the consequences of headaches. If headaches are consistently reinforced then treatment might focus on rearranging contingencies such that the level of reinforcement is maintained but reinforcement is no longer contingent on headache behavior. This approach is obviously time consuming and necessitates working with the individuals who are providing reinforcement to the patient (usually the spouse). Wilbert Fordyce's book (1976) is a valuable source of information with respect to assessing and managing chronic pain behavior from an operant perspective.

Of course, whether the individualized approach to headache management described above is superior to simply administering relaxation training is unknown. The research literature shows that techniques such as relaxation are sufficient for alleviating the headaches of a significant proportion of the chronic headache population. Such approaches are no panacea, however, and some patients remain virtually unimproved after treatment. It seems probable that an approach like the one outlined here, that seeks to understand the controlling variables for the problem behavior and then use this information to guide treatment, should be more effective than the rather superficial, symptomatic approaches described in the research literature. Obviously, individualized approaches are more difficult to evaluate empirically as they result in different patients being treated by different techniques for different periods of time. Hopefully, however, such approaches will be investigated in future research.

SUMMARY

The concept of a "tension headache" is a vague one and has been given different meanings by different authors. Whether tension headaches and migraines are qualitatively distinct, as implied by the headache classification systems, or merely represent opposite poles on a continuum is debatable, but recent research favors the latter model.

While clinicians have argued for the existence of a particular personality profile that predisposes individuals to suffer from headaches, the evidence for such an assertion is quite unconvincing. More importantly, the alleged mechanism of tension headaches—excessive tension in the muscles of the head and neck—has received minimal empirical support. Hence, studies comparing EMG levels at rest, in response to stress, and during poststress recovery, between tension headache sufferers and matched controls, have often failed to find significant group differences. Within-subject comparisons looking at the relationship between EMG and head pain have also failed to support the hypothesized association. Even more condeming for the old muscular model have been the results of studies showing that training clients to increase frontalis EMG is as effective a treatment for headaches as training them to decrease frontalis EMG. Unfortunately, researchers have not been able to come up with clear alternatives to a muscular mechanism although the results of some studies suggest that the mechanism may be vascular and similar to that of migraine headaches.

A number of individual clinic-based behavioral treatment procedures seem to be quite effective for tension headaches. Such procedures include EMG feedback training, relaxation training, stress-coping training, transcendental meditation, hypnotic analgesia, and digital temperature feedback training. The evidence is strongest for EMG feedback training and relaxation training, particularly the former. Most of the treatment techniques appear to be equally effective but cognitively orientated stress-coping training might be superior to alternatives. Why the various techniques are effective is not certain. The work of Holroyd and his colleagues, however, suggests that biofeedback works because subjects are implicitly encouraged to alter the cognitive and behavioral responses to headache-eliciting situations.

Recent studies have also indicated the value of "cheaper" forms of treatment. Hence, there is now some evidence to support the efficacy of group approaches, and minimal-therapist-contact home-based approaches.

Studies suggest that the most likely respondent to behavioral treatment for headaches is a young, female patient with no depressive symptoms, and discontinuous head pain, who practices relaxation regularly at home.

Much of the behavioral headache research has been methodologically weak, and the deficiencies identified in this chapter and elsewhere will, hopefully, be remediated in future research.

A framework for an individualized approach to headache management, based on an understanding of the variance in headaches, was outlined. It was recommended that research begin evaluating such approaches rather than remaining focused on single techniques which take no account of the idiosyncrasies of the presenting headache problem.

REFERENCES

Ad Hoc Committee. (1962). Classification of headache. *Journal of the American Medical Association, 179,* 717–718.

Anderson, C. D., & Franks, R. D. (1981). Migraine and tension headache: Is there a physiological difference? *Headache, 21,* 63–71.

Anderson, N. B., Scott, L. P., & Olson, T. W. (1981). Within-subject analysis of autogenic training and cognitive coping training in the treatment of tension headache pain. *Journal of Behavior Therapy and Experimental Psychiatry, 12,* 219–223.

Andrasik, F., Blanchard, E. B., Arena, J. G., Saunders, N. L., & Barron, K. D. (1982a). Psychophysiology of recurrent headache: Methodological issues and new empirical findings. *Behavior Therapy, 13,* 407–429.

Andrasik, F., Blanchard, E. B., Arena, J. G., Teders, S. J., Teevan, R C., & Rodichok, L. D. (1982b). Psychological functioning in headache sufferers. *Psychosomatic Medicine, 44,* 171–182.

Andrasik, F., Blanchard, E. B., Edlund, S. R., & Attanasio, V. (1983). EMG biofeedback treatment of a child with muscle contraction headache. *American Journal of Clinical Biofeedback, 6,* 96–102.

Andrasik, F., & Holroyd, K. A. (1980). A test of specific and nonspecific effects in the biofeedback treatment of tension headache. *Journal of Consulting and Clinical Psychology, 48,* 575–586.

Andrasik, F., Holroyd, K. A., & Abell, T. (1979). Prevalence of headache within a college student population: A preliminary analysis. *Headache, 19,* 384–387.

Arena, J. G., Blanchard, E. B., Andrasik, F., & Dudek, B. C. (1982). The headache symptom questionnaire: Discriminant classificatory ability and headache syndromes suggested by a factor analysis. *Journal of Behavioral Assessment, 4,* 55–69.

Bakal, D. A. (1982). *The psychobiology of chronic headache.* New York: Springer.

Bakal, D. A., Demjen, S., & Kaganov, J. A. (1981). Cognitive behavioral treatment of chronic headache. *Headache, 21,* 81–86.

Bakal, D. A., & Kaganov, J. A. (1977). Muscle contraction and migraine headache: Psychophysiologic comparison. *Headache, 17,* 208–215.

Basmajian, J. V. (1978). *Muscles alive.* Baltimore, MD: Williams & Wilkins.

Belar, C. D., Sutton, E. P., & Wilson, E. (1983). Tension headache patients: A comparison of a recruited subject sample and a clinic based subject sample. *Headache, 23,* 240–242.

Bille, B. (1962). Migraine in school children. *Acta Paediatrica, 51*(Suppl. 136), 14–151.

Blanchard, E. B., Andrasik, F., Arena, J. G., Neff, D. F., Jurish, S. E., Teders, S. J., Barron, K. D., & Rodichok, L. D. (1983a). Nonpharmacologic treatment of chronic headache: Prediction of outcome. *Neurology, 33,* 1596–1603.

Blanchard, E. B., Andrasik, F., Appelbaum, K. A., Evans, D. D., Jurish, S. E., Teders, S. J., Rodichok, L. D., & Barron, K. D. (1985a). The efficacy and cost effectiveness of minimal-theraputic contact, non drug treatments of chronic migraine and tension headache. *Headache, 25,* 214–220.

Blanchard, E. B., Andrasik, F., Evans, D. D., Neff, D. F., Appelbaum, K. A., & Rodichok, L. D. (1985b). Behavioral treatment of 250 chronic headache patients: A clinical replication series. *Behavior Therapy, 16,* 308–327.

Blanchard, E. B., Andrasik, F., Neff, D. F., Saunders, N. L., Arena, J. G., Pallmeyer, T. P., Teders, S. J., Jurish, S. E., & Rodichok, L. D. (1983b). Four process studies in the behavioral treatment of chronic headache. *Behaviour Research and Therapy, 21,* 209–220.

Blaszczynski, A. P. (1984). Personality factors in classical migraine and tension headache. *Headache, 24,* 238–244.

Borgeat, F., Hade, B., Elie, R., & Larouche, L. M. (1984). Effects of voluntary muscle tension increases in tension headache. *Headache, 24,* 199–202.

Boudewyns, P. A. (1982). Assessment of headache. In F. J. Keefe & J. A. Blumenthal (Eds.), *Assessment strategies in behavioral medicine* (pp. 167–180). New York: Grune & Stratton.

Bruhn, P., Olesen, J., & Melgaard, B. (1979). Controlled trial of EMG feedback in muscle contraction headache. *Annals of Neurology, 6,* 34–36.

Budzynski, T. H., Stoyva, J. H., Adler, C. S., & Mullaney, D. J. (1973). EMG biofeedback and tension headaches: A controlled outcome study. *Psychosomatic Medicine, 35,* 484–496.

Chesney, M. A., & Shelton, J. L. (1976). A comparison of muscle relaxation and electromyogram feedback treatments for muscle contraction headache. *Journal of Behavior Therapy and Experimental Psychiatry, 7,* 221–225.

Cohen, R. A., Williamson, D. A., Monguillot, J. E., Hutchinson, P. C., Gottlieb, J., & Waters, W. F. (1983). Psychophysiological response patterns in vascular and muscle contraction headaches. *Journal of Behavioral Medicine, 6,* 93–107.

Cox, D. J., Freundlich, A., & Meyer, R. G. (1975). Differential effectiveness of electromyograph feedback, verbal relaxation instructions, and medication placebo with tension headaches. *Journal of Consulting and Clinical Psychology, 43,* 892–898.

Dalessio, D. J. (1972). *Wolff's headache and other head pain.* New York: Oxford University Press.

Daly, E. J., Donn, P. A., Galliher, M. J., & Zimmerman, J. S. (1983). Biofeedback applications to migraine and tension headaches: A double-blinded outcome study. *Biofeedback and Self-Regulation, 8,* 135–152.

Diamond, S., Medina, J., Diamond-Falk, J., & Deveno, T. (1979). The value of biofeedback in the treatment of chronic headache: A five-year retrospective study. *Headache, 19,* 90–96.

Domino, E. (1973). Neuropsychopharmacology of nicotine and tobacco smoking. In W. Dunn (Ed.), *Smoking behavior: Motives and incentives* (pp. 5–31). Washington, DC: Winston.

Drummond, P. D. (1985). Predisposing, precipitating and relieving factors in different categories of headache. *Headache, 25,* 16–22.

Drummond, P., & Lance, J. (1984). Clinical diagnosis and computer analysis of headache symptoms. *Journal of Neurology Neurosurgery and Psychiatry, 47,* 128-133.

Ekbom, K., Ahlborg, B., & Schele, R. (1978). Prevalence of migraine and cluster headache in Swedish men of 18. *Headache, 18,* 9–19.

Epstein, L. H., & Abel, G. G. (1977). An analysis of biofeedback training effects for tension headache patients. *Behavior Therapy, 8,* 37–47.

Epstein, L. H., Hersen, M., & Hemphill, D. P. (1974). Music feedback in the treatment of tension headache: An experimental case study. *Journal of Behavior Therapy and Experimental Psychiatry, 5,* 59–63.

Eysenck, H. J., & Eysenck, S. B. G. (1976). *Manual of the Eysenck Personality Questionnaire.* London: Hodder & Stroughton.

Featherstone, H. J. (1985). Migraine and muscle contraction headaches: A continuum, *Headache, 25,* 194–198.

Feuerstein, M., Bush, C., & Corbisiero, R. (1982). Stress and chronic headache: A psychophysiological analysis of mechanisms. *Journal of Psychosomatic Research, 26,* 167–182.

Figueroa, J. L. (1982). Group treatment of chronic tension headaches. *Behavior Modification, 6,* 229–232.

Fordyce, W. E. (1976). *Behavioral methods for chronic pain and illness.* St. Louis: Mosby.

Gannon, L. R., Haynes, S. N., Safranek, R., & Hamilton, J. (1981). A psychophysiological investigation of muscle-contraction and migraine headache. *Journal of Psychosomatic Research, 25,* 271–280.

Haber, J. D., Kuczmierczyk, A. R., & Adams, H. E. (1985). Tension headaches: Muscle overactivity or psychogenic pain. *Headache, 25,* 23–29.

Harper, R. G., & Steger, J. C. (1978). Psychological correlates of frontalis EMG and pain in tension headache. *Headache, 9,* 215–218.

Harrison, R. H. (1975). Psychological testing in headache: A review. *Headache, 14,* 177–185.

Haynes, S. N., Cuevas, J., & Gannon, L. R. (1982). The psychophysiological etiology of muscle-contraction headache. *Headache, 22,* 122–132.

Haynes, S. N., Gannon, L. R., Cuevas, J., Heiser, P., Hamilton, J., & Katranides, M. (1983). The psychophysiological assessment of muscle-contraction headache subjects during headache and nonheadache conditions. *Psychophysiology, 20,* 393–399.

Haynes, S. N., Griffin, P., Mooney, D., & Parise, M., (1975). Electromyographic biofeedback and relaxation instructions in the treatment of muscle contraction headaches. *Behavior Therapy, 6,* 672–678.

Henryk-Gutt, R., & L. Rees, W. (1973). Psychological aspects of migraine. *Journal of Psychosomatic Research, 17,* 141–153.

Hoelscher, T. J., & Lichstein, K. L. (1984). Behavioral assessment and treatment of child migraine: Implications for clinical research and practice. *Headache, 24,* 94–103.

Holmes, D. S., & Burish, T. G. (1983). Effectiveness of biofeedback for treating migraine and tension headaches: A review of the evidence. *Journal of Psychosomatic Research, 27,* 515–532.

Holroyd, K. A., & Andrasik, F. (1982). Do the effects of cognitive therapy endure? A two-year follow-up of tension headache sufferers treated with cognitive therapy or biofeedback. *Cognitive Therapy and Research, 6,* 325–334.

Holroyd, K. A., Andrasik, F., & Noble, J. (1980). A comparison of EMG biofeedback and a credible pseudotherapy in treating tension headache. *Journal of Behavioral Medicine 3,* 29–39.

Holroyd, K. A., Andrasik, F., & Westbrook, T. (1977). Cognitive control of tension headache. *Cognitive Therapy and Research, 1,* 121–133.

Holroyd, K. A., Penzien, D. B., Hursey, K. G., Tobin, D. L., Rogers, L., Holm, J. E., Marcille, P. J., Hall, J. R., & Chila, A. G. (1984). Change mechanisms in EMG biofeedback training: Cognitive changes underlying improvements in tension headache. *Journal of Consulting and Clinical Psychology, 52,* 1039–1053.

Hursey, K. G., Holroyd, K. A., Penzien, D. B., & Holm, J. E. (1985). The influence of pain state on physiological reactivity of tension headache sufferers. *Headache, 25,* 79–84.

Hutchings, D. F., & Reinking, R. H. (1976). Tension headaches: What form of therapy is most effective? *Biofeedback and Self Regulation, 1,* 183–190.

Jacob, R. G., Turner, S. M., Szekely, B. C., & Eidelman, B. H. (1983). Predicting outcome of relaxation therapy in headaches: The role of depression. *Behavior Therapy, 14,* 457–465.

Kaganov, J. A., Bakal, D. A., & Dunn, B. E. (1981). The differential contribution of muscle contraction and migraine symptoms to problem headache in the general population. *Headache, 21,* 157–163.

Kremsdorf, R. B., Kochanowicz, N. A., & Costell, S. (1981). Cognitive skills training versus EMG biofeedback in the treatment of tension headaches. *Biofeedback and Self-Regulation, 6,* 93–102.

Kudrow, L., & Sutkus, B. J. (1979). MMPI pattern specificity in primary headache disorders. *Headache, 19,* 18–24.

Lake, A. E. (1981). Behavioral assessment considerations in the management of headache. *Headache, 21,* 170–178.

Levine, B. A. (1984). Effects of depression and headache type on biofeedback for muscle-contraction headaches. *Behavioral Psychotherapy, 12,* 300–307.

Levy, L. M. (1983). An epidemiological study of headache in an urban population in Zimbabwe. *Headache, 23,* 2–9.

Martin, M. J. (1966). Tension headache, a psychiatric study. *Headache, 6,* 47–54.

Martin, P. R. (1980). Behavioral management of headaches: A review of the evidence. *International Journal of Mental Health, 9,* 88–110.

Martin, P. R. (1983). Behavioral research on headaches: Current status and future directions. In K. A. Holroyd, B. Schlote, & H. Zenz (Eds.), *Perspectives in research on headache.* Lewiston, New York: Hogrefe.

Martin, P. R. (1985). Classification of headache: The need for a radical revision. *Cephalalgia, 5,* 1–4.

Martin, P. R., & Mathews, A. M. (1978). Tension headaches: Psychophysiological investigation and treatment. *Journal of Psychosomatic Research, 22,* 380–399.

Martin, P. R., & Nathan, P. R. (1987). Differential prevalence rates for headaches: A function of stress and social support? *Headache, 27,* 329–333.

Martin, P. R., Nathan, P. R., & Van Keppel, M. (1985). *Functional analysis of chronic headaches and its relationship to treatment.* Paper presented at Seventh National Conference of Australian Behaviour Modification Association, Perth, Australia.

Meichenbaum, D. H. (1974). *Cognitive behavior modification.* Morristown, NJ: General Learning Press.

Merskey, H. (1972). Personality traits of psychiatric patients with pain. *Journal of Psychosomatic Research, 16,* 163.

Moffett, A. M., Swash, M., & Scott, D. F. (1974). Effect of chocolate in migraine: A double-blind study. *Journal of Neurology Neurosurgery and Psychiatry, 37,* 445–448.

Nikiforow, R., & Hokkanen, E. (1978). An epidemiological study of headache in an urban and a rural population in Northern Finland. *Headache, 18,* 137–145.

Norton, G. R., & Nielson, W. R. (1977). Headaches: The importance of consequent events. *Behavior Therapy, 8,* 504–506.

O'Brien, M. D. (1971). Cerebral blood changes in migraine. *Headache, 10,* 139–143.

Ogunyemi, A. O. (1984). Prevalence of headache among Nigerian University students. *Headache, 24,* 127–130.

Ostfeld, A. M., & Wolff, H. G. (1958). Identification, mechanisms and management of the migraine syndrome. *Medical Clinics of North America, 42,* 1497–1509.

Passchier, M. S., van der Helm-Hylkema, H., & Orlebeke, J. F. (1984). Psychophysiological characteristics of migraine and tension headache patients. Differential effects of sex and pain state. *Headache, 24,* 131–139.

Paulin, J. M., Waal-Manning, H. J., Simpson, F. O., & Knight, R. G. (1985). The prevalence of headache in a small New Zealand town. *Headache, 25,* 147–151.

Peck, C. L., & Kraft, G. H. (1977). Electromyographic biofeedback for pain related to muscle tension. *Archives of Surgery, 112,* 889–895.

Philips, C. (1976). Headache and personality. *Journal of Psychosomatic Research, 20,* 535–542.

Philips, C. (1977a). A psychological analysis of tension headache. In S. Rachman (Ed.), *Contributions to medical psychology* (Vol. 1). Oxford: Pergamon Press.

Philips, C. (1977b). The modification of tension headache pain using EMG biofeedback. *Behaviour Research and Therapy, 15,* 119–129.

Philips, C., & Hunter, M. (1982, January). Headache in a psychiatric population. *Journal of Nervous and Mental Disorders,* pp. 34–41.

Pikoff, H. (1984). Is the muscular model of headache still viable? A review of conflicting data. *Headache, 24,* 186–198.

Pritchard, D. W., & Wood, M. M. (1983). EMG levels in the occipitofrontalis muscles under an experimental stress condition. *Biofeedback and Self-Regulation, 8,* 165–175.

Raczynski, J. M., & Thompson, J. K. (1983). Methodological guidelines for clinical headache research. *Pain, 15,* 1–18.

Reinking, R. H., & Hutchings, D. (1981). Follow-up to: "Tension headaches: What form of therapy is most effective?" *Biofeedback and Self-Regulation, 6,* 57–62.

Sachs, H., Sevilla, F., Barberis, P., Bolis, L., Schoenberg, B., & Cruz, M. (1985). Headache in the rural village of Quiroga, Ecuador. *Headache, 25,* 190–193.

Schlutter, L. C., Golden, C. J., & Blume, H. G. (1980). A comparison of treatments for prefrontal muscle contraction headache. *British Journal of Medical Psychology, 53,* 47–52.

Schnarch, D. M., & Hunter, J. E. (1979). Personality differences between randomly selected migrainous and non-migrainous people. *Psychotherapy; Theory, Research and Practice, 16,* 297–309.

Schwartz, G. E., Brown, S. L., & Ahern, G. L. (1980). Facial muscle patterning and subjective experience during affective imagery: Sex differences. *Psychophysiology, 17,* 75–82.

Scott, D. S. (1979). A comprehensive treatment strategy for muscle contraction headaches. *Journal of Behavior Therapy and Experimental Psychiatry, 10,* 35–40.

Serratrice, E., Serbanesco, F., & Sambuc, R. (1985). Epidemiology of headache in elderly—correlations with life conditions and socio-professional environment. *Headache, 25,* 85–89.

Sherman, R. A. (1982). Home use of tape recorded relaxation exercises as initial treatment for stress related disorders. *Military Medicine, 147,* 1062–1066.

Sillanpaa, M. (1976). Prevalence of migraine and other headache in Finnish children starting school. *Headache, 16,* 288–290.

Sillanpaa, M. (1983). Changes in the prevalence of migraine and other headaches during the first seven school years. *Headache, 23,* 15–19.

Steger, J. C., & Harper, R. G. (1980). Comprehensive biofeedback versus self-monitored relaxation in the treatment of tension headache. *Headache, 20,* 137–142.

Stephens, R. (1977). Psychophysiological variables in cigarette smoking and reinforcing effects of nicotine. *Addictive Behavior, 2,* 1–7.

Sternbach, R. A., Dalessio, D. J., Kunzel, M., & Bowman, G. E. (1980). MMPI patterns in common headache disorders. *Headache, 20,* 311–315.

Sternbach, R. A., & Timmermans, G. (1975). Personality change associated with reduction of pain. *Pain, 1,* 177–181.

Teders, S. J., Blanchard, E. B., Andrasik, F., Jurish, S. E., Neff, D. F., & Arena, J. G. (1984). Relaxation training for tension headache: comparative efficacy and cost-effectiveness of a minimal therapist contact versus a therapist-delivered procedure. *Behavior Therapy, 15,* 59–70.

Thompson, J. K., & Adams, H. E. (1984). Psychophysiological characteristics of headache. *Pain, 18,* 41–52.

Thompson, J. K., & Figueroa, J. L. (1983). Critical issues in the assessment of headache. *Progress in Behavior Modification, 15,* 81–111.

Tunis, M. M., & Wolff, H. G. (1953). Studies on headache: Long-term observations of the reactivity of the cranial arteries in subjects with vascular headache of the migraine type. *Archives of Neurology and Psychiatry, 70,* 551–557.

Turkat, I. D., & Adams, H. E. (1982). Covert positive reinforcement and pain modification: A test of efficacy and theory. *Journal of Psychosomatic Research, 26,* 191–201.

Waranch, H. R., & Keenan, D. M. (1985). Behavioral treatment of children with recurrent headaches. *Journal of Behavior Therapy and Experimental Psychiatry, 16,* 31–38.

Waters, W. E. (1973). The epidemiological enigma of migraine. *International Journal of Epidemiology, 2,* 189–194.

Werder, D. S., & Sargent, J. D. (1984). A study of childhood headache using biofeedback as a treatment alternative. *Headache, 24,* 122–126.

Williamson, D. A. (1981). Behavioral treatment of migraine and muscle contraction headaches: Outcome and theoretical explanations. *Progress in Behavior Modification, 11,* 163–201.

Williamson, D. A., Monguillot, J. E., Jarrell, H. P., Cohen, R. A., Pratt, J. M.,

& Blouin, D. C. (1984). Relaxation for the treatment of headache: Controlled evaluation of two group programs. *Behavior Modification, 8,* 407–424.

Winkler, R. C. (1978). *Self management procedures for chronic headache.* Paper presented at the 1st Australian Conference on Behaviour Modification, Sydney, Australia.

Ziegler, D. K., Hassanein, R., & Hassanein, K. (1972). Headache syndromes suggested by factor analysis of symptom variables in a headache prone population. *Journal of Chronic Diseases, 25,* 353–363.

12

Behavioral Aspects of Seizure Disorders

Björn Ellertsen, Hallgrim Klöve

Department of Clinical Neuropsychology
University of Bergen, Norway

David I. Mostofsky

Department of Psychology
Boston University

Because the consequences of the epileptic disruptions may affect any or all of the disease, illness, or predicament components the particular involvement of behavioral considerations must be correspondingly considered (Mostofsky, 1981). By far the greatest concern for psychology relates to the complex social and interpersonal functioning that faces the person suffering from a chronic seizure disorder. Research from different fields of psychology has significantly contributed to improve our understanding of the epileptic patient's unique psychosocial situation, as well as the role of personality factors in epilepsy or its contribution to cognitive functioning among those suffering from the disorder. Psychology has also had a substantial influence in the development of nonpharmacologic treatment approaches in epilepsy. The nature and extent of these different types of contributions will be discussed in the chapter that follows.

EVALUATION AND ASSESSMENT

The special multifactorial condition of the epilepsies has created separate domains in which evaluations and assessments must be considered. These considerations have been discussed in detail elsewhere (Mostofsky, 1982), but it is perhaps noteworthy at this time to indicate the major points of that discussion. On the one hand assessment may be concerned with the disorder itself—its manifestation, characteristics, and so on. One may also be concerned about the technologies available for assessment of epileptic disorders—for example, the validity or reliability of self-report measures. Not least, one may choose to assess personality and other behavioral aspects of the patient with the condition, either alone or in the context of his/her family and situational environment. Insofar as organized assessment efforts comprise a major element of the overall neurological management of the patient, it becomes important to have well-identified goals for the application of the assessment results (e.g., a reduction in medication, or the design of alternative work/study responsibilities).

Psychosocial aspects of epilepsy have been discussed thoroughly in numerous publications. In 1981, Carl B. Dodrill conducted a computer search based on the keywords "epilepsy," "social factors," and "emotions" (Dodrill, 1986). More than 5,000 titles were thus generated, leading Dodrill to comment that this literature seemed to cover most aspects of human psychology, rather than specific problems relating to epilepsy. According to Dodrill, the causes of psychosocial problems in epilepsy can be classified into two main categories:

1. Epilepsy is characterized by abnormal brain functioning during seizures, and quite often also between seizures (although to be sure not all EEG abnormalities qualify for meeting the sufficient diagnostic criteria for epilepsy, nor will clinical seizures necessarily occur with every instance of EEG abnormality). The abnormal brain activity is correlated with impairment of adaptive abilities, broadly defined. There is a strong correlation between degree of epileptic problems, IQ, and adaptive abilities.
2. Both the epileptic patients and other people often regard the patient as "different" from others. Even today, the epileptic patient suffers as the result of a number of superstitions and negative associations, many of which may be internalized by the patient as well.

Dodrill (1986) divided the literature on psychosocial factors in epilepsy into four categories of "clusters":

1. emotional aspects
2. problems in interpersonal relations
3. problems regarding job and economy
4. problems regarding medical treatment of epilepsy

A number of studies of emotional problems in epilepsy, and of the so-called epileptic personality have been published. In many of these studies, the Minnesota Multiphasic Personality Inventory (MMPI) has been employed. Most studies utilizing this inventory report a general elevation of all clinical scales of the MMPI, with scale 2 (Depression) and 8 (Schizophrenia) most elevated (Dodrill, 1986). It must be noted that the elevation of the Schizophrenia scale in these cases usually reflect "unusual bodily symptoms," which of course are present in epilepsy, and do not necessarily reflect psychopathology. MMPI does not seem to be a sensitive instrument for differentiating epilepsy from other chronic somatic diseases whether neurologic or nonneurologic (Kløve & Doehring, 1962; Matthews, Dikmen & Harley, 1977; Matthews & Kløve, 1968; Warren & Weiss, 1969). All groups are characterized by depressive symptoms, worrying, anxiety, and unusual somatic symptoms all of which are reflected in the MMPI profiles.

In a well-controlled study, Dodrill (1986) compared epileptic patients with a group of healthy persons, matched with regard to sex, age, and sociocultural variables. This study is of particular value since the normative data on the basis of which the MMPI scales originally were constructed have been questioned by many authors. Revised MMPI norms are now available (Colligan, Osborne, Swenson, & Offord, 1983), but an alternative to their use in research is the incorporation of control groups, as done by Dodrill. His findings were in agreement with earlier studies comparing groups of epileptic patients with the MMPI normative data, that is, the profiles were generally elevated in the epileptic group, as compared to controls, with the most pronounced elevation on scales 2 and 8. MMPI studies on diagnostic subgroups of epileptics have shown that emotional problems are most pronounced in patients with known neurologic etiology, as compared to those with unknown etiology (Matthews & Kløve, 1968). A correlation between number of seizures and degree of emotional problems was also reported. The relationship between age of onset, type of seizures and degree of emotional problems is, however, complicated.

The "epileptic personality" has been a concept within medicine for many years. However, there have been dramatic changes in the description of the epileptic patient, reflecting changes in the opinion of both physicians and the public concerning epilepsy. Typical descriptions that have been offered until recently are apathy, slow-wittedness, and incompetence. After the introduction of effective antiepileptic drugs, descriptions have emphasized impulsiveness, aggression, and violence that in some cases may be observed in temporal lobe epilepsy. Blumer and Benson (1975) concluded that the "epileptic personality" is far from characteristic of all epileptic patients. It may be noted here that the popular certainty of the TLE triad (hypergraphia, hyperreligiosity, and hyposexuality) is also not an invariant accompaniment to the condition. Certain characteristic personality traits do, however, seem to be associated with chronic involvement of temporal-limbic structures.

Different investigators have reported that between 5 and 35 percent of patients evaluated with regard to possible epilepsy have pseudoepileptic seizures in addition to their epileptic seizures or as their primary diagnosis. This differential diagnosis has been a challenge to neurologists and neuropsychologists, resulting in a number of studies. Again, the MMPI has been widely used in order to try and find crucial differentiating variables. A study by Wilkus, Dodrill, and Thompson (1984) reported 85 percent correct classification of epilepsy versus pseudoepilepsy, based on MMPI-criteria. However, Dodrill (1986) concludes that this field of research still is in need of further studies and that there still are uncertainties and unsolved questions. Indeed, the topic of pseudoseizures remains somewhat confusing both conceptually and terminologically and has not been resolved to the satisfaction of either neurology or psychology (Williams & Mostofsky, 1982).

Clinical experience and numerous studies show that epilepsy strongly affects family and peer relations. The degree and type of problems, however, may vary considerably between subjects. It is therefore of importance to screen this area in which separate case before treatment and counseling is started. The Washington Psychosocial Seizure Inventory (WPSI) was developed for the purpose of such screening of psychosocial problems in epilepsy and it has been demonstrated that this inventory is suitable both for research and for general clinical screening purposes (Dodrill, Batzel, Queisser, & Temkin, 1980; Dodrill, 1983).

The medical treatment of epilepsy offers challenges which require special knowledge and competence. As a consequence, specialized medical centers for epilepsy can be found in many countries, including Norway and the United States. However, follow-up by local physicians and other health workers, once diagnostic evaluation and start of pharmacologic treatment is concluded, is often poor. Although blood serum levels of medication should be evaluated on a regular basis, this is often not the case. Equally troubling is patient compliance in taking medication. It has been suggested that as many as 25–50 percent of all epileptic patients treated pharmacologically do not take their medication as prescribed (Peterson, McLean, & Millingen, 1982). Obviously, both follow-up, counseling, and interventions targeted to foster compliance represent interesting challenges for psychologists.

Large numbers of epileptic patients have been evaluated by neuropsychologists since psychologic testing of neurologic patients became common practice in the 1940s. A number of publications have presented findings regarding cognitive functioning, memory functions, psychomotor and sensory-motor functions in different types of epilepsy. It may safely be concluded that neuropsychologic evaluation of epileptic patients represents a valuable part of the general screening, and also of the long-term follow-up. The neuropsychologist confronted with the task of evaluating an epileptic patient is faced with a multifactorial problem, that is, the patient has a brain dysfunction which may be so minimal that no cognitive deficit of consequence can be identified, or so serious that the consequences may be substantial indeed and, in addition to epilepsy may be accompanied by multiple CNS handicaps. In addition, the patient's seizures may cause impaired functioning, at least for periods of time. Finally, the patient's medication may affect concentration, memory, and motor functions. Ideally, the neuropsychologic evaluation should make it possible to sort out these different problems.

A basic question in neuropsychologic research with epileptic patients has been whether the seizures as such, or the underlying neuropathology are main determinants with regard to the degree of impaired function. This question has been elucidated in a series of studies performed by Kløve and Matthews (1974), who utilized an extensive neuropsychologic test battery, including the measurement of psychometric intelligence (WAIS) and the Halstead neuropsychologic test battery. In one investigation four groups matched with regard to sex, age, and education were studied. One group consisted of patients with known brain pathology and a second group consisted of patients with epilepsy and known brain pathology. These two groups were matched with regard to etiology of pathology. A third group consisting of patients with unknown etiology and epilepsy was matched with group two with regard to diagnoses. A fourth group consisted of healthy subjects, and served as a "normal" control group. It was found that epilepsy was associated with significantly poorer performance on the intelligence test and on the neuropsychologic tests, as compared to normal controls. Performance was more impaired in both groups with known etiology as compared with epilepsy with unknown etiology. Thus, epilepsy per se does not seem to be associated with more pronounced impairment of cognitive functions than the impairment observed in a group of patients with comparable neuropathology. In another study, different diagnostic categories among the epilepsies were compared with regard to neuropsychologic functioning (Kløve & Matthews, 1974). Again, patients with known etiology showed most impaired functions. In addition, patients with psychomotor seizures performed better than patients with major motor seizures, regardless of etiologic variables. In a third study (Kløve & Matthews, 1974) it was demonstrated that there is a significant correlation between degree of cognitive impairment and early age of onset in patients with major motor seizures.

The main conclusion from studies of emotional, psychosocial, and neuropsychologic factors in epilepsy is that a wide range of methods for the evaluation of patients has been developed and validated. Although a number of the studies published may be criticized for the lack of detailed description of diagnostic criteria, or for the study of heterogenous groups of patients, it seems reasonable to conclude that the methods are valuable as research tools in the study of groups of patients with epilepsy. A note of caution should, however, be made with regard to the use of these methods in clinical work. Generalization of group findings to a single case is always problematic, particularly when the number of factors contributing is as high as in epilepsy. In evaluating an epileptic patient, psychologic defense mechanisms and coping strategies, as well as environment factors, are of crucial importance in addition to data obtained through psychosocial screening, personality evaluation, and neuropsychologic evaluation. With this caution in mind, we conclude by recommending a broad screening of all patients presenting with epileptic symptomatology. This screening should consist of personality evaluation, psychosocial evaluation, and neuropsychologic testing.

TREATMENT

Epilepsy may appear to be an organically objective neurologic disorder which is effectively treated with drugs. However, the diagnosis covers a wide variety of more or less complex seizure disorders and, as noted above, the differential diagnosis between epilepsy and functional seizures may be complicated. Accordingly, it is not surprising that as many as 60 percent of all epileptic patients may not be effectively treated pharmacologically (De Vivo, 1983). These patients are often described as drug resistant or medically intractable. Even for those for whom it is claimed that they are "controlled" by anticonvulsant drug programs, there is little consensus as to what constitutes the criterion for "control." Quite often, the physician's estimate is at variance with the expectations of the patient or his or her family. It should also be noted that, although clinically effective, all antiepileptic drugs have disturbing side effects and tardive and other long-term effects, such as sedation, impaired learning capabilities, and various somatic effects. In light of these facts, any procedure which may prove to be a valuable adjuvant in epilepsy should be seriously evaluated. It is, however, our impression that the resistance against alternatives to pharmacologic treatment is irrationally strong. We shall return to this point after a discussion of treatment procedures based on psychologic theory and research.

Mostofsky and Balaschak (1977) reviewed a number of treatment strategies which they classified as psychobiologic. The techniques in question were subclassified as "reward management" (represented by conditioning and behavior therapy models), "self-control" (represented by cognitive and psychodynamic models), and "psychophysiologic methods" (represented by habituation and biofeedback models). It was concluded that behavioral therapies offer substantial promise for the clinical management of seizure problems. A number of well-controlled studies have further elucidated some of the methods discussed by Mostofsky and Balaschak. There is a growing literature in both journal and handbook publications that points to the effective utilization of behavior modification and relaxation procedures for seizure control. Less attention appears to have been paid to the psychophysiologic methods. We wish to correct that imbalance by focusing on that class of treatment in this section of the chapter.

Before proceeding with a discussion of psychophysiologic treatment methods, two early studies done by Efron (1956, 1957) may serve to illustrate the rather astounding effect of conditioning therapy in a patient with psychomotor seizures. It was discovered that a powerful unpleasant odor presented during her aura would abort the seizure (the odor of undiluted jasmine was most effective) and Efron was able to subject this phenomenon to second-order conditioning. He transferred the effect of the olfactory stimulus to a bracelet through numerous copresentations of the odor and the sight of the bracelet. Ultimately, the seizures could be aborted by the mere visualization of the bracelet. This and other observations raised the question whether abnormal EEG activity could be conditioned, similar to responses in the autonomic nervous system, via classical conditioning mechanisms. The Efron study is notable in that one may detect features that are not only of the conditioning variety, but also some features that suggest the role of cognitive and psychophysiological variables. Stevens, Millstein and Dodds (1967) tried to condition paroxysmal EEG spikes to mild electric shocks in 18 patients. They concluded that spontaneous epileptiform EEG transitions have only little influence on an ongoing behavior or subjective state and only with great difficulty can it be conditioned to serve as "internal signals." Animal research done by Wyler, Robbins, and Dodrill (1979), Janowsky, Laxer, and Rushmer (1980) and Myslobodsky, Mintz, Lerner, and Mostofsky (1983) have further supported this conclusion. In these studies, acquisition and elicitation of epileptic seizures was paired with auditory or visual signals, in order to see whether seizures later could be triggered by the signal only. The kindling technique, that is, daily subconvulsive electric stimulation of brain structures (usually amygdala) resulting in the development of an epileptic focus, was employed.

A different approach to the treatment of epilepsy has been developed by Francis M. Forster and his co-workers (Forster, 1977). This approach was termed "extinction treatment of sensory induced epilepsy." Daube (1966) presented an excellent review of the sensory epilepsies. These seizures may be elicited by visual stimuli such as changes in light intensity, flickering light, geometric patterns, reading, or specific stimulus configurations such as a painting. Auditory elicited seizures may follow changes in sound, rhythmic patterns, or music. Patients with sensory-induced epilepsy are often found to be self-stimulating. In the earliest papers on the topic of extinction treatment, it was suggested that sensory-induced epilepsy was a conditioned reflex which could be experimentally extinguished (which is the historic background for the terms reflex epilepsy and extinction treatment). This point of view was later abandoned, but the term extinction treatment prevails. In order to use the technique, two requirements must be met:

1. A clear, definable, and physical, seizure precipitant.
2. Definite changes in the patient's EEG immediately preceding the clinical seizure.

Basically, two different treatment strategies have been developed. The first is to stimulate the patient repeatedly with a stimulus modified sufficiently so as not to provoke a seizure, but nonetheless sufficiently similar to the seizure-precipitating stimulus as possible. The patient is then repeatedly stimulated as the stimulus is gradually made more similar to the original stimulus. As soon as the stimulation results in epileptogenic changes in the EEG, the stimulation is stopped and the procedure is started over again. The second method is to expose the actual seizure-precipitating stimulus and remove it as soon as the characteristic epileptogenic EEG changes occur.

Data from a 5-year-old boy with major motor seizures, who was found to be pattern-sensitive (geometric patterns such as brick walls would elicit seizures) may serve to illustrate the typical change in sensitivity observed during extinction treatment. It was established that the patient's EEG would show characteristic changes immediately following slide presentation of geometric patterns. The critical change was a 8.5 Hz wave followed by a spike. Treatment consisted of repeated stimulation of the patient with a pattern that would provoke a seizure, and automatically stop the stimulation as soon as his EEG changed. When the EEG returned to base level, the procedure was repeated. Figure 12.1 shows that the patient's sensitivity to the stimulus gradually decreased. When the treatment was started he was unable to watch the stimulus for more than a few seconds, but after one month of training, twice a week, he was able to look at it for several minutes. More important, there was a generalization to his everyday situations consisting of a 70 percent reduction in number of seizures (Ellertsen & Kløve, 1976). Similar changes in stimulus sensitivity and occurrence of seizures have been observed in patients with flicker-induced seizures.

Unlike extinction treatment, which is restricted to sensory-induced seizures, a treatment approach developed by M. B. Sterman and his co-workers has been shown to be clinically effective in broader categories of epileptic patients. This treatment technique was developed on the basis of animal research. In studying behavioral correlates of specific EEG characteristics in animals, this research group identified a 12–14 Hz pattern, developed over the sensorimotor cortex in animals trained to withhold a conditioned motor response. This activity was termed the sensorimotor rhythm (SMR) and it was decided to attempt conditioning of this EEG pattern (Wyrwicka & Sterman, 1968; Sterman, Wyrwicka, & Roth, 1969). The SMR was found to be easily trained as an instrumental response, and was behaviorally found to be related to attentive immobility. Figure 12.1 illustrates the relationship between occurrence of SMR activity, behavior, and EMG activity in deep neck muscles in a cat. The figure shows two EEG signals: the upper recording is from the sensory-motor cortex. This signal is filtered in a highly tuned 12–14 Hz band-pass filter and output from the filter is shown in the channel between the EEG signals. Below the EEG channels the integrated EMG signal from neck muscles is shown. At the bottom the marker channel shows reinforcement of SMR. The figure shows that no SMR was present while the animal was moving. The animal then sits quietly, EMG activity is reduced, and SMR appears.

It was accidentally observed that animals overtrained in this response were resistant to drug-induced seizures (Sterman, LoPresti, &

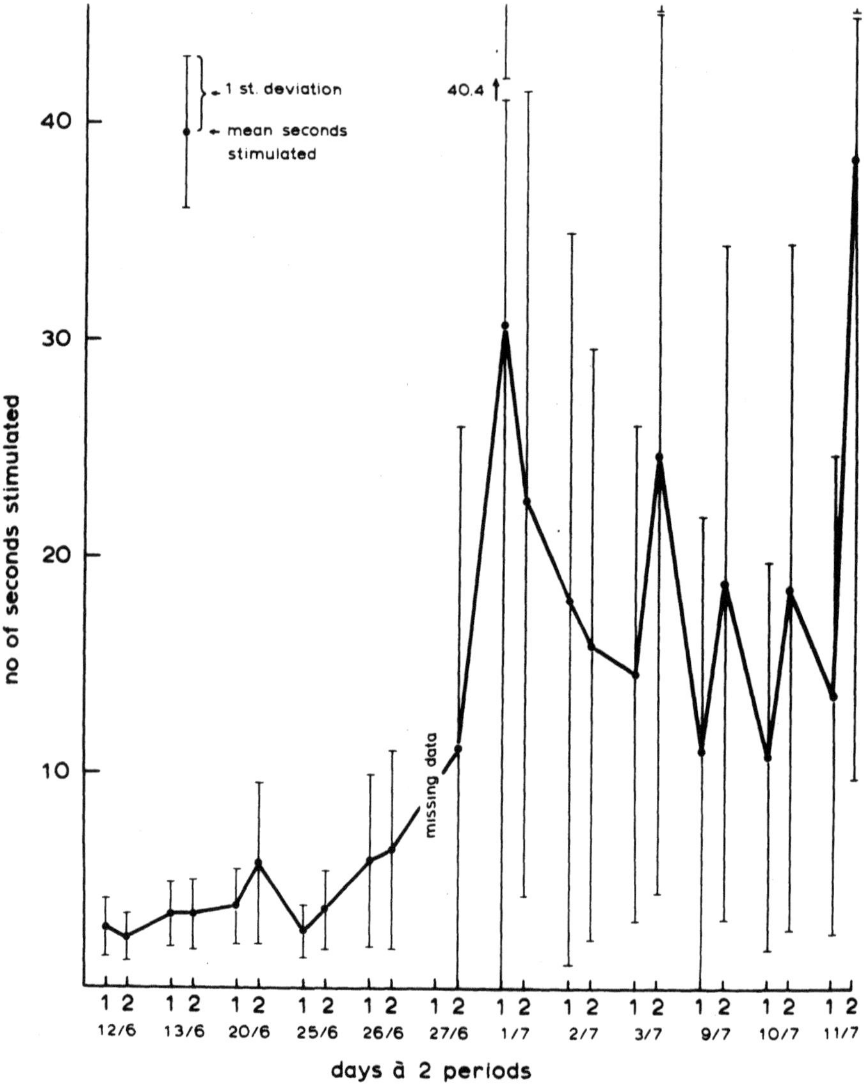

FIGURE 12.1. Mean stimulus time from each treatment period (30 min.), each day in a pattern senstive boy.

Fairchild, 1969). Sterman (1986) discussed this protective effect of SMR conditioning. It has been demonstrated that SMR is intrinsically generated by ventrobasal thalamic neurons (Sterman & Bowersox, 1981) in a similar manner as alpha rhythms, which earlier were shown to be the product of gated thalamocortical discharges. Therefore, thalamic discharge is released due to a withdrawal or attenuation of

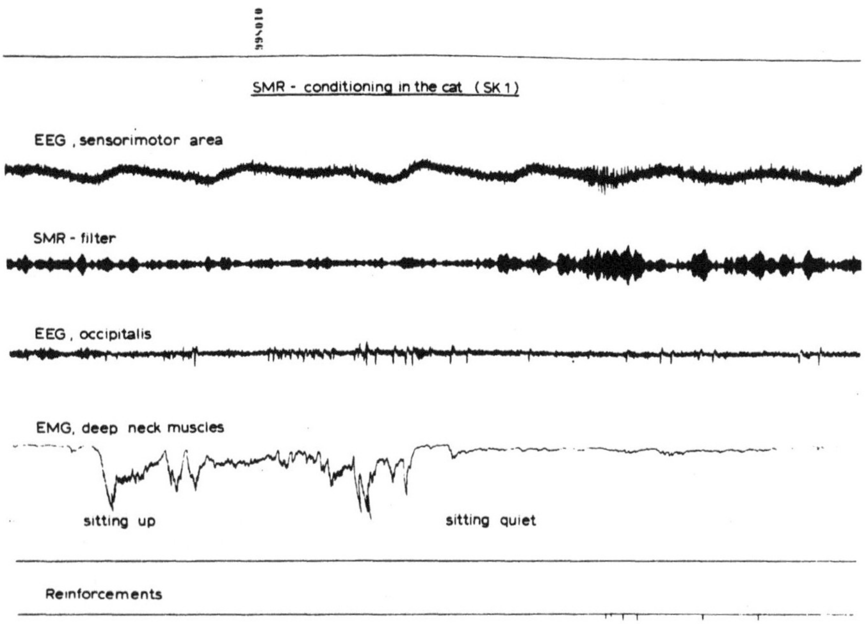

FIGURE 12.2. Polygraphic recording from SMR conditioning in cat. EEG from sensorimotor and occipital cortex, EMG from deep neck muscles, SMR-filter output, behavior, and reinforcements are indicated.

afferent activity in the sensorimotor pathways, produced experimentally by SMR conditioning (Sterman, 1986). Somatosensory pathway lesions (Shouse & Sterman, 1979), immobilization (Sterman & Kovalesky, 1979) and antiepileptics (Sterman & Kovalesky, 1983) produce the same effects, including raised seizure thresholds. On the other hand, studies of experimental epilepsy have demonstrated abnormal alterations in thalamocortical discharges, resulting in abnormal cortical rhythmic activity (Gloor, Pellegrini, & Kostopoulus, 1979; Shouse, 1986). These and other findings have led Sterman to propose the working hypothesis that manipulations which normalize these aberrant EEG patterns must also attenuate the disturbances in thalamocortical regulation, thereby facilitating normal sensorimotor function and increased seizure threshold (Sterman, 1986).

Thus, the clinical application of SMR training in epileptic patients is based on extensive basic research, which, of course, cannot be replicated with normal humans. The accumulated data offers clear and dramatic support for the meaningful clinical utilization of such a treatment alternative. It is likely that disorders other than epilepsy may also benefit from this treatment strategy (Lubar & Deering, 1981). It is, in our opinion, surprising that a treatment procedure that is founded on extensive basic research, and which has been validated in a series of well-controlled clinical studies, has received relatively little acceptance throughout the world community of epileptologists and allied agencies and institutions.

The first SMR biofeedback treatment of an epileptic patient was carried out by Sterman and Friar (1972). The patient suffered from frequent, intractable major motor seizures. She showed a clear acquisition of the conditioned sensorimotor EEG response and an abrupt cessation of seizures followed. This first single-case report has later been replicated in a number of studies performed in different laboratories. Taken together, the studies report at least 50 percent seizure reduction in patients treated with SMR biofeedback. These effects have never been questioned in the literature. However, alternative explanations regarding the therapeutic factors have been suggested, among them nonspecific placebo effects, changes in medication compliance due to the regular attention given to the patient, and so on. However, most studies performed during the last 10 years have included monitoring of medication blood levels and, in addition, the nonspecific placebo effect has been controlled for in several studies. A study by Lantz and Sterman (1988) may serve to illustrate such a recent methodologic development in the field. Twenty-four chronic, drug refractory epileptic patients were divided into three groups. For all groups the patients tabulated seizures for six weeks prior to the experimental intervention. One group was then given SMR biofeedback training, according to the procedures developed by Sterman and his co-workers. The second group served as a yoked control group and was given "sham feedback" throughout the six-week treatment period, whereas the third group served as a tabulation control group. All groups tabulated seizures for six weeks after the experimental period, and the two control groups were then given SMR feedback training, again followed by a six-week tabulation period. Thus, the experimental design was very strong with regard to identification of therapeutic factors. In addition, all patients were tested neuropsychologically and given the MMPI before experimental intervention.

It was found that seizure reduction was strongly associated with acquisition of the EEG training task. It was also found that baseline psychologic testing was able to predict treatment outcome to some extent. Successful patients scored better on a test indicative of general intelligence, and worse on tests involving strong motor components. They also had fewer psychosocial problems. The finding on motor tests is interesting in light of the fact that sensorimotor cortex and thalamocortical pathways are closely related to the SMR phenomenon (Lantz & Sterman, 1988).

Although the evidence regarding clinical effects of SMR enhancement training is substantial, there is still debate regarding the critical role of SMR. During training, patients are given feedback on the occurence of SMR, but this feedback is automatically withheld if slow-wave (2–7 Hz) or beta (20–25 Hz) activity is present over the sensorimotor cortex. Thus, one might speculate whether inhibition of certain frequencies plays an important role instead of, or in addition to, the SMR conditioning. Regardless of this issue (which presently is being studied in detail) the clinical efficacy of the SMR biofeedback treatment procedure is unquestionable. It is also important to underscore that this treatment approach has no negative side effects. In light of these facts and the sound scientific foundation on which the treatment procedures were developed, it is reasonable to conclude that SMR biofeedback training has proved worthy as an important adjuvant in the treatment of epileptic patients and therefore deserves increased serious attention among clinicians working with epilepsy.

CONCLUSIONS

We began by asserting that psychologic research significantly has contributed to improve our understanding of different aspects of epilepsy, and has been an important element in the development of treatment techniques. The contributions come from different fields of psychology, especially physiological psychology, social psychology, personality psychology, and neuropsychology. The research has been performed both by experienced clinical psychologists and by experimentally oriented psychologists. It is our conviction that both the methods of evaluation (as part of screening and follow-up) and the treatment methods significantly contribute to improve patient care. As mentioned several times, a number of epileptic patients represent diagnostic and treatment "problems." In such cases we strongly recommend psychosocial, personality, and neuropsychologic evaluation as part of a broader screening. We also recommend the use of extinction treatment procedures in sensory-induced epilepsy and SMR biofeedback treatment, not only for the medically intractable patient alone. The behavioral medicine approaches to epilepsy are in rapid development. It has not been the purpose of this chapter to give an exhaustive or completely updated overview, but rather to emphasize some approaches which are of clinical importance, and which can give emphasis to further research in the field.

REFERENCES

Blumer, D., & Benson, D. F. (1975). Personality changes with frontal and temporal lobe lesions. In D. F. Benson & D. Blumer (Eds.), *Psychiatric aspects of neurologic disease* (pp. 151–170). New York: Grune & Stratton.

Colligan, R. C., Osborne, D., Swenson, W. M., & Offord, K. (1983). *The MMPI: A contemporary normative study*. New York: Praeger Publishers.

Daube, J. R. (1966). Sensory precipitated seizures: A review. *Journal of Nervous and Mental Disease, 141*(5), 524–539.

DeVivo, D. C. (1983). How to use other drugs (steroids) and the ketogenic diet. In P. L. Morselli, C. E. Pippenger, & C. E. Penry (Eds.), *Antiepileptic drug therapy in pediatrics*. New York: Raven Press.

Dodrill, C. B. (1983). Psychosocial characteristics of epileptic patients. In A. A. Ward, Jr., J. K. Penry, & D. Purpura (Eds.), *Epilepsy*. New York: Raven Press.

Dodrill, C. B. (1986). Psychosocial consequences of epilepsy. In S. B. Filskov & T. J. Boll (Eds.), *Handbook of clinical neuropsychology* (Vol. 2, pp. 338–363). New York: John Wiley & sons.

Dodrill, C. B., Batzel, L. W., Queisser, H. R., & Temkin, N. R. (1980). An objective method for the assessment of psychological and social difficulties among epileptics. *Epilepsia, 21*, 125–135.

Efron, R. (1956). The effect of olfactory stimuli in arresting unciate fits. *Brain, 79*, 267–282.

Efron, R. (1957). The conditioned inhibition of unciate fits. *Brain, 80*, 251–262.

Ellertsen, B., & Kløve, H. (1976). Clinical application of biofeedback training in epilepsy. *Scandinavian Journal of Behaviour Therapy, 5*, 133–144.

Forster, F. M. (1977). *Reflex epilepsy, behavioral therapy and conditional reflexes*. Springfield, IL: Charles C. Thomas.

Gloor, P., Pellegrini, A., & Kostopoulus, G. K. (1979). Effects of changes in cortical excitability upon the epileptic bursts in generalized penicillin epilepsy of the cat. *Electroencephalography and Clinical Neurophysiology, 46*, 274–289.

Janowsky, J. S., Laxer, K. D., & Rushmer, D. S. (1980). Classical conditioning of kindled seizures. *Epilepsia, 21*, 393–398.

Kløve, H., & Doehring, D. G. (1962). MMPI in epileptic groups with differential etiology. *Journal of Clinical Psychology, 18*, 149–153.

Kløve, H., & Matthews, C. G. (1974). Neuropsychological studies of patients with epilepsy. In R. M. Reitan & L. A. Davison (Eds.), *Clinical neuropsychology: Current status and applications* (pp. 237–265). New York: John Wiley & Sons.

Lantz, D., & Sterman, M. B. (1988). Neuropsychological assessment of subjects with uncontrolled epilepsy: effects of EEG feedback training. *Epilepsia, 29*, 163–171.

Lubar, J. F., & Deering, W. M. (1981). *Behavioral approaches to neurology* (pp. 5–20). New York: Academic Press.

Matthews, C. G., Dikmen, S., & Harley, J. P. (1977). Age at onset and psychometric correlates of MMPI profiles in major motor epilepsy. *Diseases of the nervous System, 38*, 173–176.

Matthews, C. G., & Kløve, H. (1968). MMPI performance in major motor, psychomotor and mixed seizure classification of known and unknown etiology. *Epilepsia, 9*, 43–53.

Mostofsky, D. I. (1981) Paroxysmal disorders of the central nervous system. In S. Turner, K. Calhoun, & H. Adams (Eds.), *Handbook of clinical behavior therapy* (pp. 447–474). New York: John Wiley & Sons.

Mostofsky, D. I. (1982). Epilepsy. In F. J. Keefe & J. A. Blumenthal (Eds.), *Assessment strategies in behavioral medicine* (pp. 181–196). New York: Grune & Stratton.

Mostofsky, D. I., & Balaschak, B. A. (1977). Psychobiological control of seizures. *Psychological Bulletin, 84*(4), 723–750.

Myslobodsky, M. S., Mintz, M., Lerner, T., & Mostofsky, D. I. (1983). Amygdala kindling in the classical conditioning paradigm. *Epilepsia, 24*, 275–283.

Peterson, G. M., McLean, S., & Millingen, K. S. (1982). Determinants of patient compliance with anticonvulsant therapy. *Epilepsia, 23*, 607–613.

Shouse, M. N. (1986). Thalamic mechanisms of state dependent kindled seizures in cats. In J. Wada (Ed.), *Kindling 3*. New York: Raven Press.

Shouse, M. N., & Sterman, M. B. (1979). Changes in seizure susceptibility, sleep time, and sleep spindles following thalamic and cerebellar lesions. *Electroencephalography and Clinical Neurophysiology, 46*, 1–12.

Sterman, M. B. (1986). Epilepsy and its treatment with EEG feedback therapy. *Annals of Behavioral Medicine, 8*, 21–25.

Sterman, M. B., & Bowersox, S. S. (1981). Sensorimotor EEG rhythmic activity: A functional gate mechanism. *Sleep, 4*(4), 408–422.

Sterman, M. B., & Friar, L. (1972). Suppression of seizures in an epileptic following sensorimotor EEG feedback training. *Electroencephalography and Clinical neurophysiology, 33*, 89–95.

Sterman, M. B., & Kovalesky, R. A. (1979). Anticonvulsant effects of restraint and pyridoxine on hydrazine seizures in the monkey. *Experimental Neurology, 65*, 78–86.

Sterman, M. B., & Kovalesky, R. A. (1983). Baseline studies and anticonvulsant drug effects on the sleep EEG power spectral profile. *Electroencephalography and Clinical Neurophysiology, 55*(2), 212–222.

Sterman, M. B., & LoPresti, R. W., & Fairchild, M. D. (1969). *Electroencephalographic and behavioral studies of monomethylhydrazine toxicity in the cat* (Tech. Rep. AMRL-TR-69-3). Dayton, OH: Air Force Systems Commands, Wright-Patterson Air Force Base.

Sterman, M. B., Wyrwicka, W., & Roth, S. (1969). Electrophysiological correlates and neural substrates of alimentary behavior in the cat. *Annals of the New York Academy of Science, 157*, 723–739.

Stevens, J. R., Milstein, V. M., & Dodds, S. A. (1967). Endogenous spike discharges as conditioned stimuli in man. *Electroencephalography and Clinical Neurophysiology, 23*, 57–66.

Warren, L. W., & Weiss, D. J. (1969). Relationship between disability type and measured personality characteristics. *Proceedings of the 77th Annual Convention of the American Psychological Association*, *4*, 773–774.

Wilkus, R. J., Dodrill, C. B., & Thompson, P. M. (1984). Intensive EEG monitoring and psychological studies of patients with pseudoepileptic seizures. *Epilepsia*, *25*(1), 100–107.

Williams, D. T., & Mostofsky, D. I. (1982) Psychogenic seizures in childhood and adolescence. In T. L. Riley & A. R. Roy (Eds.), *Pseudoseizures* (pp. 169–184). Baltimore: Williams and Wilkins.

Wyler, A. R., Robbins, C. A., & Dodrill, C. B. (1979). EEG operant conditioning for control of epilepsy, *Epilepsia*, *20*(3), 279–286. Wyrwicka, W., & Sterman, M. B. (1968). Instrumental conditioning of sensorimotor cortex EEG spindles in the waking cat. *Physiology and Behavior*, *3*, 702–707.

13

Sleep Disorders: Their Prevalence and Behavioral Treatment

Leon C. Lack

Flinders University of South Australia
Bedford Park, South Australia

Steven J. Thorn

Noarlunga Health Services
Noarlunga, South Australia

THE HEALTH PROBLEMS OF SLEEP/ WAKE DISORDERS

Approximately one-third of our life, or over 23 total years of a 70-year life span, is spent—for reasons which still elude the scientific community—in a recumbent, unconscious state we call sleep. Those who have busy lifestyles and wish for more hours in the day may resent it. Those who are trying to escape life's demands may covet it. But despite our feelings about sleep—so aptly named "The Gentle Tyrant" by Wilse B. Webb (1975)—it usually exerts its influence over us every night. Since it is going to occur sooner or later, most of us would simply prefer it to occur in a trouble-free and efficient way. Like rainy weather we want it to be over and done with quickly but effectively. We are not amused by nighttime awakenings and restless, light sleep in a similar way to our annoyance at weather which drizzles off and on inordinately. Taking this weather analogy further we would prefer our days to be sunny rather than overcast as we would prefer our minds to be alert and productive rather than foggy and lethargic. Unfortunately, we do not live in a Camelot where the weather is ideal and sleep/wake processes work perfectly. Most of us experience disturbed, unsatisfying sleep and subsequent daytime dysphoria occasionally and some experience it quite frequently. However, how much of a problem is this imperfect sleep/wake pattern and does it have any health repercussions?

Disturbed sleep may be viewed as a health problem in its own right. In a survey of over one million Americans "insomnia" was found to be the 12th most frequent health problem among men and the 6th most frequent among women (Hammond, 1964). Insomnia has been reported as the third most common complaint in general medical practice behind headache and gastrointestinal problems (Lugaresi et al., 1983). Five percent of adult medical patients present with complaints of insomnia (Regestein & Reich, 1978). Enough people perceive that they have a substantial sleep problem to make hypnotic drugs a common medical prescription. Surveys have found between 2–9 percent of the population reported using hypnotic drugs frequently. There is little doubt that many people's quality of life is adversely affected by frequently disturbed sleep and its concomitants of anxiety, frustration, negative mood, lethargy, and sleepiness.

Many researchers have found an association between psychological distress, psychiatric symptoms, and insomnia. Those identified as insomniacs or those with self-reported frequent sleep troubles also show increased psychopathology, as measured, for example, in elevated ratings on the MMPI (Carskadon et al., 1976; Johns, Gay, Masterton, & Bruce, 1971; Kales et al., 1978; Kales et al., 1984; Karacan, Ilaria, Ware, Thornby, & Chambliss, 1978; Mellinger, Balter, & Unlenhath, 1985). Conversely, those who have been identified as psychiatric patients or who were suffering anxiety or depression were much more likely to have a disturbed sleep pattern (Hetta, Almquist, Liljenberg, & Rous, 1987; Weiss, Kasinoff, & Baily, 1962). It is unclear from these studies whether a causal connection can be established between sleep disturbance and psychological disturbance, if indeed, causal attribution is a useful construct in this area. While some researchers have stressed that "psychopathology is the primary etiology of chronic insomnia . . ." (Kales et al., 1978), it would also seem plausible that chronic insomnia arising primarily from nonpsychopathological factors would be a stressor which could exacerbate or even produce a psychological disturbance.

A more useful model may be derived from control systems theory in which sleep disturbance and psychological disturbance feed back on each other in a positive way, resulting in a vicious circle of increasing psychological and sleep disturbance. A negative feedback control system leads to a homeostatic state while a positive feedback arrangement leads to instability and, sooner or later, a challenge to the tolerance limits of the system. If those limits are exceeded, psychobiological breakdown is the result. This model would predict that since sleep and psychological parameters are two interacting elements of the same system, reducing disturbance in one will reduce disturbance in the other. This prediction has strong support from successful antidepressive therapies which usually improve sleep as well. There is also some support from clinical sleep research which showed improved MMPI profiles following successful behavioral treatment of sleep onset insomnia (Shealy, Lowe, & Ritzler, 1980).

Sleep disturbance has also been linked with physical health. Those who report cardiac disease, hypertension, or diabetes also report greater frequency of difficulties initiating and maintaining sleep than those who are disease-free (Hetta et al., 1987). Several survey studies have found more hospitalizations and physical illness symptoms such as cardiovascular, musculoskeletal, gastrointestinal, respiratory, and skin disorders among those identified as insomniac or sleep-disturbed than in good sleepers (Bixler, Kales, Soldatos, Kales, & Healey, 1979; Johns, Egan, Gay, & Masterson, 1970; Mellinger, Balter, & Unlenhuth, 1985; Urponen, Vuori, Hasan, & Partinen, 1987). Longitudinal studies have investigated the mortality associated with insomnia and abnormal reported sleep lengths. Hammond (1964), in a one year follow-up of approximately one million Americans, found an increased mortality ratio of 1.32 in men reporting insomnia. From the same base sample Hammond and Garfinkel (1969) and Kripke, Simons, Garfinkel, and Hammond (1979) reported on later follow-ups that death rates were consistently higher for those reporting shorter than six hours sleep or longer than nine hours sleep compared with 7–8 hour sleepers. This differential mortality rate was present in respondents free of serious disease in the original survey. Men and women reporting less than four hours sleep were 2.8 times and 1.48 times respectively more likely to die than 7–8 hour sleepers over a six-year period. After controlling for age and hypnotic pill taking, "insomniac" men and women were respectively 34 percent and 17 percent more likely to die over the six-year period. Reporting less than five hours or more than ten hours nightly sleep was almost as predictive of mortality as a medical history of diabetes, coronary heart disease, stroke, or hypertension. Wingard, Berkman, and Brand (1979) in a similar but smaller study also found an increased mortality rate in short and long sleepers even after controlling for age, sex, smoking, alcohol consumption, physical activity, and weight-to-height ratio. Although the mechanism linking increased mortality to insomnia or unusual sleep lengths still needs to be investigated, the salient point here is that sleep disturbance and abnormalities have reliable physical health sequelae.

MEASUREMENT ISSUES

Before discussing studies of the prevalence of sleep disorders a few measurement problems need to be addressed. How can the prevalence of sleep disorders be assessed in the population? Ideally, we would obtain a large (N = 1000–2000) sample representative of sex, age groups from childhood to the most elderly, occupation, socioeconomic level, and other relevant demographic and health status variables. All aspects of sleep including subjective qualitative and time estimate measures and the whole range of objective polysomnographic (PSG) variables including EEG, ECG, EMG, plasma O_2 saturation, respiration activity, EOG, and movement data would be measured over a minimum of seven nights in the subject's normal sleep environment. Such a study has not been conducted nor is it likely to be until further technological advances of ambulatory monitoring are made and problems of subject compliance after selection are overcome. In any case, such a study would be extremely costly.

With the much lower resources practically available less ideal solutions are attempted. Resources have been spent on a relatively small number of subjects (50–100) measured comprehensively in the research laboratory or home environment with PSG. Because subjects are not selected randomly or representatively, the large drawback of these studies is their dubious generalizability to the population. Sleep/wake diaries are much less expensive and can be collected from larger samples (300–600) somewhat more representative of the general population. However, the measures are based on subjective estimates and although usually correlate significantly with PSG measures (Bixler, Kales, Leo, & Slye, 1973; Carskadon et al., 1976) a large source of variance is idiosyncratic to the subject. Furthermore, some important sleep disorders such as sleep apnea, nocturnal myoclonus, and narcolepsy require PSG for reliable diagnosis as they all may manifest similar symptoms of daytime sleepiness and vague impressions of disrupted nighttime sleep. Therefore, a tradeoff exists between large sample sizes generalizability on the one hand and objectively measured small samples on the other hand.

The use of survey questionnaires shifts this tradeoff even further towards large sample size and generalizability. Quite comprehensive sleep/wake questionnaires have been administered to random and representative samples of up to 31,000 in Finland (Partinen, Kapio, Koskenvua, & Langinvainio, 1983) and 5,700 in San Marino (Lugaresi et al., 1983). One survey in the United States included over one million respondents but contained only one general question about the presence of sleep difficulty (Hammond, 1964). Although sleep questionnaires have been shown to have reasonable test-retest reliability (Ellis et al., 1981), they usually have little or no correlation with PSG measures obtained in the laboratory. This is not surprising, given that most survey questions ask respondents for judgments of a sleep parameter average over a long period of time and PSG studies are usually only a small sample of sleep episodes. In any case subjective evaluations of sleep are important clinical parameters on their own and may not be appropriately identified with presently available PSG measures. One's subjective evaluation of sleep is what determines whether treatment is sought from a health professional. This chapter first considers the most common sleep disorders of initiating and maintaining sleep. Studies to evaluate the prevalences of these disorders have usually been questionnaire surveys, while a few have been sleep/wake diary studies.

A number of studies have been published that have given percentages of the population reporting various types of sleeping problems. Many of the studies were not designed to assess sleep specifically, but were general health surveys including one or more questions about sleep. Some were as general as "Do you suffer from sleeplessness" (Hammond, 1964). Other studies have used somewhat more specific questions about the intensity of general sleeping difficulty by using more than two (Yes, No) response alternatives such as "no trouble, not much trouble, a lot of trouble" (Balter & Bauer, 1975). A more common way to elicit more specific descriptions of sleeping problems is to use several different frequency descriptors such as never, seldom, sometimes, often, all the time" (Karacan et al., 1976).

Often it is the case that health surveys only include a question about general sleeping difficulty. These questions are not very informative because they will elicit responses resulting from a wide variety of causes and which require quite different treatments. For example, respondents to a general sleep difficulty question may be suffering frequent daytime sleepiness simply because their lifestyle and responsibilities do not allow sufficient sleep time. Alternatively, they may be suffering daytime sleepiness because their sleep is interrupted hundreds of times during the night by sleep apneic episodes or nocturnal myoclonus. They may be largely unaware of these interruptions which bring the sleeper into lighter stages of sleep or into a brief awakening, but which rarely result in conscious awareness of wakening. Reliable confirmation of these sleep pathologies requires polysomnography. However, the most common reason for affirming a sleeping problem is in not being able to sleep when it is intended. This may involve difficulty getting to sleep, waking during the night, and awakening before intending to in the morning but not being able to get back to sleep. These have been classified as disorders of initiating and maintaining sleep (DIMS). These are questions about wakefulness which are accompanied by awareness and memory functions and thus should result in reliable estimates. More informative sleep surveys include separate questions for each of these types of sleep and daytime symptoms as well as a measure of intensity of difficulty with the use of frequency descriptions.

PREVALENCE OF DIMS

The authors found 61 published studies of sleep surveys covering the 25-year period from 1962 to 1987.[1] The publications varied in their informativeness from a simple percentage of the sample responding "yes" or "no" on a single question about sleep difficulty to studies including a variety of questions about sleep, daytime sleepiness, and hypnotic drug use, using multiple response alternatives and including an analysis of age, gender, and other demographic variables. Sample sizes varied from 55 to 1,064,000 with a median sample size of 1,245.

More studies have been reported from the United States than any other country. However, sleep questionnaire studies have also been reported from several European or European-derived populations including the United Kingdom, France, Belgium, Sweden, Finland, Italy, Greece, Canada, and Australia. This emphasis on European-based and North American populations probably reflects the relative populations of sleep researchers. Cross-cultural comparisons of reported sleeping difficulties would seem to be a fruitful area of research for studying the potential effects of lifestyle, diet, climate, and the social constructs or attitudes towards sleep. To the author's knowledge only one study (Domino et al., 1985) has compared sleep characteristics

[1] The reference list may be obtained from the first author of this chapter.

between countries using the same questionnaire. The seven countries included in the study were also from North American and European-derived populations and the study was largely descriptive rather than analytical. Of interest would be a comparison of more diverse cultures such as from Africa, Asia, Latin America, and South Pacific Islands, including urban, rural, and aboriginal cultures from these regions. Such comparisons may provide a test of the notion that the individual's perception of sleep difficulty is influenced by society's attitude or conception of what is considered to be "normal" sleep. More specifically is the incidence of reported sleep difficulty smaller in cultures which have no concept or very loosely defined notion of "normal" sleep? In other words, to what extent are "sleep difficulties" a culturally generated phenomenon?

The 61 studies were included if they reported results from a general question about sleeping difficulty or at least one specific question including: (a) difficulty falling asleep, (b) difficulty staying asleep, (c) awakening before intended and unable to resume sleeping, (d) use of hypnotic drugs, and (e) daytime sleepiness. Responses to these questions were either with a Yes/No alternative or with multiple response alternatives such as (a) "never," (b) "seldom" or "rarely," (c) "sometimes" or "occasionally," (d) "frequently" or "often," and (e) "always" or "almost all the time." If a study used frequency descriptors other than those above or fewer than five response alternatives, an attempt was made to fit percentage data to the closest of the five alternatives. Studies reporting data in the form of estimated days per week or month of experiencing a sleep difficulty were also fitted to the estimated closest alternative of the five above. For example, two to four times per week was considered to be a "frequent" difficulty. Because the response "yes" and descriptors "sometimes" and "frequently" were commonly used, we analyzed the percentages relevant to those possible responses. Any studies were included which could yield a percentage of the population responding with at least "sometimes," "yes," and at least "frequently" or "often."

Unweighted averages were calculated on each sleep question for each of the three types of frequency descriptors. Table 13.1 shows for each sleep question the number of studies included (*N*), the simple mean percentage of those studies and standard deviation in brackets, and the median percentage for each of the three response categories. The response of "yes" to the various sleep difficulties and related questions yielded mean and median percentages which were, in all cases, intermediate between the percentage answering at least "sometimes" and the percentage answering at least "frequently." For example, in the first question about general sleeplessness or difficulty sleep-

Table 13.1.
Unweighted Average Percentages of All Studies (*N*) Having Any of the Three Response Descriptors for the Sleep Difficulty and Related Survey Questions

Survey Questions		Response Descriptors: "Sometimes" or More Often		"Yes"		"Frequently" or More Often	
General DIMS	N	13		6		18	
Mean (S.D.) %		32.8	(13.9)	21.3	(6.4)	10.8	(4.0)
Median %		35		20		12.7	
Difficulty Falling Asleep	N	6		11		20	
Mean (S.D.) %		32.2	(13.7)	23.6	(8.2)	12.8	(5.9)
Median %		32.3		23		12.2	
Difficulty Maintaining Sleep	N	7		12		19	
Mean (S.D.) %		40.6	(19.5)	26.5	(16.6)	11.1	(6.5)
Median %		45.5		21.5		10.2	
Early Morning Awakening	N	6		9		12	
Mean (S.D.) %		32.8	(19.5)	15.4	(10.9)	10.2	(7.3)
Median %		28.5		15.0		6.6	
Hypnotic Drug Use	N	18		5		16	
Mean (S.D.) %		13.7	(7.8)	10.5	(11.8)	5.1	(2.4)
Median %		10.7		6.6		4.3	
Daytime Sleepiness	N	3		13		12	
Mean (S.D.) %		56.1	(18.2)	22.6	(13.6)	12.1	(7.3)
Median %		58.6		18.8		10.3	

ing a mean of 32.8% and median of 35% across 13 studies answered at least "sometimes," a mean of 21.3% and median of 20% from six studies answered "yes," and a mean of 10.8% and median of 12.7% from 18 studies answered at least "frequently." For most questions the difference in means between "sometimes" and "yes" percentages and the difference between "yes" and "frequently" were significant ($p < .05$) using independent samples t-tests. For all questions the difference between at least "sometimes" and at least "frequently" were significantly ($p < .01$) different. Thus, reliable differences in percentages of respondents are obtained to different frequency descriptors used in questionnaire studies.

It is most likely that the averages across all studies are more reliable estimates than those derived from any one study alone. For example, the data for the category of frequent difficulty in falling asleep were derived from 20 studies representing an aggregate sample size of 32,111. The gender and personality characteristics of interviewers and exact wording of questions has been shown to affect the response rate to questions. Whereas these factors can easily bias the results of a small study, they are likely to be balanced out in the present metaanalysis. It also appears that the median values are very similar to the means for each category and that the standard deviations are usually considerably less than the mean values. This indicates that the distributions of percentage values generally are not highly skewed nor dispersed. Thus the inherent advantages of meta-analysis and favorable distributions obtained in this analysis gives one confidence that the average percentages shown in Table 13.1 are very good estimates of the population parameters for these questions.

Taking the response to "frequently" or more often as a more serious indication of sleeping difficulty it can be seen in Table 13.1 that the mean percentages reporting frequent or more often difficulty with (a) sleeping in general, (b) falling asleep at night, (c) staying asleep at night, and (d) waking before intended in the morning, are all between 10–13 percent. The reported use of hypnotic drugs may be taken as an indicator of sleeping difficulty. The fact that the percentages reporting hypnotic drug use are less for each frequency descriptor (e.g., frequent hypnotic use in 5.1% overall) suggests that hypnotic drug use may be an indication of a more serious sleep problem. Daytime sleepiness is often the result of insufficient sleep resulting from difficulty getting to sleep or staying asleep. Frequent daytime sleepiness is reported by a mean of 12.1 percent from 12 studies. Thus about one out of eight in the population reports at least frequent daytime sleepiness.

Gender Differences

Questionnaire studies. Forty-three out of the 61 considered studies reported a comparison of male and female responses to at least one of the six types of sleep difficulties and related questions. For each type of question we counted the number of studies reporting (a) a significantly higher percentage for females, (b) no gender difference, and (c) a significantly lower percentage for females than males. Table 13.2 shows the number of studies counted for each gender comparison on each type of question. There are clearly more studies which found more reported difficulty by females for general sleep difficulties, specific difficulty in falling asleep, and greater reported use of hypnotic drugs. The gender difference is not as clear in the case of difficulty maintaining sleep at night. There are two studies that found more reported sleep maintenance difficulty by males (Gerard, Collins, Dore, & Exton-Smith, 1978; Lack, Miller, & Turner, 1988) and more studies finding

Table 13.2.
Gender Analysis Showing the Number of Studies with More Females Reporting Difficulty than Males (F > M), no Significant Difference (F = M), and Fewer Females Reporting Difficulty (F < M)

Question	F > M	F = M	F < M
General DIMS	16	5	1
Falling Asleep Difficulty	11	7	0
Difficulty Maintaining Sleep	7	9	2
Early Morning Awakening	3	6	1
Hypnotic Drug Use	14	3	0
Daytime Sleepiness	2	8	1

no gender difference than finding greater difficulty reported in females. With respect to early morning awakening and daytime sleepiness there are no clear gender differences. Thus, of the six question types, three show a clear indication of more reported sleep difficulties among females, one shows a trend in that direction and two show no gender differences.

Polysomnographic studies. While most questionnaire and survey studies have found that females report more sleeping difficulty than males, laboratory polysomnographic (PSG) studies have not found this difference. Six laboratory conducted studies have compared males and females on a full range of conventional PSG variables (Bixler, Kales, Jacoby, Soldatos, & Vela-Bueno, 1984; Monroe, 1969; Reynolds et al., 1985; Spiegel, 1981; Webb, 1983; Williams, Karacan, & Hursch, 1974). These studies have found a few gender differences but differences in the opposite direction expected from the survey studies. Males, particularly in the older age groups, tend to show more awakenings, more light Stage 1 sleep, more stage shifts, and less delta wave sleep—a pattern suggestive of more disrupted and less efficient sleep. One may be tempted to explain this apparent discrepancy by the fact that questionnaire and PSG correlations are usually low. However, by itself, a low correlation (e.g., between reported difficulty falling asleep and PSG recorded sleep onset latency) suggests an inconsistency in one or both measures or that the two are measuring quite different things. In any case, a low correlation does not explain this discrepancy. A low correlation could also exist with PSG differences between males and females equal to those in survey studies or with females showing even more apparent sleep difficulty in the laboratory than is apparent from surveys.

Three other possibilities for the apparent gender discrepancies between questionnaire and PSG studies seem more likely:

1. The PSG studies using relatively small, highly selected samples of males and females may have been less representative of the whole population of males and females than the survey studies. In most of the laboratory studies only healthy males and females free of chronic health problems, sleep problems, or medication were included in the study. It may be the case that these criteria excluded a greater percentage of females, particularly in the older age groups, resulting in relatively more healthy females in the sample than males.

2. It has been found that the incidence of sleep apnea in otherwise healthy individuals without reported sleep problems is high (35–40%) and somewhat higher in males than females, particularly in the older age groups (Carskadon & Dement, 1981; Kripke & Ancoli-Isreal, 1983). More sleep apneic males than females could account for the somewhat greater number of awakenings and Stage 1 sleep and decreased delta wave sleep in the males as a group. Although this possibility could explain the more disrupted PSG sleep of males, it could not, however, explain the very much higher incidence in females of reported sleep problems such as difficulty falling asleep. Furthermore, studies of healthy seniors have not always found more apneic activity among men than women. In fact, a recent PSG study of 40 healthy seniors that found less delta wave sleep and more awakenings in the men found that somewhat fewer males reached the apneic/hyponeic index of 5.0 than females (Reynolds et al., 1985).

3. It may be the case that in sleep questionnaires females overestimate their sleep difficulties, or males underestimate them or both biases occur. In a recent telephone survey of 510 respondents in the Adelaide, South Australia population, gender differences were examined in the various areas of sleep difficulty (e.g., falling asleep, staying asleep, etc.) with questions that differed in degree of specificity and evaluative connotation (Ruler & Lack, 1988). For example, questions about falling asleep included a general, negatively connotative question ("Do you have a problem falling asleep at night?"), general neutral question ("Does it take you a while to fall asleep?"), and a specific, neutral question ("How long did it take you last night to fall asleep?"). The general, negatively worded question produced the largest gender difference which was approximately the same as those found in the past surveys. With the specific, neutral question there was no gender difference. A significant interaction effect between gender and question type indicated that the gender difference in sleep surveys is dependent on the type of question used in the survey. An issue which

could not be resolved by the above study is which type of question and which gender gives responses closer to PSG data? It has been shown that specific questions regarding the previous night's sleep are more highly correlated with that night's PSG data than general questions about the same aspect of sleep (Webb, 1983). Therefore, it seems probable that if the specific question about the previous night's sleep onset latency is relatively valid, then it is the negatively connotative, general question above which elicits response bias in males, females, or both. Gender stereotypes in the culture make it more likely for females and less likely for males to report a health-related "problem." One recent study has found a higher correlation in females than in males between subjective and objective measures of sleep (Hoch et al., 1987). Therefore, the best guess is that the often-reported gender difference in sleep questions, particularly about falling asleep, arises mainly from fewer males reporting a "problem" than is reasonable given their degree of sleep disturbance, particularly in the older age groups. In any case, the Ruler and Lack study (1988) suggests that the gender differences commonly found in surveys, at least with respect to "problems" of falling asleep, should not necessarily be taken as indicating that there is a difference in sleep onset latency between males and females in the general populations.

Age Effects

Questionnaire studies. Thirty-four out of the 61 reviewed studies reported an analysis of age effects for at least one of the types of sleep questions. We considered only age effects from young adulthood to old age. Generally, most sleep surveys of the adult population have found increases in most types of sleep problems across this age range.

However, there is some controversy about the amount of sleep difficulty in adolescents relative to the adult population. Welstein, Dement, Redington, Guilleminault, and Mitler (1983), in a large (N = 6,340) telephone survey, including all ages from 6 years to 93 years, found the largest percentage of reported sleep difficulty in children and adolescents, the lowest in young adults, and then a gradual increase with age. They considered the possibility that the children and adolescents may have conformed more than the adults to perceived demand characteristics of the telephone survey and were therefore more likely to report a sleeping difficulty. Nevertheless, they suggested that children's and adolescents' sleep should be investigated more closely. Recent questionnaire studies of adolescents and university students in Australia using Welstein's et al. (1983) questions and more detailed questions confirmed the high rate of reported sleep difficulty, particularly in falling asleep, and long sleep onset latencies (mean = 20 minutes) and daytime sleepiness (Bearpark & Michie, 1987; Henschel & Lack, 1987; Lack, 1986). These studies have pointed to the delayed sleep and waketimes on weekends and the possibility that many adolescents have delayed circadian rhythms such that it is difficult for them to fall asleep early enough on weeknights to get sufficient sleep before necessary early awakenings on weekdays. The resultant chronic sleep loss would lead to daytime sleepiness and reduced school achievement. This "sleep" problem arises not from a weakness in the sleep mechanism but from its time and placement in the 24-hour day. Therapies should be directed toward management of lifestyle and regularity of bed and waketimes throughout the week.

Apart from the particular problems of adolescents, we considered the change of reported sleep problems across age in the adult population. We counted for each of the six types of sleep related questions the number of studies which generally found increases of reported difficulty with age, no change across age, and decreases with age. These figures are shown in Table 13.3. It can be seen that virtually all of the sleep problems show significantly more studies finding increased problems with age. The most consistent changes are in maintaining nighttime sleep and with waking too early in the morning. This trend with age is perhaps somewhat less clear, although still significant with a sign test, with regards to the problem of falling asleep in which five out of 15 studies found either no change or decreased problem with age.

PSG studies. All of the PSG studies that have investigated age effects confirm an increase in the number of nighttime awakenings, total time awake, and early morning awakenings, but none have found an increase with age in recorded sleep onset latency (SOL) or latency to

Table 13.3.
Age Analysis Showing the Number of Studies Finding Increased Percentages of Older Subjects Reporting Difficulty, No Significant Age Effect or Decreases with Age

Question	Increases	No Change	Decreases
General DIMS	13	1	1
Falling Asleep Difficulty	10	3	2
Difficulty Maintaining Sleep	15	1	0
Early Morning Awakening	8	2	0
Hypnotic Drug Use	19	0	0
Daytime Sleepiness	0	3	4

Stage 2 sleep. This inconsistency with the survey studies may arise from the lighter sleep and less delta wave sleep in the first sleep cycle of the elderly which could result in the subjective impression of longer SOL. There is also the tendency in older individuals to go to bed and to get up earlier than younger people. Contributing to this tendency may be generally advanced (earlier) circadian rhythms in older people as recently suggested by chronobiologic studies (Czeisler, Kronauer, Rios, Sanchez, & Rogacz, 1986; Czeisler, Rios, et al., 1986; Zepelin, 1983). This would also contribute to more early morning premature awakening problems in older people.

The explanation given earlier for the discrepancy between questionnaire and PSG studies regarding gender differences may also apply to the above discrepancy in age effects. The selection criteria for most of the PSG studies (i.e., healthy, good sleepers) eliminates from consideration those who have obvious sleep difficulty such as in falling asleep and may result in a less representative older sample than in the younger sample. Waking during the night, on the other hand, apparently is not as obvious and may be so pervasive with aging that there are more awakenings even in older people who consider themselves relatively good sleepers—the subjects in the PSG studies. In summary, the picture which emerges from both survey and polysomnographic studies regarding the effects of age is an increase in nighttime awakenings, more time awake, less time in delta wave sleep, generally lighter sleep, and earlier awakenings. With regards to falling asleep the survey studies and PSG studies do not agree; however, one suspects that in the general population there is somewhat more difficulty in falling asleep for the elderly than in the younger adult population. Whether these changes with age should be considered pathological will be discussed later after the question of daytime sleepiness and sufficient sleep is addressed.

Daytime sleepiness. A surprising result in Table 13.3 is that reports of daytime sleepiness do not increase with age. In fact, four studies (although there are too few to be significant) found decreases of reported daytime sleepiness (Addison, Thorpy, & Roth, 1987; Broughton & Roberts, 1985; Lack, 1986; Lack, Miller, & Turner, 1988), three found no change (Lavie, 1981; Lavie, Zomer, Peled, & Rubin, 1985; McGhie & Russell, 1962), and no survey found increases with age. This is surprising because other survey and diary studies have found increasing daytime napping reported in the elderly and more "objective sleepiness" in the elderly, as measured by the multiple-sleep latency test (MSLT) (Carskadon, Van Den Hoed, & Dement, 1980). Taken together we are left with the apparent paradox that the elderly can more easily fall asleep during the day and do so more frequently, yet appear to experience less subjective sleepiness. Perhaps it is simply because the elderly can more readily take naps to quell the onset of sleepiness that they are bothered less and actually experience less time of sleepiness during the day. Unfortunately, this attractively parsimonious explanation, to the authors' knowledge, has never been tested. Alternatively, this paradox may only be apparent since there appears to be little correlation between sleep tendency and subjective sleepiness (Seidel et al., 1984).

Increased nighttime arousals and daytime naps would also be consistent with recent chronobiologic studies in humans and rats, which suggests that as well as a relative advance of the circadian system with aging, there is a reduction of amplitude (Czeisler, Kronauer, et al., 1986; Van Gool & Mirmiran, 1986). This would lead to an increase of nighttime arousal and decrease of daytime arousal compared to young adults, which would be manifest in lighter nighttime sleep with less SWS and increased sleep tendency during the day. This increased sleep tendency is seen in more naps and quicker sleep onsets in the MSLT procedure during the day. One would also expect it to be seen in increased subjective sleepiness. As suggested earlier sleepiness may not increase because of compensatory naps. However, the suggestion of a decrease in subjective sleepiness and an increase in perceived sufficiency of sleep (Lack, Miller, & Turner, 1988; Ruler & Lack, 1988) seem to indicate that despite the decreased efficiency of sleep in the elderly, sufficient sleep is more likely to be obtained in the elderly. Indeed, because the elderly spend more time in bed, they are more likely to obtain enough sleep to satisfy their sleep need. Extra time in bed in excess of their sleep need will result in longer SOL, more awakenings, early morning awakening, and even reduced SWS. Their reduced sleep "efficiency" which is measured as total sleep time divided by time in bed (TIB) will be artificially reduced by an excessive TIB. Therefore, two changes which occur with aging, a reduced amplitude of the circadian system, and increased time in bed would both lead to a reduction of sleep "efficiency" but still allow sufficient sleep to be obtained to avoid excessive daytime sleepiness.

Hypnotic drug use. Probably the most dramatic change with aging of the sleep-related questions is the increased use of hypnotic drugs. As seen in Table 13.3, all 19 studies that analyzed age effects of hypnotic drug use found an increase with age. For example, Balter and Bauer (1975) found in the survey ($N = 2{,}552$) that those obtaining a hypnotic prescription in the previous year went from 2% of 18–44-year-olds to 7.5% of 60–74-year-olds. More recently Partinen et al. (1983) in

Finland ($N = 31{,}140$) found that sleeping pill use went from 1% in young adults to 9.3% in the elderly. If hypnotic drug use is taken as an indicator of disturbed sleep, these results support the notion that more older people experience disturbed sleep than younger people. The increased use of hypnotic drugs is probably a response to these perceptions of sleep.

If these were acute changes of sleep within an individual they would usually be associated with increased daytime sleepiness, dysphoric mood, and feelings of insufficient sleep. In this circumstance the use of hypnotic drugs would be sensible if the improvement of sleep alleviated the aversive daytime symptoms. However, these daytime symptoms do not seem to accompany the reduction of sleep efficiency with aging. If older people generally do obtain sufficient sleep to meet their sleep need, there is little positive benefit to daytime wakefulness which can be gained from hypnotic drugs. Furthermore, hypnotic drugs often produce detrimental side effects. Drugs with medium to long elimination half-lives produce significant daytime sedation resulting in less efficient daytime behavior than without the hypnotic drug (Moskowitz & Linnoila, 1987; Oswald, 1979; Roehrs, Kribbs, Zorick, & Roth, 1986). This daytime sedation would be particularly problematic and even dangerous to the elderly whose cognitive functioning may be already impaired by the effects of other drugs or the onset of senility. Hypnotics with short half-lives have less or no daytime sedation effects but tend to develop rapid tolerance effects, significant drug withdrawal effects including REM sleep rebound and insomnia rebound, and increased likelihood of drug dependence (Lupolover, Dazzi, & Ward, 1982). There are other possible health detriments of hypnotic drug use which should also be considered. Kripke, Ancoli-Isreal, Mason, and Messin (1983) reported a statistical analysis of sleep habits and hypnotic drug use related to mortality rates for the duration of an 8-year period in over 800,000 Americans. The mortality ratio of those who frequently took sleeping pills was 100 percent higher than those who never took pills. When all other variables such as age, sex, reported insomnia, and chronic illnesses were statistically controlled the mortality ratio for frequent hypnotic pill users was still significantly higher (50%) than nonpill users. How the increased mortality is associated with pill use has not been determined. It could derive from an interaction with sleep apnea; increased possibility of suicide; automobile or other accidents; or even possible health detriments from the suppression of delta wave sleep. In any case, this increased mortality ratio along with the immediate detrimental side effects of hypnotic drugs should provide strong enough contraindications to avoid hypnotic drugs for the purpose of "improving" sleep, particularly in the elderly. In fact, Reynolds, Kupfer, Hoch, and Sewitch (1985) suggest for many reasons that hypnotic drugs should only rarely be prescribed for the elderly. It seems ironic that it is the older population that receives most of the hypnotic prescriptions. It is also ironic that one of the strongest messages in this chapter to medical practitioners for the improvement of the health and well-being, particularly of the elderly, is to curtail or at least reduce their practice of prescribing hypnotic drugs.

DISORDERS OF EXCESSIVE SOMNOLENCE

We have already discussed the prevalence of the symptom of daytime sleepiness as reported in a number of questionnaire surveys. In studies that required simply a yes/no response to whether daytime sleepiness was experienced ($N = 13$ studies) the mean and median percentages responding "yes" were 22.6% and 18.8% respectively. Greater severity of a sleepiness problem would be indicated in those surveys which measured the frequency of the problem. In those studies ($N = 12$) the mean and median percentages of those experiencing daytime sleepiness at least frequently were 12.1% and 10.3% respectively. These figures are comparable to those experiencing frequent difficulties initiating and maintaining sleep. This is not to suggest, however, that sleepiness arises solely from difficulties in falling or staying asleep. Indeed, chronic insomniacs tend to be no more sleepy (although frequently more tired) than good sleepers (Dorsey & Bootzin, 1987; Seidel et al., 1984). Furthermore, excessive daytime sleepiness is often a problem for many who report no problems in falling or staying asleep. This latter group includes those who suffer from "voluntarily" curtailed sleep, narcolepsy, sleep apnea, and nocturnal myoclonus.

Restricted Sleep

It may seem strange that people would restrict their sleep to such an extent that they carry with them throughout the day an increased sleep pressure. This is most apparent as overwhelming sleepiness developing during quieter times in the day such as at a sedentary desk job, in a dull lecture or meeting, reading in a quiet library, driving along a familiar route, or relaxing in front of the television. At best this condition simply reduces one's efficiency and subsequent productivity; at worst it could be dangerous and life imperiling. In these individuals sleep duration is reduced because they have been more attracted to alternative activities than to sleep or have taken on voluntarily or not so voluntarily too many time-consuming responsibilities to leave them enough time for sufficient sleep. Because these individuals chronically restrict their sleep, they have such sleep pressure that they are unlikely to report problems falling or staying asleep. These individuals will often not recognize this sleep pressure because they frequently use stimulants such as caffeine and nicotine which tend to counteract the sleep pressure. It is interesting that several surveys have failed to find a correlation between reported amount of chronic caffeine consumption and amount of sleeping difficulty (Broughton & Roberts, 1985; Hicks, Hicks, Reyes, & Cheers, 1983; Kales et al., 1984). One survey (Shirlow & Mathers, 1985) found a positive correlation between amount of caffeine consumption and probability of sleep problems at least sometimes, but one survey (Lugaresi et al., 1983) actually found that fewer poor sleepers then good sleepers consumed coffee. It may be the case that if a balance is maintained between daily caffeine amount and level of sleep pressure that sleep difficulties may not necessarily be related to the amount of caffeine consumed on a regular basis. However, if these stimulants are consumed before bedtime they will delay sleep onset and will tend to disrupt sleep and increase the following day's sleep pressure (Brezinova, 1974; Karacan et al., 1975; Okuma, Matsuoka, Matsue, & Toyomura, 1982). A vicious circle of increasing caffeine and nicotine consumption to combat increasing sleep pressure can easily develop and lead to caffeinism and health risks associated with cigarette smoking. It seems likely that these behaviors are reinforced in many cases by the stimulants' effect of reducing sleepiness, and that the alternative way of reducing sleepiness by obtaining more sleep could facilitate the reduction of caffeine and nicotine consumption. Therefore, the issue of adequate sleep also relates to other important health behaviors.

Narcolepsy

In comparison with the other disorders of sleep narcolepsy is a relatively debilitating disorder. Four symptoms may accompany the disorder of which periodic overwhelming daytime sleepiness is always present. The rapid development of sleepiness invariably produces a sleep episode which is usually brief (10–25 minutes) and effective at relieving sleepiness at least temporarily. Daytime bouts of sleepiness may vary in number from one or two to a dozen. Sleep onsets are more likely to occur during periods of reduced arousal and relaxation, but may occur at unexpected and inappropriate times such as during conversations or while driving an automobile. Cataplexy or sudden paralysis of the skeletal muscle system frequently is present in cases of narcolepsy. Catapletic episodes are more likely to be triggered, paradoxically, during periods of heightened arousal, particularly from positive or negative affect. Even though they may last only seconds to minutes they are potentially more dangerous than sleep attacks as they are less predictable or controllable. Hypnogogic hallucinations and sleep paralysis are also frequently a part of the narcoleptic tetrad of symptoms and usually occur at the onset or termination of the normal night sleep period. They are unlikely to be physically dangerous since they usually occur when the narcoleptic is in bed. Nevertheless, the vivid, dream-like experiences of the hallucination are often interpreted as reality and can be very disturbing. Similarly, the experience of total skeletal paralysis can be disconcerting and when it frequently accompanies hypnogogic hallucinations it can be particularly frightening. The nighttime sleep architecture of the narcoleptic is also frequently distorted showing REM sleep onset, reduced delta wave sleep, and more arousals from sleep (Roth, 1980).

Only a few studies have tried to estimate the incidence of narcolepsy in the population. Since it is comparatively rare and since a reliable diagnosis relies substantially on laboratory recording, it has been difficult to get confident estimates from sleep surveys in the population. Estimates have often been based, instead, on replies to advertisements and electronic media appeals. These, of course, rely upon rather ad hoc assumptions about the size of the exposed public and the likelihood that a potential narcoleptic candidate would actually contact the researchers. The wide range of estimates (a 40-times difference) is probably the result of the variety of estimation techniques and crude assumptions inherent in some of the techniques. The authors found 10 publications that state their best estimates of the incidence of narcolepsy in the general population. They ranged in their estimates from .004% to .16% with a mean of .067% and median of .045%. So it appears that the best estimate of the incidence of narcolepsy would be about .05% or five out of 10,000. Therefore, it appears from this best estimate that narcolepsy is about 200 times less prevalent in the population than the disorders of initiating and maintaining sleep.

It is felt that narcolepsy, which is chronic, without cure and largely genetically determined, involves a disorder of the REM sleep mechanism. Sleep attacks and nighttime sleep periods frequently show REM sleep onset. Cataplexy and sleep paralysis are seen as uncontrolled outbreaks of the skeletal muscle inhibition of REM sleep. The hypnogogic hallucinations symptom is interpreted as a dream episode triggered by the REM sleep mechanism at sleep onset and perhaps before the narcoleptic has perceived that sleep has begun. Medical symptomatic treatment for severe cases consists of a drug cocktail, methylphenidate, to reduce sleep attacks and tricyclic antidepressants to reduce the auxillary symptoms of cataplexy, hypnogogic hallucinations, and sleep paralysis (Roth, 1980). The antidepressants are thought to be effective because of their REM sleep-suppressing capacity. The difficulty in monitoring drug effects and titrating the dosages to the appropriate level to minimize daytime attacks but not to interrupt nighttime sleep, as well as the adverse side effects of these drugs, makes their use with this chronic condition problematic.

Nondrug alternatives or adjuncts to drug therapy have been found to have significant practical benefit (Kales, Kales, & Soldatos, 1982; Roth, 1980; Sours, 1963). The narcoleptic and his or her family and associates usually need counseling and information regarding the nature of the disorder to dispel unfounded impressions of the narcoleptic as being lazy, unmotivated, or negligent. Social support organizations can be important for rectifying the narcoleptic's self-image and for providing moral support in coping with the severe inconveniences and potential dangers of the condition. Behavioral management strategies have also been shown to be of benefit in controlling the effects of the condition. This would involve the careful monitoring of the symptoms on a daily basis and the development of strategies such as the scheduling of short naps at convenient times in order to minimize the practical inconveniences which can be generated by the narcoleptic symptoms. In other words, through careful attention to the precursors of symptoms it is possible, to some extent, to avoid and constrain the symptoms to less dangerous or more convenient times in the day.

Sleep Apnea

Of all the sleep disorders sleep apnea syndrome has probably received the most medical attention and recent media notoriety. Apart from the cataplectic attacks of narcolepsy, sleep apnea is the most dramatic disorder associated with sleep and potentially is the most lethal. It is suggested to be linked with deaths during sleep in the elderly and sudden infant death syndrome. In an extreme case of obstructive sleep apnea the apneic may experience hundreds of lengthy (>45 seconds) total breathing obstructions, blood oxygen desaturations, and sleep interruptions each night. Typically, upon falling asleep there is a decrease of muscle tone which, particularly in an obese, male, heavy snorer, results in a collapse of the pharyngeal airway upon inspiration and total blockage to breathing despite vigorous respiratory effort (Kripke, Ancoli-Isreal, & Okudaira, 1982). As the blockage continues for 20, 40, 60 seconds there is a progressive and marked drop of blood oxygen saturation, sometimes as low as 30–40 percent normal, and an increase of blood carbon dioxide level. At some point the brain's arousal center is activated to awaken the sleeper sufficiently to result in a return of muscle tone, removal of the obstruction, and return of breathing. Blood gases return to normal and the apneic returns to sleep usually without full awareness or recall of the episode the following morning. The return to sleep, however, triggers another episode and a subsequent repeat of the same process which may number in the hundreds each night.

Even though the sleep apneic may accumulate a normal amount of total sleep time, the quality of the sleep is not normal. The 90-minute sleep cycles are so disrupted they are no longer evident. Delta wave sleep and REM sleep rarely have a chance to develop and are virtually absent. By default they are replaced by light Stage 1 sleep. This type of sleep apneic usually suffers morning headache and tiredness and excessive sleepiness during the day. Bonnet (1985) has simulated this disrupted sleep pattern in normals with multiple periodic awakenings throughout the night. The effect of this disruption procedure in terms of subsequent sleepiness and performance is approximately equivalent to halving the total sleep time. Thus, the obstructive apneic, despite a generous sleep period time of 8–10 hours, effectively suffers chronic sleep loss and excessive daytime sleepiness. This would explain the rapid sleep onset, rapid return to sleep with each episode, and deficient memory of the apneic episodes. The daytime sleepiness not only reduces the quality of life, but it poses a danger in many situations.

Associated with severe obstructive sleep apnea are several life-threatening medical conditions such as hypertension, angina, and several cardiac irregularities (Kripke et al., 1982). This condition is rightly perceived by the medical profession as potentially serious with high morbidity and probably increased mortality. Treatments for extreme cases have included tracheostomy, UVPP, tonsillectomy, and other surgical interventions. Nonsurgical alternatives and adjunct procedures have included tongue restraining devices and CPAP (continuous positive airway pressure).

Severe obstructive sleep apnea has grabbed the attention of the medical profession, partly because of its serious medical complications and interventions. However, medical practitioners have also been alerted to the importance of proper diagnosis and potentially lethal consequences of misdiagnosis. Given the symptoms of daytime sleepiness and only the vague impression of disrupted nighttime sleep the medical practitioner may suggest a hypnotic drug. The contraindicating evidence to drug therapy of loud snoring and irregular breathing may not be available because there is no bed partner to offer the evidence or the medical practitioner simply may not investigate the possibility. If a hypnotic drug is prescribed and taken, its effect would be a reduced sensitivity of the respiratory centers, extended apneic episodes, and greater O_2 desaturations. The patient would have even less memory of the episodes but no alleviation of daytime sleepiness. Therefore, he may escalate the drug dose in an attempt to gain sufficient sleep. This process would quickly become life threatening. Alcohol exacerbates an apneic condition on its own. Coupled with hypnotic drugs its effects are compounded and present a particularly lethal condition for the obstructive sleep apneic. To the knowledge of the authors, this scenario, although plausible, has not been investigated sufficiently to determine its prevalence. Kripke et al. (1979, 1983) and Kripke, Ancoli-Isreal, Mason, and Kaplan (1986) have suggested that the increased mortality rates of those with extremely short or long sleep duration and hypnotic pill use may be explained, partly, as due to central sleep apnea (often reported short sleep duration) and obstructive sleep apnea (often reported long sleep duration).

Since, by definition, sleep apnea is the cessation of breathing during sleep, the two main ways in which breathing may cease have been taken as two subcategories of the same disorder. Obstructive apneic episodes have already been described. Central sleep apnea refers to the cessation of breathing effort, presumably at the behest of a central neural mechanism. Mixed apneic episodes may also occur with a cessation of breathing effort followed by the development of an obstruction upon the resumption of breathing effort. However, because the apneic mechanisms appear to be quite different it may be prudent to consider the possibility that they may have different sequelae and prevalence within the population. The definition of a single sleep apnea disorder may be masking fundamental distinctions between the two types of apnea.

A second consequence of considering sleep apnea basically a unitary disorder is to have defined sleep apnea solely in terms of apneic episodes regardless of type. Irregular breathing with occasional pauses of perhaps 5–15 seconds have always been accepted as a normal feature in Stage 1 and REM sleep and to a less extent in light Stage 2 sleep. The task for earlier clinicians and researchers was to set a criterion for the amount of breathing cessation necessary to constitute a classification of sleep apnea. An apneic episode was defined as a cessation of breathing for at least 10 seconds. The sleep apneic index (SAI) was defined as the average number of episodes per hour across the sleep period. The criterion for sleep apnea was set at an apneic index of five per hour or at least 30 episodes in a nighttime sleep period.

Prevalence of Sleep Apnea

The criterion apneic index of 5 for sleep apnea was based on laboratory studies with relatively young subjects. It seemed to appropriately pick out the few more extreme cases of disturbed respiration in sleep. However, some studies found an apparently alarming rate of sleep apnea in the elderly (65 years plus). In otherwise healthy, asymptomatic elderly subjects Ancoli-Israel, Kripke, Mason, and Messin (1981) and Carskadon and Dement (1981) found in 24 and 40 subjects respectively 38% to have Apneic indexes of 5.0 or greater. Since then another 10 studies have reported the results on the same type of population and a total of 238 out of 941 (or 25.3%) were found to have an apneic index of at least 5.0 or by this criterion, would have sleep apnea. Since sleep apnea is considered a serious disorder, it would be considered a major health problem to have over a quarter of the elderly population with this disorder. Since younger populations contained much smaller percentages of apneics, it appears that apnea develops with aging. If anything like the medical and behavioral difficulties associated with severe obstructive sleep apnea were associated with apnea in the elderly, it would be a major contributor to their mortality rates. The reduced longevity of males may be explained, in part, by their higher incidence of sleep apnea particularly the obstructive type. The higher mortality rates in hypnotic pill users may arise partly from the dangerous interaction with sleep apnea (Kripke et al., 1986). The fact that sleep apnea was found to reside insidiously within apparently healthy elderly did nothing to lessen the concern and warnings of some researchers. With no suspicion of respiratory difficulty from clinical symptoms medical practitioners would have no strong reason to warn patients against the use of hypnotics or alcohol.

All of this concern is predicated on the assumption that sleep apnea, as defined by an apneic index of five or more, is a serious disorder with significantly increased morbidity and mortality. The available evidence does not support this assumption. In healthy, asymptomatic elderly those with SAI>5 did take more naps, but they did not differ from those with SAI<5 in PSG measured nocturnal awake time, total sleep time, snoring, excessive daytime sleepiness, satisfaction with sleep, and use of sleeping pills (Ancoli-Israel et al., 1983; Kripke et al., 1983). In a group of 35 healthy elderly people, Prinz, Smallwood, Giblin, Ralph, and Vitiello (1984) found none to have a drop of oxygen saturation below 80%. These subjects were compared with four sleep apneic patients who had SAI>5, as well as the other symptoms of morning headaches, snoring, and excessive daytime sleepiness, and who all had O_2 saturations drop below 75% during sleep recording nights. Out of 28 healthy men, 50–72 years old, Smyth, Giblin, and Lee (1981) found six (28%) to have SAI>5. However, the mean drop of SaO_2 was only 6.7% ± 5% with the maximum single reduction being 21%. Dickel, Sassin, and Mosko (1986) found nine out of 20 elderly (45%) to have a SAI>5, but no subject showed a SaO_2 drop of more than 15%. In a critical review of the sleep apneic index as a diagnostic criterion Berry, Webb, and Block (1984) reported that the SAI of 5.0 failed to discriminate healthy subjects in terms of heart disease, hypertension, obesity, sinus problems, or daytime sleep tendency. A three-year longitudinal study found no higher risk in those with SAI>5. Krieger and Kurtz (1987) recorded 20 healthy, older subjects (mean age of 67 years) and found six (30%) to have SAI>5. At a seven-year follow-up two of the non-SAS subjects had died and seven more had chronic health problems (64%), while four of the six SAS subjects (67%) had similar health problems. Thus, this small longitudinal study showed no difference in health risk based on the SAI criterion alone. Thus, the SAI criterion by itself seems unable to identify a condition of illness at least in a normal elderly population.

Berry et al. (1984), Block, Boysen, Wynne, and Hunt (1979), and Prinz et al. (1984) have been critical of the SAI criterion for sleep apnea syndrome. Since increased irregularity of breathing and apneic episodes are a common phenomenon in the elderly, with no associated morbidity, they should be considered a benign concomitant of aging. Apneic episodes are more likely to occur in Stage 1 sleep (Smyth et al., 1981). Kreiger (1985) suggested that apneic episodes in Stage 1 sleep may be an extension of the periodic and irregular breathing of young subjects in Stage 1 sleep. The increased apnea in the aged may be a consequence of increased Stage 1 sleep which is associated with generally lighter sleep of the aged and increasing number of nocturnal arousals which are usually followed by periods of Stage 1 sleep. Bonnet, Dexter, and Arand (1987) found that apneic episodes were decreased in number with the use of the short acting benzodiazepine, triazolam, presumably because the number of awakenings and amount of Stage 1 was reduced with the hypnotic. This viewed apneic episodes in the healthy elderly as a result of increased Stage 1 sleep from lighter and more disrupted sleep, rather than the episodes being a cause of the more disrupted sleep of the elderly. This distinction has yet to be adequately tested.

The question now is "what is the prevalence of the type of sleep apnea which does have significant morbidity?" Three studies have tried to identify sleep apneics on the basis of multiple criteria in addition to SAI>5. From 120 consecutive chest clinic patients among whom one would expect more SAS, Shapiro, Catterall, Oswald, and

Flenley (1981) found only three (2.5%) significant obstructive sleep apneics. From all admissions to a general hospital ($N = 2{,}518$), Franceschi, Smirne, Zamproni, Crippa, and Ferini-Strambi (1983) found 28 (1.11%) to have excessive daytime sleepiness. Of these, 25 (1%) were shown with PSG to have sleep apnea, mainly obstructive. Most of these were obese, 15 had morning headache, and all snored. Gislason, Almquist, Boman, Eriksson, and Taube (1987) conducted a study to estimate the prevalence of sleep apnea among Swedish men. They received 3,201 postal questionnaires (80% response rate) regarding sleep and daytime sleepiness. From these, 166 (5.1%) reported habitual snoring and excessive daytime sleepiness. Sixty-one of these 166 were investigated with PSG and 15 found to have an SAI>5. If this rate of 15/61 is assumed for the 166, then 41 out of 3,201 or 1.3% would be estimated to be sleep apneic in the Swedish male population. The highest estimated rate was 2.0% for the 50–59 year age group. Broughton and Roberts (1985), in a survey questionnaire of 493 males and 238 female working adults aged 20–77 years, found 5.1% reporting excessive daytime sleepiness and habitual snoring. If 24% of these, as in the Gislason et al. (1987) study were found to have an SAI>5, then the estimate for sleep apnea would be about 1%. Lavie (1983) used the same methodology as Gislason et al. (1987) of selecting samples of subjects for PSG who were selected by a questionnaire response to excessive daytime sleepiness or frequent nocturnal awakenings. From his base sample of 1,502 industrial workers in Israel he estimated that, at a minimum, 1% and perhaps most likely about 3.5% of the population would have SAI>5, as well as the other subjective complaints of sleep apnea. In a recent questionnaire study in Sweden, Hetta et al. (1987) estimated the prevalence of sleep apnea syndrome to be 1.1%. Therefore, there is a fair degree of consesus about the prevalence of sleep apnea which includes the criteria of SAI>5 plus the subjective symptoms of snoring and excessive daytime sleepiness. This type of apnea is more likely to be the obstructive type and show decreases of blood oxygen saturation to below 75%. Most of the studies estimate the prevalence at around 1% with the highest estimate at 3.5%

Even though extreme obstructive sleep apnea syndrome would appear to have a high morbidity with its nightly marked O_2 desaturations, hypertension, and cardiac irregularities, its mortality rate is still in doubt. Partinen, Jamieson, and Guilleminault (1986) followed 60 patients with severe obstructive SAS over at least six years. Of 37 who received medical and weight reduction treatment four had died, of which two died for reasons unrelated to the sleep apnea. Of 23 who had been tracheostomized only one had died. The authors concluded that it still was not clear from the study that OSAS is a particularly dangerous condition. Nevertheless, the poor quality and inefficient sleep, morning headache, and excessive daytime sleepiness suffered by the OSAS patient, as well as the unbearable snoring suffered by bed partners are quite enough reasons to seriously consider treatment of OSAS.

The medical and surgical treatments of OSAS have already been mentioned. The efficacy of drug treatments is still uncertain. The surgical treatments have often resulted in dramatic alleviation of the OSAS but create their own risks and problems. Other physical interventions, such as the use of a tongue-retaining device or CPAP, produce significant improvement when used by a patient, but often have unreliable patient compliance. More recent studies have explored behavioral treatments. It has been suggested that weight reduction should help to reduce OSAS and that behavior therapists could play a useful role in facilitating that process. Snoring and obstructive apneic episodes are much more likely to occur on the back in the supine position rather than on the side (Cartwright, Ristanovic, Jaski, & Lloyd, 1987). Orr, Rundell, Jones, Fixley, and Clark (1986) and Lloyd, Cartwright, Kravitz, and Ristanovic (1987) have had considerable success using a conditioning procedure to get OSAS patients to shift from their backs to their sides. Lloyd et al. (1987) used a back position alarm device in the patient's own home which sounded an alarm for supine positions. Subjects learned within one night to avoid back sleeping and also showed a significant reduction (50%) of sleep apneic index.

Other researchers have explored the possibility of respiration control during sleep using conditioning procedures. The first step in this endeavor has been to demonstrate that sleepers can elicit a deep breath response to an external discriminative stimulus. Badia et al. (1984) conditioned subjects to produce a deep breath response during sleep to a tone stimulus. The probability of response was high ($p > .9$) and latency short (< 10 seconds) without arousal from Stage 1, 2 and REM sleep, the sleep stages most likely to have apneic episodes. The next step will be to determine if the discriminative stimulus can be generalized from the external tone to the internal cue of a cessation of breathing in order to avoid lengthy central apneic episodes. EMG biofeedback training to increase parapharyngeal muscle tone and free the blockage during obstructive apneic episodes may be another fruitful area of research into behavioral treatments of sleep apnea.

Nocturnal Myoclonus

Nocturnal myoclonus or, as Coleman et al. (1983) have suggested, "periodic movements in sleep (PMS)" is the occurrence of periodic leg movements during sleep. They can be conveniently recorded from

EMG electrodes on the anterior tibialis muscle. The movements consist of leg flexions occurring in bursts of 3–30 leg jerks. A common criterion defining PMS has been 40–90 of these bursts during the sleep period or a movement index (MI) of five or more bursts per hour (Kripke et al., 1982). PMS, as does sleep apnea, usually occurs in the lighter stages of sleep. The bursts of movements are often but not always associated with arousals from sleep. The briefer arousals (less than a minute) are more common and usually not remembered the following morning. The lengthier arousals may extend to hours and be a cause of sleep maintenance insomnia and excessive sleepiness the following day. As a result of this sleep loss, the following sleep may have less light sleep, fewer lengthy arousals, and fewer PMS episodes. This night-to-night variability may account for the night-to-night variability of PMS within the patient as noted by Kripke et al. (1982).

The prevalence of PMS has been estimated by many of the same studies which also investigated sleep apnea in healthy asymptomatic populations. Interestingly, the estimates for PMS using the MI>5 criterion are approximately the same as sleep apnea using the SAI>5 criterion. PMS also shows a dramatic increase with age. Bixler et al. (1982), in a sample of 100 healthy workers in a medical complex, found no PMS in the 18–30-year-olds, 2.6% in the 31–49-year-olds, and 16.1% in the 50–74-year-olds. George, Ancoli-Israel, and Kripke (1985) found 21% PMS in 18 30–40-year-old women, but 41% PMS in 106 women over 65 years of age. A total of seven studies measured the prevalence of PMS in healthy asymptomatic older subjects (>60 years) using PSG. Out of a total of 374 subjects in these studies, 144 (38.5%) were found to have PMS.

However, as was the case in the healthy elderly of sleep apnea defined only by SAI>5, PMS defined only by MI>5 seems not to be associated with any specific morbidity. Ancoli-Isreal, Kripke, and Mason (1983) found in their 145 seniors no differences between PMS and nonsleep-disordered groups in sleep satisfaction, reported total sleep time, sleep complaints, excessive daytime sleepiness, snoring, leg twitches, and weight. The PMS group did wake up earlier and had less TST but apparently with no daytime consequences. Coleman et al. (1983) followed up 14 PMS patients after 1–9 years. The four oldest patients showed increases in the total number of movements and the arousal index. However, total sleep time and nocturnal wake time did not change and sleepiness/alertness did not vary with the severity of PMS from the previous night. Therefore, at least in healthy elderly there seem to be no adverse consequences specifically associated with PMS as defined by the conventional criterion. Whether the criterion movement index can be increased to a point that does significantly identify a specific morbidity remains to be tested. One would imagine that there must be a great enough amount of PMS that would disrupt sleep sufficiently to produce some adverse daytime effects. In the meantime, the available evidence suggests that, in most cases, PMS is a relatively benign phenomenon of aging.

SUMMARY OF SLEEP DISORDER PREVALENCES

There are a variety of other disorders associated with sleep and waking which are not covered in this chapter. Other adult disorders are relatively rare or have received insufficient research attention to provide an informative review.

The insomnias and disorders in initiating and maintaining sleep appear to be the most prevalent problem throughout the community. If "frequent trouble" falling asleep or maintaining sleep is taken as the criterion for a sleep disorder, this afflicts about 10% of the general adult population. Narcolepsy is a relatively serious disorder but is present in only about .05% of the population. Sleep apnea, more specifically obstructive sleep apnea syndrome accompanied by heavy snoring, excessive daytime sleeping, significant O_2 desaturations, cardiac irregularities, and hypertension seems to be present in perhaps about 1 percent of the population. Periodic movements in sleep are relatively common (about 38%) in the elderly but appear to be mainly benign. The prevalence of morbid PMS (if indeed such a condition exists) is yet to be determined. Thus, leaving aside PMS for the present "insomnia" is about 10 times more prevalent than obstructive SAS and 200 times more prevalent than narcolepsy.

BEHAVIORAL TREATMENT OF INSOMNIA

Behavioral approaches to the treatment of narcolepsy and sleep apnea have been discussed already. Because (a) the insomnias are the most common sleep disorder, (b) compared with most of the other sleep/wake disorders the insomnias have etiologies with relatively important psychological and behavioral factors, and (c) most past behavioral research applied to sleep disorders has been with respect to disorders in initiating and maintaining sleep, the following section of this chapter discusses behavioral treatments for insomnia.

There are many biological, psychological, and environmental factors which can contribute to insomnia and many nonpharmacological considerations for its treatment or management. For example, the misconception that everyone must obtain at least eight hours of sleep may be the main anxiety of an individual who needs, in fact, only six hours of sleep. Another misconception that sleep should be one long period of unconsciousness may contribute to the anxiety of an older individual who experiences several brief nocturnal awakenings. If these awakenings were interruptions of deep sleep, it would be an understandable concern. On the other hand, if these awakenings were perceived as normal manifestations of the light and less efficient sleep that occurred periodically (approximately every 90 minutes) through the total sleep period, there would be much less cause for concern. Thus, information about the nature of sleep and counseling can play an important role in the treatment of insomnia. Another example of a nonpharmacological treatment might be the use of bright light exposure in the morning for sleep onset insomniacs (Lingjaerde, Bratlid, & Hansen, 1985; Morris, Lack, & Dawson, 1990). For a broad review of the diagnosis and behavioral approach to insomnia see Montgomery and Trinder (1986). The following section will focus specifically on the more extensively researched behavioral treatments for insomnia.

Anxiety Reduction Approaches

Various forms of relaxation training constitute the behavioral treatment that has received most attention in the literature. These have included training procedures such as progressive muscle relaxation, autogenic training, transcendental meditation, hypnosis, and biofeedback. The initial application of these treatments was based upon the premise that excessive arousal at bedtime was responsible for delayed sleep onset. This is supported by studies showing poor sleepers to have higher levels of physiological arousal than good sleepers prior to and during sleep (Monroe, 1967; Johns, Gay, Masterton, & Bruce, 1971; Freedman & Sattler, 1982), higher emotional arousal as measured by symptom check lists and self-report inventories (Coursey, Bucksbaum, & Frankel, 1975; Freedman & Sattler, 1982; Haynes, Follingstead, & McGowan, 1974; Nicassio & Bootzin, 1974) and higher levels of cognitive activity at bedtime (Roth, Kramer, & Lutz, 1976; Kales, Caldwell, Preston, Healey, & Kales, 1976; Borkovec, 1979). However, the findings relating to the higher physiological arousal have not been consistently replicated, and the possibility remains that the elevated levels of anxiety and cognitive activity are an epiphenomenon of insomnia. These observations, together with the fact that a functional relationship has yet to be demonstrated between sleep improvement and a reduction in arousal, leaves the mediational role of arousal open to conjecture. Nonetheless, the hypothesis that excessive arousal at bedtime was responsible for insomnia provided theoretical justification for the use of arousal-reducing procedures.

Progressive muscle relaxation. This procedure, developed by Jacobson (1938), involves the systematic tensing and relaxing of progressively more muscle groups until a low level of general muscle tension is able to be achieved at will. A considerable body of evidence exists to indicate that even abbreviated forms of this procedure are effective in reducing muscular tension and autonomic arousal (Paul, 1969; Paul & Trimble, 1970). These empirical data, coupled with the arousal model of insomnia, have meant that progressive relaxation has been the most extensively researched nonpharmacological treatment for this clinical problem.

The first study to include a control group was conducted by Borkovec and Fowles (1973). They randomly assigned female students with moderate sleeping difficulties to either progressive relaxation, hypnotic relaxation, self-relaxation, or no-treatment control conditions. Subjective measures of sleep indicated that both the active treatments and the self-relaxation control were equally superior to no-treatment, thus raising the possibility that nonspecific factors, such as expectancy, were responsible for the improvement.

Steinmark and Borkovec (1974) utilized a counterdemand strategy to control for expectancy in their attempt to evaluate this hypothesis. The results of their study indicated that progressive relaxation and single-item desensitization equally produced significant reductions in sleep onset latency during the counterdemand period (when subjects were told not to expect improvement). The placebo and waiting-control conditions did not. However, during the final phase of the study when positive expectations were encouraged, subjects in the quasidesensitization placebo condition reported improvement equivalent to that achieved by the treatment groups. Global estimates at five-month follow-up indicated that the treatment conditions had made additional gains and that the placebo subjects had regressed somewhat. These results clearly demonstrate the powerful influence positive expectations may have on self-reports of sleep behavior. Consequently, this data both accentuates the need for corroboration of self-reports of sleep improvement and reinforces Kazdin's (1979) call to attend closely to such nonspecific treatment factors in outcome studies.

Recognizing the need for reliability checks on self-report measures, Nicassio and Bootzin (1974) obtained reports from household members concerning the subject's sleep onset latency in their comparison of progressively relaxation, autogenic training, and self-relaxation. Using severe insomniacs drawn from the general population, they found progressive relaxation and autogenic training equally effective in reducing self-reports of sleep onset latency, with reports from household members and pupillography measures of restedness providing convergent validation of their superiority over no-treatment. In addition, the results of the study showed that contrary to Borkovec and Fowles' (1973) finding, self-relaxation (scheduling time to relax during the day and in bed before sleep) did not achieve a significant group mean reduction in sleep onset latency. Nicassio and Bootzin (1974) argued that the different populations sampled may account for this discrepant finding, and concluded that actual training in relaxation is required for severe, chronic insomniacs to obtain some benefit.

Research has consistently demonstrated the superiority of progressive relaxation over placebo and/or no-treatment in reducing self-reported sleep onset latency. In addition, progressive relaxation has been found to achieve significantly greater improvement than placebo in objectively defined EEG sleep (Freedman & Papsdorf, 1976; Borkovec & Weerts, 1976; Borkovec, Grayson, O'Brien, & Weerts, 1979). However, Borkovec and Weert's (1976) findings should be interpreted cautiously as all groups improved during the counterdemand period, with no significant difference between groups. The superiority of progressive relaxation was evident only during the positive demand period for the onset of Stage 1 sleep. The absence of effects on Stage 2 sleep limits conclusions regarding the impact of relaxation on the complaint of insomnia. This is highlighted by Hauri and Olmstead's (1983) finding that the insomniac's subjective experience of being asleep correlates best with the beginning of the first 15-minute period of uninterrupted Stage 2 sleep. Borkovec et al. (1979) considered that the failure to find a significant EEG effect for relaxation over placebo and no treatment in the Borkovec and Weert's (1976) study, may have been due to the fact that subjects without objective deficits had been included in the study in sufficient numbers so as to confound the results. They arbitrarily categorized subjects as pseudoinsomniacs or idiopathic insomniacs on the basis of discrepancies between EEG and self-report estimates of sleep onset latency. Their results showed that progressive relaxation reduced both EEG defined Stage 2 sleep onset latency and subjective estimates of time taken to fall asleep for idiopathic insomniacs. Progressive relaxation also decreased the complaint of insomnia for those subjects without an objective deficit at pretreatment.

Although the data indicates that progressive relaxation can achieve group mean reductions in sleep onset latency of about 45 percent (Borkovec, 1982), the mechanism by which this occurs is far from clear. The evidence suggests that muscle-tension release may play some important role (Borkovec, Kaloupek, & Slama, 1975; Borkovec & Hennings, 1978; Borkovec et al., 1979). However, it seems unlikely that muscle tension release achieves its effectiveness through reducing autonomic hyperarousal. The failure to find any relationship between sleep improvement and a relaxation-induced decline in physiological activity (Borkovec et al., 1979; Borkovec & Fowles, 1973; Coursey, Frankel, Gaarder, & Mott, 1980; Haynes, Sides, & Lockwood, 1977; Hauri, 1981; Freedman & Papsdorf, 1976; Lick & Heffler, 1977) suggests that researchers must consider alternative hypotheses to account for the moderate, yet consistent success of progressive muscle relaxation treatment. Given that progressive relaxation involves the focusing of attention on the internal sensations generated by muscle-tension release, and away from worrisome thoughts and images incompatible with sleep, cognitive factors may prove to be a critical target for future clinical research.

Biofeedback. Of the relatively few controlled experiments which have examined the efficacy of this procedure, most have employed frontalis electromyograph (EMG) biofeedback.

Freedman and Papsdorf (1976) compared EMG biofeedback with progressive relaxation and a contact control in which subjects practiced physical exercises in the belief that they would promote relaxation. According to EEG data, subjects in both treatment groups made approximately equivalent gains over the control group. However, global estimates at a two-month follow-up indicated that this improvement had not been maintained for most subjects.

Relying on self-report, Haynes et al. (1977) found that EMG feedback and taped passive relaxation instructions were equally effective and both were significantly more effective than a self-relaxation control. However, as this study failed to assess the credibility of any of the conditions, the data are open to question. Further equivocal support for the effectiveness of EMG biofeedback was provided by Coursey et al. (1980). They claimed that while biofeedback did not reduce the group mean significantly, three of the six subjects in this condition made significant improvement (50% decrease in laboratory sleep onset latency). Although methodological problems and incomplete data analysis make it difficult to interpret the results of this study, it does serve to highlight the need to match treatment to the client rather than assume that insomnia arises from a unitary source (Coates & Thoresen, 1981). This point has also been emphasized in several studies comparing EMG, theta, and sensori motor rhythm (SMR) biofeedback. In the first comparison Hauri (1981) found that neither SMR feedback nor EMG training were effective treatments. However, when the subjects were categorized in a post hoc analysis according to appropriateness for SMR (low anxiety) and EMG training (high anxiety), significant objective effects became evident. This outcome has been essentially replicated by Hauri, Percy, Hellekson, Hartmann, and Russ (1982). They found that tense insomniacs made objective improvement only under EMG/theta biofeedback training, whereas nontense subjects improved only under SMR feedback.

Interestingly, all subjects in the Hauri et al. (1982) study reported improvement in their sleep diaries irrespective of the type of biofeedback administered or whether it was considered to be appropriate or inappropriate for an individual. Hauri et al. (1982) speculated on the basis of this finding that some general effect, not specific to the biofeedback parameter, operated on self-reports of home sleep improvement. They suggested the revival of hope or the relatively intensive interaction between staff and patient as factors which may possibly account for this changed phenomenology. Similarly, Nicassio, Boylan, and McCabe (1982), who found false biofeedback to be as effective as EMG biofeedback and progressive relaxation in reducing reported sleep onset latency, suggest that increased confidence in one's ability to cope (and thus reduced anxiety) arising from the therapeutic experience could explain the perceived improvement.

Although the mechanism by which biofeedback achieves its effect is of interest, the fact that the procedure requires relatively expensive equipment and considerable training sessions to attain the same moderate levels of improvement achieved by relaxation, suggests that this is not the treatment of choice for most clients.

Cognitive relaxation strategies. Schultz and Luthe (1959) provided informal case study evidence for the effectiveness of autogenic training, a procedure they developed which utilizes self-suggestion and imagery to bring about a state of low physiological arousal compatible with sleep. Nicassio and Bootzin (1974) conducted the first evaluation of autogenic training that included control groups. Utilizing self-report data, they found that both autogenic training and progressive muscle relaxation were significantly more effective than self-relaxation (scheduled time to relax) or no-treatment. These improvements, confirmed by household members, were maintained at six-month follow-up. In addition, Nicassio and Bootzin (1974) claimed to provide convergent data from an analysis of photographed pupils to support the efficacy of these procedures.

Coursey et al. (1980) employed the more widely accepted EEG measure to provide an objective index of the effectiveness of autogenic training, electromyograph biofeedback, and electrosleep therapy.

While none of the insomniacs receiving low-current intracranial electrical stimulation (electrosleep therapy) improved on all-night laboratory EEG sleep records or daily home sleep logs, approximately one-half of the subjects treated by the two relaxation procedures showed marked improvements. However, the group mean reduction in sleep onset latency did not reflect this improvement in either the autogenic or biofeedback condition.

Meditation is another procedure which utilizes the individual's ability to produce imagery and to concentrate. This involves the focusing of attention on undifferentiated or repetitive stimulation, a process found to reduce cortical excitation and the metabolic rate (Woolfolk, 1975). This procedure was compared with progressive relaxation in a sample of nonstudent adult insomniacs by Woolfolk, Carr-Kaffashan, McNulty, and Lehrer (1976). Subjects in the meditation treatment were sequentially instructed to focus passively on the physical sensations associated with their breathing silently, to repeat the mantra "in" and "out," and to focus upon a specific image. Subject's reports of sleep onset latency indicated that both meditation and progressive relaxation were superior to no-treatment (waiting list control) and that these treatments were equally effective. Woolfolk et al. (1976) argue that this result, coupled with the demonstrated efficacy of autogenic training, suggested that attention focusing procedures facilitated sleep onset in insomniacs. Unfortunately their data do not allow an unequivocal conclusion to be drawn, as subject's expectations of improvement from being offered an "active" treatment may have accounted for the group differences.

Woolfolk and McNulty (1983) attempted to overcome this problem in their component analysis of relaxation procedures by utilizing a counterdemand strategy and assessing subject's expectations pre- and posttreatment. While subjects trained in attention focusing rated this treatment least positively, it was as effective as the muscle tension release conditions in reducing reports of sleep onset latency during the period when improvement would not have been expected. Importantly, subjects receiving this imagery training also showed significantly greater reductions in nocturnal awakenings during the counterdemand period, the complaint of nocturnal awakenings being regarded as severely debilitating. Thus it appears that visual attention focusing plays a role in the relaxation treatment of onset and maintenance insomnia, perhaps by directing attention away from obsessive and arousing mentation.

The final treatment strategy to be considered as a cognitive procedure is paradoxical intention. As it relates to insomnia, this involves instructing the insomniac to try to remain awake as long as possible.

By changing the cognitive focus in the direction of trying not to fall asleep, it is hypothesized that thoughts maintaining anxiety about the inability to sleep will be reduced and sleep onset facilitated. Ascher and Efran (1978) provided case study reports on the effectiveness of this procedure with five outpatients who had been unsuccessfully treated for insomnia with progressive muscle relaxation and systematic desensitization. Utilizing an A-B design with a single subject, Relinger, Bornstein, and Mungas (1978) reported that time series analysis revealed significant improvement during the counterdemand phase. Recognizing the methodological problems inherent in such a design, Relinger and Bornstein (1979) employed a multiple baseline design across subjects. While the procedure resulted in substantial reductions in sleep onset latency for all subjects, of more importance is the demonstration of functional control as evidenced by the sequential improvement in subject sleep behaviors only after treatment had been focused directly upon each individual. Further evidence for the effectiveness of this procedure was provided by Ascher and Turner (1979) who found paradoxical intention to be superior to both a credible quasidesentization placebo control (Steinmark & Borkovec, 1974) and a no-treatment control. In a multivariate outcome study with severe insomniacs, Turner and Ascher (1979a) found paradoxical intention to be as effective as progressive relaxation and stimulus control therapy, all of which were significantly superior to the above-mentioned placebo control and a no-treatment control. However, results have shown paradoxical intention to be inferior to these treatment modalities in two subsequent studies (Turner & Ascher, 1982; Lacks, Bertelson, Gans, & Kunkel, 1983) thus necessitating further research using convergent measures.

Habit-Restructuring Approach

The second major behavioral approach to treatment is based on an operant analysis of sleep and insomnia in which falling asleep is conceptualized as an instrumental act emitted to produce reinforcement (sleep). This, together with the stimulus control work of Brown (1965), led Bootzin (1972) to hypothesize that the bedroom contained cues (i.e., discriminative stimuli) for sleeping. On this basis, Bootzin suggested that difficulty sleeping may be due to inadequate stimulus control. He speculated that strong discriminative stimuli for sleep may not become established because the person retires to bed when there is a low probability of sleep (through not being tired because of an erratic sleep schedule or daytime napping). In addition, bed and bedtime may become cues for activities incompatible with sleep (reading, watching television, problem solving, worrying, especially about falling asleep). As such, Bootzin (1972) developed a stimulus control procedure for the treatment of insomnia.

Stimulus control instructions. Bootzin's procedure was designed to reassociate the bed, as a cue or discriminative stimulus, with sleep, and to help the insomniac acquire a consistent sleep rhythm. His instructions were:

1. Lie down intending to go to sleep *only* when you are sleepy
2. Do not use your bed for anything except sleep; that is, do not read, watch television, eat, or worry in bed. Sexual activity is the only exception to this rule. On such occasions the instructions are to be followed afterward when you intend to go to sleep
3. If you find yourself unable to fall asleep, get up and go into another room. Stay up as long as you wish and then return to the bedroom to sleep. Although we do not want you to watch the clock, we want you to get out of bed if you do not fall asleep immediately. Remember, the goal is to associate your bed with falling asleep quickly. If you are in bed more than about 10 minutes without falling asleep and have not gotten up, you are not following this instruction
4. If you still cannot fall asleep, repeat step 3. Do this as often as is necessary through the night
5. Set your alarm and get up at the same time every morning irrespective of how much sleep you get during the night. This will help your body to acquire a consistent sleep rhythm
6. Do not sleep during the day.

Evaluation of stimulus control therapy. The success experienced by the subject of Bootzin's (1972) initial case study (using only the first four instructions) led to the complete procedure being offered to a total of 31 clients over a period of time (Bootzin & Nicassio, 1978). These severe, chronic insomniacs reduced their average reported sleep onset latencies from 85 to 36 minutes through stimulus control treatment. Such reports of the treatment's success were followed by a number of more systematic and better controlled investigations.

Utilizing college students as subjects, Zwart and Lisman (1979) compared stimulus control, temporal control, noncontingent control (subjects arose from bed a fixed number of times within 20 minutes of retiring), stimulus countercontrol (subjects stayed in bed to read or watch television, etc., if unable to sleep) and no-treatment conditions. During the counterdemand period, only subjects receiving stimulus control and stimulus countercontrol instructions significantly reduced their reports of sleep onset latency. Under positive demand conditions, however, all treated groups reported equal improvement in comparison to the no-treatment group. While this study indicates that stimulus control procedures are effective for moderate insomnia, the success of the countercontrol group, which violated the associative aspects of the stimulus control treatment, raises doubts as to the validity of the theoretical mechanism proposed to account for its efficacy. This is also questioned by the Haynes et al. (1974) finding that insomniacs did not engage in significantly more sleep incompatible behavior in the bedroom than did noninsomniacs. As such, Zwart and Lisman (1979) suggest that the effectiveness of stimulus control treatment is most parsimoniously explained by its ability to contingently disrupt sleep incompatible activities and/or cognitions that occur prior to sleep onset.

Although the critical study required to determine its theoretical mechanism has yet to be conducted, comparative investigations have clearly demonstrated the stimulus control procedure to be as effective or superior to progressive relaxation, EMG biofeedback, and paradoxical intention in reducing self-reported sleep onset latency. Bootzin and Nicassio (1978) point out that in absolute terms, 57% of these stimulus control subjects averaged less than 25 minutes a night to fall asleep after training, whereas only 29% of progressive relaxation subjects, 27% of self-relaxation, and 22% of no-treatment control subjects achieved this criterion. Although Hughes and Hughes (1978) found stimulus control to be as effective as relaxation, EMG biofeedback, and pseudo-biofeedback, they acknowledge that the stimulus control subjects may have been disadvantaged by having only two sessions with a therapist, while relaxation subjects received four and biofeedback eight sessions. Turner and Ascher (1979a, 1982) compared stimulus control, progressive relaxation, and paradoxical intention with placebo and no-treatment control groups. In their first study, they found all active treatments to be more effective than desensitization placebo and no-treatment, with no significant difference between treatments. In the subsequent study, only stimulus control and progressive relaxation proved to be effective in comparison to no-treatment.

Lacks et al. (1983) similarly reported that paradoxical intention was not an effective treatment when they also compared it with stimulus control, progressive relaxation, and desensitization placebo. Unlike Turner and Ascher (1979a, 1982), however, they included the counterdemand strategy in their design. Lacks et al. (1983) found stimulus control to be significantly more effective during the period when expectancy effects should have been minimal. Importantly, stimulus control remained superior to all other conditions during the positive demand period and at follow-up. This finding is of significance because differences between behavioral treatments under counterdemand instructions have disappeared during the positive-demand period in a number of studies (Carr-Koffashan & Woolfolk, 1979; Shealy, 1979; Steinmark & Borkovec, 1974; Zwart & Lisman, 1979).

In addition to the stimulus control groups statistically significant superiority over the other treatments, Lacks et al. (1983) also report that subjects receiving these instructions made the most clinically significant gains. The percentage of stimulus control subjects who showed improvement was 93% ($n=15$), with the percentage for the other groups (including placebo) ranging from 57% to 68%. As a group, stimulus control subjects reduced their perceived time to fall asleep by 50% from 75 min. to almost 30 min., while considerably smaller improvements were reported for the other groups (range = 18% – 23% decrease). Finally, in terms of the number of nights per week that insomnia was experienced (SOL > 30 mins.) stimulus control subjects had an average reduction of two full nights per week as compared to about one-half a night reduction for the other groups. Lacks et al. (1983) conclude on the basis of their data that stimulus control is the treatment of choice regardless of severity level.

Several studies have addressed the issue of clinical, as opposed to statistical, significance more directly by employing a single subject design; an experimental design which Hersen and Barlow (1976) maintain is more appropriate for this purpose. Haynes, Price, and Simons (1975) used an A-B-A-B design in their attempt to determine the clinical efficacy of the stimulus control procedure. All four subjects showed improvement under treatment conditions but only two showed any movement in the direction of return to baseline values during the reversal phase. While a number of factors may be responsible for this, the fact that the study failed to demonstrate an unambiguous reversal effect limits any conclusions that might be proposed regarding a functional relationship between stimulus control therapy and reported reductions in sleep onset latency. This, together with the ethical consideration of withdrawing treatment from a patient so as to demonstrate experimental control, indicates that single-subject reversal designs are not as useful as the multiple baseline across subject's design. This allows the effect of an intervention to be demonstrated by showing changes across separate individuals, when, and only when, a treatment intervention is introduced (Kazdin & Kopel, 1975).

Using this design, Turner and Ascher (1979b) divided six chronic insomniacs into two groups of three subjects each. After a 10-day baseline period, subjects one, two, and three were given stimulus control instructions while subjects four, five, and six followed the desensitization placebo regime. Subjects in the stimulus control group showed improvement in self-reported sleep onset latency, drug intake, and on a number of other measures. During this period, subjects receiving the placebo treatment experienced only modest reductions in sleep onset latency. When transferred to stimulus control therapy, two of these three subjects reported concomitant improvements in sleep. Five of the six subjects achieved onset of sleep in less than 30 minutes—the criterion for clinical significance. Importantly, reductions in dosage of sleeping medication occurred only after the introduction of stimulus control therapy.

It would appear on the basis of the studies reviewed, that stimulus control instructions can effect clinically and statistically significant reductions in reported sleep onset latency. Indeed, according to Borkovec (1982), studies employing the stimulus control program have averaged 70% group mean reductions in subjective reports of sleep onset latency; a level not achieved by other behavioral procedures. However, Borkovec (1982) also points out that this is far from an ideal outcome, for, as with the other treatments already mentioned, some insomniacs fail to benefit at all from the intervention. This again raises the question of the appropriateness of a particular treatment for an individual. As an example, it may be that stimulus control treatment is not suitable for clients who find it more aversive to get out of bed than to wait 30 minutes to fall asleep. Similarly, stimulus control instructions may be relatively ineffective by themselves for an insomniac with high levels of somatic tension and who requires training in relaxation and stress management. Sleep onset insomniacs who have a delayed circadian temperature rhythm may also require bright light stimulation in the mornings (Morris, Lack, & Dawson, 1990).

It is apparent from the literature that only by conducting a thorough assessment and tailoring treatment to meet the clients' needs, can a clinician maximize the probability of a successful outcome for that client. Notwithstanding this, the data indicates that clinicians should consider the stimulus control procedure as an important component of the interventions they design. The procedure is relatively easy to teach, requires minimal therapist time to administer and can facilitate rapid and dramatic reductions in subjective reports of sleep onset latency. This procedure, in conjunction with the other behavioral treatments discussed, provides the clinician with an efficacious means of assisting clients presenting with primary insomnia.

SUMMARY

Sleep disorders can lower the quality of our lives and they also have been linked to serious psychiatric and physical health problems. An unstable positive feedback model suggests that poor health can lead to poor sleep but poor sleep can, in turn, exacerbate poor health. Sleep disorders may, therefore, be a major contribution to an individual's poor health. The extent to which sleep disorders are a community health problem is dependent on the prevalences of these disorders in the population. Measuring the prevalence has generally been attempted using large sample questionnaire surveys or small sample polysomnographic (PSG) studies. Neither method is ideal. Nevertheless, a meta-analysis was conducted on all studies using survey questionnaire or sleep/wake diaries in the expectation that averages of the most prolific source of data would yield the most reliable prevalence estimates. Frequent difficulty with sleep in general or more specifically with falling asleep, staying asleep, awakening too early, or daytime sleepiness was reported by 10–12% of the population. Frequent use of hypnotic drugs was reported by 5% of the population. Although more women than men reported frequent difficulties with sleep and hypnotic drug use, PSG studies find few gender differences except more awakening and lighter sleep in men. This apparent discrepancy was suggested to be due to nonrepresentative PSG samples and response bias in surveys on the part of males in underestimating sleeping difficulties. The greatest effects of age were increases in nighttime and early morning awakening and hypnotic drug use. However, an apparent decrease in daytime sleepiness with age suggests that older individuals are more likely to get adequate sleep despite more numerous awakenings and that hypnotic drugs are, therefore, inappropriate and potentially dangerous for the elderly.

Causes of excessive daytime sleepiness may include restricted sleep, narcolepsy, sleep apnea, and nocturnal myoclonus. Adequate, instead of restricted, sleep should be obtained by attention to lifestyle factors such as reducing excessive responsibilities and keeping a regular sleep/wake pattern. Narcolepsy is a debilitating form of excessive sleepiness which afflicts about 0.05% of the population. Behavioral management considerations can form an effective adjunct to drug treatment in the control of sleep attacks and cataplectic seizures. Sleep apnea poses definitional problems. Defined only in terms of the number of breathing cessations it is extremely prevalent in the elderly population (about 25%); however it appears to be benign with no illness consequences. The more severe obstructive sleep apnea is strongly associated with numerous health problems including hypertension, cardiac abnormalities, and dangerous oxygen desaturations. But this form of sleep apnea has a prevalence of about 1% of the population. Nocturnal myoclonus or periodic movements in sleep increases dramatically with age but also appears relatively benign.

A variety of behavior therapies for the most prevalent sleep disorders of insomnia were described and evaluated. These included progressive muscle relaxation, biofeedback, cognitive relaxation strategies, and stimulus control therapy. While all therapies were shown to provide some benefit it was concluded that stimulus control therapy was most efficacious, particularly for sleep onset insomnia.

REFERENCES

Addison, R. G., Thorpy, M. J., & Roth, T. (1987). A survey of the United States public concerning the quality of sleep. *Sleep Research, 16*, 244.

Ancoli-Isreal, S. Kripke, D. F., & Mason, W. (1983). Prevalence of sleep apnea and PMS in seniors: An update. *Sleep Research, 12*, 221.

Ancoli-Isreal, S., Kripke, D. F., Mason, W., & Messin, S. (1981). Sleep apnea and nocturnal myoclonus in a senior population. *Sleep, 4*, 349–458.

Ascher, L. M., & Efran, J. S. (1978). Use of paradoxical intention in a behavioral program for sleep onset insomnia. *Journal of Consulting and Clinical Psychology, 46*(3), 547–550.

Ascher, L. M., & Turner, R. M. (1979). Paradoxical intention and insomnia: An experimental investigation. *Behaviour Research and Therapy, 17*(4), 408–411.

Badia, P., Harsh, J., Balkin, T., Cantrell, P., Klemport, A., O'Rourke, D., & Schoen, L. (1984). Behavioral control of respiration in sleep. *Psychophysiology, 2*, 494–500.

Balter, M. B., & Bauer, M. L. (1975). Patterns of prescribing and use of hypnotic drugs in the United States. In A. D. Clift (Ed.), *Sleep disturbance and hypnotic drug dependence* (pp. 262–293). Amsterdam: Excerpta Medica.

Bearpark, H. M., & Michie, P. T. (1987) Prevalence of sleep/wake disturbances in Sydney adolescents. *Sleep Research, 16*, 304.

Berry, D. T. R., Webb, W. B., & Block, A. J. (1984). Sleep apnea syndrome: A critical review of the Apnea Index as a diagnostic criterion. *Chest, 86*(4), 529–531.

Bixler, E. O., Kales, A., Jacoby, J. A., Soldatos, C. R., & Vela-Bueno, A. (1984) Nocturnal sleep and wakefulness: Effects of age and sex in normal sleepers. *International Journal of Neuroscience, 23*, 33–42.

Bixler, E. O., Kales, A., Leo, L. A., & Slye, T. (1973). A comparison of subjective estimates and objective sleep laboratory findings in insomniac patients. *Sleep Research, 2*, 143.

Bixler, E. O., Kales, A., Soldatos, C. R., Kales, J. D., & Healey, S. (1979). Prevalence of sleep disorders in the Los Angeles metropolitan area. *American Journal of Psychiatry, 136*, 1257–1262.

Bixler, E. O., Kales, A., Vela-Bueno, A., Jacoby, J. A., Scarone, S., & Soldatos, C. R. (1982). Nocturnal myoclonic activity in a normal population. *Research Communications in Chemical Pathology and Pharmacology, 35*(1), 129–140.

Block J., Boysen, P., Wynne, J., & Hunt, L. (1979) Sleep apnea, hypopnea and oxygen desaturation in normal subjects. *New England Journal of Medicine, 300*, 513–517.

Bonnet, M. H. (1985). Effect of sleep disruption on sleep, performance, and mood. *Sleep, 8*, 11–19.

Bonnett, M. H., Dexter, J. R., & Arand, D. (1987). The effect of triazolam in increasing sleep apnea. *Sleep Research, 16*, 310.

Bootzin, R. R. (1972). A stimulus control treatment for insomnia. *Proceedings of the American Psychological Association*, pp. 395–396.

Bootzin, R. R., & Nicassio, P. M. (1978). Behavioral treatments for insomnia. In M. Hersen, R Eisler, & P. Miller (Eds.), *Progress in behavior modification*. New York: Academic Press.

Borkovec, T. D. (1979). Pseudo (experiential) - insomnia and idiopathic (objectived) insomnia: Theoretical and therapeutic issues. In H. J. Eysenck & S. Rachman (Eds.), *Advances in behaviour research and therapy 2* (pp. 27–55). London: Pergamon Press.

Borkovec, T. D. (1982). Insomnia. *Journal of Consulting and Clinical Psychology, 50*(6), 880–895.

Borkovec, T. D., & Fowles, D. C. (1973). Controlled investigation of the effects of progressive and hypnotic relaxation on insomnia. *Journal of Abnormal Psychology, 82*, 153–158.

Borkovec, T. D., Grayson, J. B., O'Brien, G. T., & Weerts, T.C. (1979). Relaxation treatment of pseudo-insomnia and idiopathic insomnia: An electroencephalographic evaluation. *Journal of Applied Behavior Analysis, 12*, 37–54.

Borkovec, T. D., & Hennings, B. L. (1978). The role of physiological attention-focussing in the relaxation treatment of sleep disturbance, general tension, and specific stress reaction. *Behaviour Research and Therapy, 16*, 7–19.

Borkovec, T. D., Kaloupek, D. G., & Slama, K. M. (1975). The facilitative effects of muscle tension-release in the relaxation treatment of disturbance. *Behavior Therapy, 6*, 301–309.

Borkovec, T. D., & Weerts, T. C. (1976). Effects of progressive relaxation on sleep disturbance: An electroencephalographic evaluation. *Psychosomatic Medicine, 38*, 173–180.

Brezinova, V. (1974). Effect of caffeine on sleep: EEG Study in late middle-age people. *British Journal of Clinical Pharmacology, 1*, 203–208.

Broughton, R., & Roberts, J. (1985). A survey of subjective sleep measures and performance in working adults. *Sleep Research, 14*, 89.

Brown, J. S. (1965). Generalization and discrimination. In D. J. Mostofsky (Ed.), *Stimulus generalization* (pp. 7–23). Stanford: Stanford University Press.

Carr-Kaffashan, L., & Woolfolk, R. L. (1979). Active and placebo effects in treatment of moderate and severe insomnia. *Journal of Consulting and Clinical Psychology, 47*, 1072–1080.

Carskadon, M. A., & Dement, W. C. (1981). Respiration during sleep in the aged human. *Journal of Gerontology, 36*, 420–423.

Carskadon, M. A., Dement, W. C., Mitler, M. M. Guilleminault, C., Zarcone, U. P., & Spiegel, R. (1976). Self-reports versus sleep laboratory findings in

122 drug-free subjects with complaints of chronic insomnia. *American Journal of Psychiatry, 133*, 1382–1388.

Carskadon, M. A., Van Den Hoed, J., & Dement, W. C. (1980). Sleep and daytime sleepiness in the elderly. *Geriatric Psychiatry, 13*(2), 135–151.

Cartwright, R., Ristanovic, R., Jaski, M., & Lloyd, S. (1987). Non-invasive treatments for sleep apnea. *Sleep Research, 26*, 321.

Coates, T. J., & Thoresen, C. E. (1981). Treating sleep disorders: Few answers, some suggestions and many questions. In S. M. Turner, K. S. Calhoun, & H. E. Adams (Eds.), *Handbook of clinical behavior therapy* (pp. 240–284). New York: Wiley.

Coleman, R. M., Bliwise, D. L., Sajben, N., De Bruyn, L., Boomkamp, A., Meun, M. E., & Dement, W. C. (1983). Epidemiology of periodic movements during sleep. In C. Guilleminault & E. Lugaresi (Eds.), *Sleep/wake disorders* (pp. 217–229). New York: Raven.

Coursey, R.D., Bucksbaum, M., & Frankel., B. L. (1975). Personality measures and evoked responses in chronic insomniacs. *Journal of Abnormal Psychology, 84*, 239–250.

Coursey, R. D., Frankel, B. L., Gaarder, K. B., & Mott, D. E. (1980). A comparison of relaxation techniques with electro-sleep therapy for chronic sleep onset insomnia. A sleep EEG study. *Biofeedback and Self Regulation, 5*, 57–73.

Czeisler, C. A., Kronauer, R. E., Rios, C. D., Sanchez, R., & Rogacz, S. (1986). Attenuated output of the endogenous circadian oscillator (X) in an 85 year old man: A case study. *Sleep Research, 15*, 267.

Czeisler, C. A., Rios, C. D., Sanchez, R., Brown, E. N., Richardson, G. S., Ronda, J. M., & Rogacz, S. (1986). Phase advance and reduction in amplitude of the endogenous circadian oscillator correspond with systematic changes in sleep-wake habits and daytime functioning in the elderly. *Sleep Research, 15*, 268.

Dickel, M. J., Sassin, J., & Mosko, S. (1986). Sleep disorders in an aged population: Preliminary findings of a longitudinal study. *Sleep Research, 15*, 116.

Domino. G., Romero, M., Blair, G., Villa Lobos, S., Suriano, T., & Bridges, A. (1985). Cross cultural aspects of sleep in the elderly. *Research on Aging, 1*(2), 195–208.

Dorsey, C., & Bootzin, R. R. (1987). Subjective and psychophysiologic insomnia: Multiple sleep latency test, sleep tendency, and personality. *Sleep Research, 16*, 328.

Ellis, B. W., Johns, M. W., Lancaster, R., Raptopoulos, R., Angelopoulos, N., & Priest, R. G. (1981). The Saint Mary's Hospital sleep questionnaires: A study of reliability. *Sleep, 4*, 93–97.

Franceschi, M., Smirne, S., Zamproni, P., Crippa, D., & Ferini-Strambi, L. (1983). Prevalence of excessive daytime sleepiness in an unselected inpatient population. In W. P. Koella (Ed.), *Sleep 1982* (pp. 315–317). Basel: S. Kanger.

Freedman, R. R., & Papsdorf, J. D. (1976). Biofeedback and progressive relaxation treatment of sleep-onset insomnia: A controlled all-night investigation. *Biofeedback and Self Regulation, 1*, 253–271.

Freedman, R. R., & Sattler, H. L. (1982). Physiological and psychological factors in sleep-onset insomnia. *Journal of Abnormal Psychology, 91*(5), 380–389.

George, B., Ancoli-Israel, S., & Kripke, D. F. (1985). Comparison of sleep apnea and periodic movements in sleep in two age groups of females. *Sleep Research, 14*, 156.

Gerard, P., Collins, K. J., Dore, C., & Exton-Smith, A. N. (1978). Subjective characteristics of sleep in the elderly. *Age and Aging, 7*, 55–63.

Gislason, T., Almquist, M., Boman, G., Eriksson, G., & Taube, A. (1987). Prevalence of sleep apnea syndrome among Swedish men—An epidemiological study. *Sleep Research, 16*, 335.

Hammond, E. C. (1964). Some preliminary findings on physical complaints from a prospective study of 1,064,004 men and women. *American Journal of Public Health, 54*, 11–23.

Hammond. E., & Garfinkel, R. (1969). Coronary heart disease, stroke, and aortic aneurysm: Factors in etiology. *Archives of Environmental Health, 19*, 167–182.

Hauri, P. (1981). Treating psychophysiological insomnia with biofeedback. *Archives of General Psychiatry, 38*, 752–758.

Hauri, P., & Olmstead, E. (1983). What is the moment of sleep onset for insomniacs? *Sleep, 6*(1), 10–15.

Hauri, O., Percy. L., Hellekson, C., Hartmann, E., & Russe, D. (1982). The treatment of psychophysiological insomnia with biofeedback: A replication study. *Biofeedback and Self Regulation, 7*(2), 223–235.

Haynes, S. N., Follingstead, D., & McGowan, W. (1974). Insomnia: Sleep patterns and anxiety level. *Journal of Psychosomatic Research, 18*, 69–74.

Haynes, S. N., Price, M. G., & Simons, J. B. (1975). Stimulus control treatment of insomnia. *Journal of Behavior Therapy and Experimental Psychiatry, 6*, 279–282.

Haynes, S. N., Sides, H., & Lockwood, G. (1977). Relaxation instructions and frontalis electromyographic feedback intervention with sleep onset insomnia. *Behavior Therapy, 8*, 644–652.

Henschel, A., & Lack. L. (1987). Do many adolescents sleep poorly or just too late? *Sleep Research, 16*, 354.

Hersen, M., & Barlow, D. H. (1976). *Single-case experimental designs: Strategies for studying behavior change*. New York: Pergamon.

Hetta, J., Almquist, M., Liljenberg, B., & Roos, B. (1987). Epidemiological aspects on relations between psychiatric and somatic symptoms and sleep disturbances. *Sleep Research, 16*, 356.

Hicks, R. A., Hicks, G. J., Reyes, J. R., & Cheers, Y. (1983). Daily caffeine use and the sleep of college students. *Bulletin of the Psychonomic Society, 21*, 24–25.

Hoch, C. C., Reynolds, C. F., Kupfer, D. J., Berman, S. R., Houck, P. R., & Stack, J. A. (1987). *Sleep Research, 16*, 205.

Hughes, R. C., & Hughes, H. H. (1978). Insomnia: Effects of EMG biofeedback, relaxation training, and stimulus control. *Behavioral Engineering, 5*(2), 67–72.

Jacobson, E. (1938). *Progressive relaxation.* Chicago: University of Chicago Press.

Johns, M. W., Egan, P., Gay, T. J. A., & Masterson, J. P. (1970). Sleep habits and symptoms in male medical and surgical patients. *British Medical Journal, 2,* 509–512.

Johns, M. W., Gay, T. J. A., Masterton, J. P., & Bruce, D. W. (1971). Relationship between sleep habits, adrenocortical activity and personality. *Psychosomatic Medicine, 33,* 499–508.

Kales, A., Bixler, E. O., Vela-Bueno, A., Cadieux, R. J., Soldatos, C. R., & Kales, J. D. (1984). Biopsychobehavioral correlates of insomnia, III: Polygraphic findings of sleep difficulty and their relationship to psychopathology. *International Journal of Neuroscience, 23,* 43–56.

Kales, A., Caldwell, A. B., Bixler, E. O., Healey, S., Kales, J. D., & Preston, T. A. (1978). Further evaluation of MMPI findings in insomnia: Comparison of insomniac patients and normal controls. *Sleep Research, 7,* 189.

Kales, A., Caldwell, A. B., Preston, T. A., Healy, S., & Kales, J. D. (1976). Personality patterns in insomnia: Theoretical implications. *Archives of General Psychiatry, 33,* 1128–1134.

Kales, A., Kales, J. D., & Soldatos, C. R. (1982). Insomnia and other sleep disorders. *Medical Clinics of North America, 66,* 971–991.

Kales, J. D., Kales A., Bixler, E. O., Soldatos, C. R., Cadieux, R. J., Kashurba, G. J., & Vela-Bueno, A. (1984). Biopsychobehavioral correlates of insomnia, V: Clinical characteristics and behavioral correlates. *American Journal of Psychiatry, 141,* 1371–1376.

Karacan, I., Ilaria, R., Ware, J. C. Thornby, J., & Chambliss, S. (1978). Is the poor sleep if insomniacs due to anxiety? *Sleep Research, 7,* 236.

Karacan, I., Thornby, J. I., Anch, M., Holzer, C. E., Warheit, G. J., Schwab, J. J., & Williams, R. L. (1976). Prevalence of sleep disturbance in a primarily urban Florida county. *Social Science and Medicine, 10,* 239–244.

Karacan, I., Thornby, J. I., Anch, A. M., Salis, P. J., Williams, R. L., Okawa, M., & Booth, G. H. (1975). Dose-response effects of coffee on the sleep of normal middle-aged men. *Sleep Research, 5,* 71.

Kazdin, A. E. (1979). Therapy outcome questions requiring control of credibility and treatment-generated expectancies. *Behavior Therapy, 10,* 81–93.

Kazdin, A. E., & Kopel, S. A. (1975). On resolving ambiguities in the multiple-baseline design: Problems and recommendations. *Behavior Therapy, 6,* 601–608.

Krieger, J. (1985). Breathing during sleep in normal subjects. *Clinics in Chest Medicine, 6,* 577–594.

Krieger, J., & Kurtz, D. (1987). Sleep apneas in normal older subjects do not worsen their long-term morbidity and mortality. *Sleep Research, 16,* 374.

Kripke, D. F., & Ancoli-Isreal, S. (1983). Epidemiology of sleep apnea among the aged: Is sleep apnea a fatal disorder? In C. Guilleminault & E. Lugaresi (Eds.), *Sleep/wake disorders: Natural history, epidemiology, and long-term evolution* (pp. 137–142). New York: Raven Press.

Kripke, D. F., Ancoli-Isreal, S., Mason, W., & Messin, S. (1983). Sleep related mortality and morbidity in the aged. In M. Chase & E. D. Weitzman

(Eds.), *Sleep disorders: Basic and clinical research* (pp. 415–429). New York: Spectrum.

Kripke, D. F., Ancoli-Isreal, S., Mason, W. J., & Kaplan, O. (1986). Sleep apnea, long and short sleep. *Sleep Research, 15*, 139.

Kripke, D. F., Ancoli-Isreal, S., & Okudaira, N. (1982). Sleep apnea and nocturnal myoclonus in the elderly. *Neurobiology of Aging, 3*(4), 329–336.

Kripke, D., Simons, R., Garfinkel, L., & Hammond, E. C. (1979). Short and long sleep and sleeping pills. *Archives of General Psychiatry, 36*, 103–116.

Lack, L. (1986). Delayed sleep and sleep loss in university students. *Journal of American College Health, 35*, 105–110.

Lack, L., Miller, W., & Turner, D. (1988). A survey of sleeping difficulties in an Australian population. *Community Health Studies, 12*, 200–207.

Lacks, P., Bertelson, A. D., Gans, L., & Kunkel, J. (1983). The effectiveness of three behavioral treatments for different degrees of sleep onset insomnia. *Behavior Therapy, 14*, 593–605.

Lavie, P. (1981). Sleep habits and sleep disturbances in industrial workers in Isreal: Main findings and some characteristics of workers complaining of excessive daytime sleepiness. *Sleep, 4*, 147–158.

Lavie, P. (1983). Sleep apnea in industrial workers. In C. Guilleminault & E. Lugaresi (Eds.), *Sleep/wake disorders: Natural History, epidemiology, and long-term evolution* (pp. 127–135). New York: Raven Press.

Lavie, P., Zomer, J., Peled, R., & Rubin, A. H. (1985). A rapid method to screen large populations for pathologic daytime somnolence. *Sleep Research, 14*, 185.

Lick, J., & Heffler, D. (1977). Relaxation training and attention placebo in the treatment of severe insomnia. *Journal of Consulting and Clinical Psychology, 45*, 153–161.

Lingjaerde, O., Bratlid, T., & Hansen T. (1985). Insomnia during the "dark period" in northern Norway. *Acta Psychiatry Scand., 71*, 506–512.

Lloyd, S. R., Cartwright, R. D., Kravitz, H., & Ristanovic, R. (1987). The diagnosis and treatment of positional sleep apnea. *Sleep Research, 16*, 386.

Lugaresi, E., Cirignotta, F., Zucconi, M., Mondine, S., Lenzi, P. L., & Coccagna, G. (1983). Good and poor sleepers: An epidemiological survey of the San Marino population. In C. Guilleminault & E. Lugaresi (Eds.), *Sleep/wake disorders: Natural history, epidemiology, and long-term evolution* (pp. 1–12). New York: Raven Press.

Lupolover, R., Dazzi, H., & Ward, J. (1982). Rebound phenomena: Results of a 10 years' (1970–1980) literature review. *International Pharmacopsychiatry, 17*, 194–237.

McGhie, A., & Russell, S. M. (1962). The subjective assessment of normal sleep patterns. *Journal of Mental Science, 108*, 642–654.

Mellinger, G. D., Balter, M. B., & Unlenhuth, E. H. (1985). Insomnia and its treatment: Prevalence and correlates. *Archives of General Psychiatry, 42*, 225–232.

Monroe, L. (1967). Psychological and physiological differences between good and poor sleepers. *Journal of Abnormal Psychology, 72*, 255–264.

Montgomery, I., & Trinder, J. (1986). Insomnia. In N. J. King & A. Remenyi (Eds.), *Health care: A behavioural approach* (pp. 87–103). Sydney: Harcourt, Brace & Jovanovich.

Morris, M., Lack. L., & Dawson, D. (1990). Sleep onset insomniacs have delayed temperature rhythms. *Sleep, 13*, 1–14.

Moskowitz, H., & Linnoila, M. (1987). Psychomotor performance during short- and long-term administration of two benzodiazepines, flurazepam and midazolem, to chronic insomniacs. *Sleep Research, 16*, 115.

Nicassio, P. M., & Bootzin, R. R. (1974). A comparison of progressive relaxation and autogenic training as treatments for insomnia. *Journal of Abnormal Psychology, 83*, 253–260.

Nicassio, P. M., Boylan, M. B., & McCabe, T. G. (1982). Progressive relaxation, EMG biofeedback and biofeedback placebo in the treatment of sleep-onset insomnia. *British Journal of Medical psychology, 55*, 159–166.

Okuma, T., Matsuoka, H., Matsue, Y., & Toyomura, K. (1982). Model insomnia by methyplphenidate and caffeine and use in the evaluation of temazepam. *Psychopharmacology, 76*, 201–208.

Orr, W. C., Rundell, O H., Jones, R. K., Fixley, M. F., & Clark, M. (1986). Modulation of central sleep apnea by sleeping position. *Sleep Research, 15*, 152.

Oswald, I. (1979, May 5). The how and why of hypnotic drugs. *British Medical Journal*, pp. 1167–1168.

Partinen, M., Jamieson, A., & Guilleminault, C. (1986). Mortality of patients with obstructive sleep apnea syndrome: A follow-up study. *Sleep Research, 15*, 153.

Partinen, M., Kaprio, J., Koskenvuo, M., & Langinvainio, H. (1983). Sleeping habits, sleep quality, and use of sleeping pills: A population study of 31,140 adults in Finland. In C. Guilleminault & E. Lugaresi (Eds.), *Sleep/wake disorders: Natural history, epidemiology, and long-term evolution* (pp. 29–35). New York: Raven Press.

Paul, G. L. (1969). Physiological effects of relaxation training and hypnotic suggestion. *Journal of Abnormal Psychology, 74*, 425–437.

Paul, G. L., & Trimble, R. W. (1970). Recorder vs. "Live" relaxation training and hypnotic suggestions: Comparative effectiveness for reducing physiological arousal and inhibiting stress response. *Behavior Therapy, 1*, 285–302.

Prinz, P., Smallwood, R., Giblin, E., Ralph, D., & Vitiello, M. (1984). Breathing dysfunction during sleep: Normative data for asymptomatic older adults in relation to sleep apnea syndrome. *Sleep Research, 13*, 158.

Regestein, Q. R., & Reich, P. (1978). Current problems in the diagnosis and treatment of chronic insomnia. *Perspectives in Biological Medicine, 21*, 232–239.

Relinger, H., & Bornstein, P. H. (1979). Treatment of sleep-onset insomnia by paradoxical instruction. *Behavior Modification, 3*, 203–222.

Relinger, H., Bornstein, P. H., & Mungas, D. M. (1978). Treatment of insomnia by paradoxical intention: A time series analysis. *Behavior Therapy, 9*, 955–959.

Reynolds, C. F. III, Kupfer, D. J., Hoch, C. C., & Sewitch, D. E. (1985). Sleeping pills for the elderly: Are they ever justified? *Journal of Clinical Psychiatry, 46*, 9–12.

Reynolds, C. F. III, Kupfer, D. J., Taska, L. S., Hoch, C. C., Sewitch, D. E., & Spiker, D. G. (1985). Sleep of healthy seniors: A revisit. *Sleep, 8*, 20–29.

Roehrs, T., Kribbs, N., Zorick, F., & Roth, T. (1986). Hypnotic residual effects of benzodiazepines with repeated administration. *Sleep, 9*, 309–316.

Roth, B. (1980). *Narcolepsy and hypersomnia.* Basel: Karger.

Roth, T., Kramer, M., & Lutz, T. (1976). The nature of insomnia: A descriptive summary of a sleep clinic population. *Comprehensive Psychiatry, 17*, 217–220.

Ruler, A., & Lack, L. (1988). Gender differences in sleep surveys. *Sleep Research, 17*, 244.

Schultz, J. H., & Luthe, W. (1959). *Autogenic training.* New York: Grune and Stratton.

Seidel, W. F., Ball, S., Cohen, S., Patterson, N., Yost, D., & Dement, W. C. (1984). Daytime alertness in relation to mood, performance, and nocturnal sleep in chronic insomniacs and non-complaining sleepers. *Sleep*, 7(3), 230–238.

Shapiro, C. M., Catterall, J. R, Oswald, I., & Flenley, D. C. (1981). Where are the British sleep apnea patients? *Lancet, 2* (8245), 523.

Shealey, R. C. (1979). The effectiveness of various treatment techniques on different degrees and durations of sleep onset insomnia. *Behaviour Research and Therapy, 17*(6), 541–546.

Shealy, R. C., Lowe, J. D., & Ritzler, B. A. (1980). Sleep onset insomnia: personality characteristics and treatment outcome. *Journal Consulting and Clinical Psychology, 48*, 654–661.

Shirlow, M. J., & Mathers, C. D. (1985). A Study of caffeine consumption and symptoms: Indigestion, palpitations, tremor, headache and insomnia. *International Journal of Epidemiology, 14*, 239–248.

Smyth, M., Giblin, E. C., & Lee, K. (1981). Prevalence of apneas and oxygen desaturation during sleep in healthy older men. *Sleep Research, 10*, 118.

Sours, J. A. (1963). Narcolepsy and other disturbances in the sleep waking rhythm: A study of 115 cases with review of the literature. Journal of Nervous and Mental Diseases, *137*, 525–542.

Spiegel, R. (1981). *Sleep and sleeplessness in advanced age.* Lancaster, England: MTP Press.

Steinmark, S. W., & Borkovec, T. D. (1974). Active and placebo treatment effects on moderate insomnia under counterdemand and positive demand instruction. *Journal of Abnormal Psychology, 83*, 157–163.

Turner, R. M., & Ascher, L. M. (1979a). Controlled comparison of progressive relaxation, stimulus control and paradoxical intention therapies for insomnia. *Journal of Consulting and Clinical Psychology, 47*(3), 500–508.

Turner, R. M., & Ascher, L. M. (1979b). A within-subject analysis of stimulus control therapy with severe sleep-onset insomnia. *Behaviour Research and Therapy, 17*(2), 107–112.

Turner, R. M., & Ascher, L. M. (1982). Therapist factor in the treatment of insomnia. *Behaviour Research and Therapy, 20*, 33–40.

Urponen, H., Vuori, I., Hasan, J., & Partinen, M. (1987). Quality of sleep in relation to health. *Sleep Research, 16*, 512.

Van Gool, W. A., & Mirmiran, M. (1986). Effects of aging and housing in an enriched environment on sleep-wake patterns in rats. *Sleep, 9*, 335-347.

Webb, W. B. (1975). *Sleep: The gentle tyrant.* Englewood Cliffs, NJ: Prentice-Hall.

Webb, W. B. (1983). Older sleep. In M. Chase & E. D. Weitzman (Eds.), *Sleep disorders: Basic and clinical research* (pp. 489–501). New York: Spectrum.

Weiss, H., Kasinoff, B., & Baily, M. (1962). An exploration of reported sleep disturbance. *Journal of Nervous and Mental Disease, 134*, 528–534.

Welstein, L., Dement, W. C., Redington, D., Guilleminault, C., & Mitler, M. M. (1983). Insomnia in the San Francisco Bay Area: A Telephone survey. In C. Guilleminault & E. Lugaresi (Eds.), *Sleep/wake disorders: Natural history, epidemiology, and long-term evolution* (pp. 78–85). New York: Raven Press.

Williams, R. L., Karacan, I., & Hursch, C. J. (1974). *Electroencephalography (EEG) of human sleep: Clinical applications.* New York: Wiley.

Wingard, D. L., Berkman, L. E., & Brand, R. J. (1979). A multivariate analysis of health practices: A nine year mortality follow-up of the Alameda County study. *American Journal of Epidemiology, 110*, 362.

Woolfolk, R. L. (1975). Psychophysiological correlates of meditation. *Archives of General Psychiatry, 32*, 1326–1333.

Woolfolk, R. L., Carr-Kaffashan, L., McNulty, T. J., & Lehrer, P. M. (1976). Meditation training as a treatment for insomnia. *Behavior Therapy, 7*, 359–365.

Woolfolk R. L., & McNulty, T. F. (1983). Relaxation treatment for insomnia: A component analysis. *Journal of Consulting and Clinical Psychology, 51* (44), 495–503.

Zepelin, H. (1983). Normal age related change in sleep. In M. Chase & E. D. Weitzman (Eds), *Sleep disorders: Basic and clinical research.* Jamaica, NY: Spectrum.

Zwart, S. A., & Lisman, S. A. (1979). Analysis of stimulus control treatment of sleep-onset insomnia. *Journal of Consulting and Clinical Psychology, 47*, 113–118.

V

OTHER ISSUES IN BEHAVIORAL MEDICINE

14

Behavioral Approaches to Exercise and Health*

Christina Lee

University of Newcastle, Australia

Neville Owen

Department of Community Medicine
University of Adelaide, Australia

Behavioral scientists have increasingly become involved in the testing of new approaches for the promotion of exercising with healthy adults. The prominent role being given to exercise in the prevention of disease has had a strong influence on the type of programs which have been tested and developed; however, there is also a growing interest in the promotion of exercise for psychological and social benefits. Although developments in this field are recent, and much work remains speculative and inconclusive, the promotion of exercise and the development of a variety of therapeutic and preventive exercise programs is proceeding rapidly. Behavioral research has much to contribute to an understanding of the development and maintenance of patterns of

* Preparation of this Australian chapter was supported in part by a grant to the second author from the Sport and Recreation Ministers' Council. It has been adapted from reviews by Owen and Lee (1984) and Lee and Owen (1986b)

regular physical exercise. Following an outline of the benefits of physical activity, applications of behavioral theories to exercise are then described, and future directions for program development, community interventions, public policy, and research are suggested.

EXERCISE AS A PREVENTIVE INTERVENTION

Programs to alter lifestyles in order to reduce the mortality and morbidity associated with coronary heart disease have proliferated over the past decades in Western developed countries (cf. Stamler, 1981; Walker, 1983). Although some studies (e.g., Sedgwick, Brotherhood, Harris-Davidson, Taplin, & Thomas, 1980) have disputed the relationship between regular exercise and decreased likelihood of heart disease, others (e.g., Blair, Cooper, Gibbons, Gettman, Lewis, & Goodyear, 1983) have found a relationship between the adoption of exercise and the reduction of heart-disease risk factors, and it is now accepted that exercise has an important role to play in heart-disease prevention and rehabilitation (Blair, 1982; Carleton & Lasater, 1983).

While much of the research in this area has focused on coronary heart disease, exercise has been shown to have other health benefits. Obesity, itself associated with heart disease risk, has been effectively treated by exercise (Brownell, 1982a, 1982b; Thompson, Jarvie, Lahey, & Cureton, 1982). Exercise appears to reduce weight not only through direct caloric cost but also by producing temporary increases in basal metabolic rate (e.g., Allen & Quigley, 1977). Epstein and Wing's (1980) meta-analytic review concluded that exercise has a reliable effect on weight loss, the size of which is directly proportional to energy expenditure. However, the rate of weight loss through exercise alone is much slower than when exercise is combined with reduced food intake.

Regular exercise may have other preventive benefits. It has been suggested that it may play a role in the management of diabetes (Martin & Dubbert, 1982a). Exercise may enhance normal health, prevent muscular injuries, control obesity, reduce risk of heart disease, ameliorate the effects of chronic respiratory and muscular problems, and alleviate disease and degenerative problems in the elderly. While much of the evidence concerning these benefits is preliminary, their existence is coming to be accepted as probable (Siscovick, LaPoste & Newman, 1985; Serfass & Gerberich, 1984).

The American College of Sports Medicine (1978) recommends that the amount of training necessary to achieve and maintain cardiorespiratory fitness in a healthy adult was 3 to 5 exercise sessions per week, each between 15 and 60 minutes' duration and at an intensity of 60–90% of maximum heart rate, or 50–85% of maximum oxygen uptake. However, Pollock et al. (1977) show that, in previously sedentary adults, the risk of injury increases markedly as running frequency increases above 3 sessions weekly and exercise periods increase from 15 minutes. This "aerobic" level of exercise may not be necessary in order to attain some other benefits of exercise, such as weight loss, increase in lean body mass, or improvements in sleeping patterns (Brownell, 1982b). It is possible that the "training effect" has been overemphasized, with a resultant high rate of injury and dropout, especially in the middle-aged and elderly, and that an emphasis on lower levels of exercise or on a more gradual buildup of intensity may be more appropriate for many sections of the population (Ryan, 1978). Luria and Koepke (1975), for example, presented evidence from a walking program for healthy adults indicating a low dropout rate and physiological effects which, although more variable than those associated with running, were quite significant for a number of individuals.

PSYCHOLOGICAL CONCOMITANTS OF EXERCISE

There are suggestions that running may sometimes be as effective as psychotherapy for problems such as mild depression and anxiety (Griest et al., 1978; Ledwidge, 1980). It has also been argued that alleviation of depression and improvement in self-confidence are important reasons for the use of exercise following myocardial infarction (Martin & Dubbert, 1982a). Folkins and Sime's (1981) review on the relationship between physical training and mental health concluded that there was evidence for a relationship between exercising and improved affect, self-concept, and work behavior, but that cognitive skills and personality traits were largely unaffected. Effects appear greatest in populations with very low initial fitness levels, such as the permanently institutionalized. However, most investigations have not controlled for the nonspecific aspects of exercise programs, such as attention and social contact (Hughes, 1984). As there is some evidence (e.g., Jasnoski, Holmes, Solomon, & Aguiar, 1981) to suggest that increases in subjective well-being following exercise training are unrelated to improvements in fitness, such nonspecific aspects may be important in producing psychological effects (Morgan, 1982; Taylor, Sallis, & Needle, 1985). Yet ideas that exercise has psychological benefits have been popularized over the past decade (e.g., Egger, 1979) and are concomitants of the increasing interest in exercise among the general community. Theoretical analyses of the psychological effects of running are also appearing with increasing frequency (e.g., Sacks & Sachs, 1981).

EXERCISE AS A SOCIAL GOAL

Changes in social organization and technological innovations have resulted in the general use of motorized transport, high levels of unemployment, decreases in working time, and reduced physical activity components in many occupations (Fitness Ontario, 1984). These social changes have led to the concept of the "leisure society" and increased governmental concern for the recreational aspects of social life. For example, the Australian Government's sport and recreation policy (Australian Labor Party, 1982) argues that government should actively assist groups and individuals to participate in sport and recreation at all levels, from international competition through noncompetitive exercise to passive recreations. Similarly, publications of the Canadian Ministry of Tourism and Recreation (e.g., Fitness Ontario, 1980) proposed particular emphasis on blue-collar workers (Allison & Coburn, 1981), increased participation in sport and leisure activities with who may be most affected by technological advances. Exercise may also provide opportunities for companionship and for the development of social networks. Social trends that are creating a society in which many individuals are oriented toward leisure rather than toward careers or work involve major redirection of attitudes and educational goals. The widespread promotion of physical exercise (Iverson, Fielding, Crow, & Christenson, 1985) can be seen as a part of this process of social change, as well as being based on a concern with therapeutic, preventive, and health-promoting goals.

PERSISTENCE WITH EXERCISE HABITS

The problems with maintenance that are common to a wide range of behaviors (Karoly & Steffen, 1980) apply equally to patterns of regular exercise (Martin & Dubbert, 1982a). Organized exercise programs generally have adherence rates of around 50% at six months (e.g., Carmody, Senner, Manilow, & Matarazzo, 1980; Lee & Owen, 1986a; Oldridge, 1982; Shephard, 1979). Despite the recent argument that behavior change rates and persistence levels in the general population may be much higher than those seen in organized intervention programs (Schachter, 1982), there is evidence for quite low rates of exercise in the general community. Recent Australian figures, for example, indicate the only 10% of adult men and 5% of adult women exercise regularly (National Heart Foundation, 1983) with a majority reporting virtually no exercise at all. Similar data exist for American populations (e.g., Stephens, Jacobs, & White, 1985). Canadian studies report rates of activity closer to 40% (Ministry of Tourism & Recreation, 1983); however, their finding that 20% of the population take up regular exercise every year without the overall percentage increasing dramatically suggests that many find this pattern hard to maintain.

Dropout rates from exercise programs (Carmody et al., 1980) resemble the rates of relapse which have been reported following interventions for addictive behaviors (Hunt, Barnett, & Branch, 1971). Some recent reviews of exercise adherence (e.g., Martin & Dubbert, 1982a, 1982b) have been so pessimistic as to conclude that efforts to encourage exercise should be concentrated on that portion of the population who are most interested in adopting exercise, and the most sedentary and least interested, ignored. Alternatively, it can be argued that more work is required at a theoretical level in an attempt to determine more effective techniques of intervention so that soundly based efforts can be made with all sections of the population.

The prevalence of adherence problems across a range of substantive areas has led to increasing interest in the issue of the maintenance of behavior change from a number of theoretical perspectives. While the issues of generalization and maintenance of behavior change were listed as an important priority in the initial development of behavior therapy (e.g., Baer, Wolf, & Risley, 1968) it is only relatively recently that there has been a strong emphasis on this area, and substantial follow-up intervals in research reports are coming to be expected (e.g., Kazdin, 1979). This increase in the frequency of assessment of maintenance of behavior change reflects both an increasing theoretical interest and the development of techniques to enhance maintenance (e.g., Karoly & Steffen, 1980; Owen, 1981; Stuart, 1982).

STAGES OF BEHAVIOR CHANGE

Behavior change is not a unitary process, and a number of stages of change can be identified. DiClemente and Prochaska (1982), for example, identify three stages: decision to change, active changing, and maintenance of the new behavior. They offer arguments derived from work on smoking cessation programs for the operation of different mechanisms at different stages of the change process, with verbal processes such as education and self-persuasion important in the first stage, and direct instruction more useful in the second and third. That there could be stages in exercise adoption has also been argued (e.g., Heinzelman & Bagley, 1970), and Dishman (1982) reviewed evidence from physical activity programs for separate processes occurring during adoption and during maintenance of the new activity.

Abrams, Elder, Lasater, and Carleton (1982) argue that behavior change should be considered in three stages: promotion of the new behavior, skills development, and maintenance. Maccoby and Alexander (1980) propose five stages: agenda setting; informing; training new behaviors; motivating and reinforcing the new behaviors; and maintenance training. This apparent variety of stages and labels is based on similar notions of change: Behavior change requires a process of producing awareness of the problem, then motivation to change, followed by instructions and initial change, and consolidated by a final stage assisting the maintenance of the new behavior (Owen, 1985a). It seems likely (e.g., Abrams et al., in press; Dishman, 1982; Olson & Zanna, 1981) that different behavior-change techniques will be effective at different stages in the change process, and for this reason Abrams et al. (1982) and Olson and Zanna (1981) have recommended a multiple approach in which all stages are addressed as targets throughout any community intervention campaign, so that individuals at all stages of readiness to change can be influenced.

APPLICATIONS OF BEHAVIORAL THEORIES TO EXERCISE PROMOTION

Attempts to increase levels of exercise have been based on various theories, and as a consequence their focus has been on various settings, behaviors, incentives for action, and individual cognitions. Given that a number of different processes may be operating at different stages of the behavior change sequence, we argue that it is most appropriate to adopt an integrative approach, based primarily on operant conditioning, learning-theory, cognitive-behavioral, and social-learning explanations (Lee & Owen, 1986b). An emphasis on variables which can be defined explicitly and on the modification of these variables appears to offer the widest scope for the design and objective evaluation of behavior-change programs; thus, a primary basis in learning theory and its more recent derivations seems most appropriate (Martin & Dubbert, 1982a).

Because the prime concern in exercise promotion is behavior change, theories which emphasize behavioral stability or dispositional variables appear of limited utility. The application of theories which deal explicitly with change in behavior will be emphasized. These include operant-conditioning and mediational learning theories, cognitive-behavioral and self-management theories, social learning theory, and models which attempt to integrate such theories in order to account for stages, processes, and contexts of change.

OPERANT AND INSTRUMENTAL CONDITIONING THEORIES

Theoretical Considerations

The past two decades have seen the extension of operant conditioning techniques to a wider range of clinical and applied problems (cf. Wilson & Franks, 1982), and an increasing emphasis on the issues of transfer and maintenance of change. Reviews by Stokes and Baer (1977), Marholin, Siegel, and Phillips (1976), and Owen (1981) have suggested a range of maintenance techniques, including the sequential modification of behavior across situations, the introduction of the exerciser to naturally occurring positive contingencies in the maintaining environment, the training of more than one example of the desired behavior, the training of the behavior under variable conditions, the use of delayed and intermittent schedules of reinforcement, the matching of stimuli in the training and maintenance environments, the training of significant others to supply reinforcement in the maintenance environment, the use of verbal responses as mediators, and specific training in generalization skills. However, there has been only limited empirical research in this area, and the extent to which these techniques are effective is not yet well established.

Theories which emphasize mediational processes to explain the effects of different conditions and schedules of reinforcement also have relevance to the understanding of applied problems in behavior change. For example, Nation and Woods (1980) review literature indicating that partial or intermittent reinforcement produces resistance to extinction and pointed out the implications of this for the development of treatment strategies to enhance persistence. They drew on Amsel and Ward's (1965) general theory of persistence, which argues that training under conditions of intermittent reinforcement produces a resistance to response disruption by nonreinforcement, and thus that responses so developed will be relatively resistant to extinction. Their theoretical analysis emphasizes an affective process, frustration, as a prime mediating mechanism in the development of behavior maintenance. From this perspective they argue that behavior-change pro-

programs should use partial reinforcement during the response acquisition phase so that extinction following this phase is slowed and the individual has an opportunity to discover natural reinforcers for the new behavior.

Applications of Operant and Instrumental Conditioning Techniques

Techniques based on these approaches are most readily applicable in settings where the behavior-change agent can control many reinforcing contingencies, such as institutional settings. Such research highlights the role played by the manipulation of incentives to exercise, and some issues for their application in less controlled settings.

Allen and Iwata (1980), for example, used a group contingency procedure to institute regular exercising in 10 intellectually disabled adults. It was established that, when free to choose, the subjects spent more time playing games than they did performing a series of calisthenics exercises. Participation in games was made contingent upon the entire group completing all calisthenics exercises correctly, and this increased calisthenics participation. Libb and Clements (1969) used an individualized token procedure with elderly psychiatric patients, who rode a stationary exercise bicycle to earn tokens. The procedure was effective for three of the four individuals. Such studies suggest that the provision of incentives to exercise could increase exercising in less restricted settings. It may be noted that, in both studies, contingencies to increase the probability of a behavior occurring were manipulated, rather than modifying the activity itself to make it more intrinsically enjoyable, or attempting to alter the setting or the participants' attitudes, any of which may have enhanced maintenance.

Another situation in which it is possible to have considerable control over contingencies and incentives is high-level sports training, which takes place in a highly structured environment. Such an approach has been attempted by Allison and Ayllon (1980), who used operant techniques to increase performance of skills in football, gymnastics, or tennis. They were able to improve performance on the specified skills, but performance returned to or near baseline when contingencies were withdrawn. Rushall and Pettinger (1969) used a number of extrinsic reinforcers to increase distance swum in training by young competitive swimmers, and found that money and sweets were equally effective in increasing training distance, while contingent attention by the coach had a small negative effect. Donahue, Gillis, and King (1980) reviewed the use of operant techniques in sport and physical education, indicating that similar techniques have been used to modify coaches' behavior, athletes' self-regulatory activities, and athletes' skills. Practical guidelines have been provided for the application of such strategies with competitors (Rushall, 1979). In general, however, such studies have not explicitly programmed for maintenance of behavior change.

In all but the most restricted of settings, it is not possible to control completely the incentives to exercise. In natural settings, incentives may be manipulated to some extent, but other determinants of action such as attitudes, beliefs, and individual skill differences must be taken into account. Researchers working in less-controlled settings have in general included techniques derived from cognitive behavioral and social-learning approaches to alter exercise patterns, sometimes in combination with the use of social psychological frameworks to influence attitudes and knowledge.

COGNITIVE-BEHAVIORAL AND SOCIAL-LEARNING THEORIES

Cognitive Behavior Modification and Self-Management

Recent developments in cognitive behavior modification and behavioral self-control have been regarded widely as potentially useful in enhancing maintenance of behavior change (e.g., Karoly & Steffen, 1980; Wilson & Franks, 1982), though some authors (e.g., Ledwidge, 1978; Skinner, 1977) have argued against their adoption.

Both approaches have as a primary aim the alteration of the way people think about their actions and the skills they have for dealing with problems. It can be argued that cognitions may be less directly under external stimulus control than more overt behaviors (e.g., Bandura, 1969). Therefore, cognitive changes may generalize more readily to settings other than those in which they have been developed, and thus the probability of maintenance of change in the natural environment will be greater than if cognitions are not affected (e.g., Owen, 1981). A high degree of control over the environment and reinforcement contingencies is of less importance with cognitive than with operant approaches. Thus, it is in naturalistic settings that cognitive behavior modification and self-control techniques have most potential.

It is argued that a cognitive change is necessary for behavior changes to be maintained (e.g., Bandura, 1969), and this implies that cognitive behavior modification may be more useful than a strictly operant approach in the production of permanent changes in behavior.

There is evidence that cognitive methods of behavior change alone are less effective than the combination of cognitive and enactive methods (Kazdin, 1980), and such a combined approach is generally used in cognitive behavior change programs.

Paralleling the development of cognitive-behavior modification has been a growing interest in self-management. It is argued that, since these behavioral approaches are technology-based, a person should be able to apply them to him or herself (e.g., Stuart, 1977). Self-management may help to produce maintained change, as the problem of transfer to new environments is lessened (e.g., Richards & Perri, 1978).

There has been considerable debate concerning definitions of self-management and the mechanisms by which it operates (e.g., Mahoney, 1976; McReynolds, Green, & Fisher, 1983), but the use of self-management techniques is increasingly widespread. The basic self-management steps of problem identification, self-monitoring, selecting a goal, altering setting events, arranging reinforcement, and using cognitive control strategies have been described and applied to a number of self-change problems (e.g., Mahoney & Thoresen, 1974; Williams & Long, 1975).

Social Learning and Self-Efficacy Theories

These theories have been used as a framework for the development of lifestyle change programs (McAlister, Farquhar, Thoresen, & Maccoby, 1976; Wilson, 1980). Social learning theory rejects the idea of unidirectional determinism of behavior by events in the environment in favor of a strongly interactionist viewpoint. Three classes of phenomena—environmental events, cognitive and other personal events, and overt behaviors—are seen as existing within a dynamic equilibrium of multidirectional reciprocal determinism. Social learning theory places particular emphasis on learning through observation, arguing that it is the most common factor of learning in day-to-day life. A social learning theory approach is similar to cognitive behavior modification in the types of technique used, but differs in explanatory emphasis. While both approaches regard the modification of cognitions as essential to maintained behavior change, social learning theory gives more detailed and explicit emphasis to the active involvement of the individual in observing events, considering them in the light of knowledge, projecting possible outcomes of various courses of actions, and actively selecting a course of action or change of view on the basis of this process (Bandura, 1977a). This analysis makes clear that cognitive behavior modification has been an important conceptual link between the operant approach and social learning theory, and has allowed for integration of techniques at a theoretical level.

A potentially useful development from social learning theory has been the construction of self-efficacy theory (Bandura, 1977b). Bandura argues that people have efficacy expectations, or highly specific beliefs, about their ability to perform certain actions or groups of related actions, and that the strength of these efficacy expectations is a major proximal determinant of behavior. Efficacy expectations are seen as arising from information from a number of sources, including the individual's previous perceived successes and failures with the activity in question, the observation of others performing that activity, linguistic information, the cognitive interpretation of physiological arousal, and knowledge of the constraints of a particular situation. Information from all sources is weighted and combined to produce an overall efficacy expectation, which in turn determines the action taken. Efficacy expectations are readily modifiable by the input of new information, and are seen as acting within the context of reciprocal determinism. Self-efficacy theory has received widespread support since its original description, and relationships between self-efficacy and behavior have been demonstrated in a range of substantive areas (Bandura, 1982). While there are some contentious issues (e.g., Lee, 1983b) for this theory it appears to have potential in the understanding of maintenance. Recent work has highlighted the importance of explicit behavioral goals and of performance feedback in the development of accurate efficacy expectations (Bandura & Schunk, 1981).

Applications of Cognitive Behavioral and Social Learning Theories

These theories have generated a range of specific techniques which have been used in exercise programs. For example, Wysocki, Hall, Iwata, and Riordan (1979) used behavioral contracting with eight college students who wished to increase their physical fitness. Students agreed to set themselves weekly exercise goals and deposited valuables with the experimenters which would be returned contingent upon their reaching those goals. This approach, a mixture of cognitive (goal setting) and operant (external reinforcement) methods, increased exercising both during the program and during a follow-up period of one year. Spevak (1982) found that self-control strategies, together with fading, booster sessions, and other operant techniques, increased maintenance at a six-month follow-up assessment. Oldridge and Jones

(1983), Turner, Polly, and Sherman (1976), and Vance (1976) also used contracts and self-control to increase exercising. Epstein, Wing, Thompson, and Griffin (1980) used a multigroup design to show that the use of behavioral contracts and of lotteries contingent on exercising produced levels of exercise higher than in standard fitness classes. Keefe and Blumenthal (1980), with three subjects, combined a changing criterion and stimulus control with a program of self reinforcement to produce increases in physical activity which they found had persisted at a nine-month follow-up. Investigations with a group suffering chronic obstructive pulmonary disease (Kaplan, Atkins, & Reinsch, 1984) found a combination of cognitive and behavioral strategies to produce greater adherence than either set of strategies alone.

Combinations of external reinforcement and the use of cognitive behavioral techniques to increase commitment to exercising appear successful, but require a considerable level of expert intervention (e.g., Vance, 1976). Further, they seem most useful with individuals who are already highly motivated and prepared to place themselves under considerable external control (Turner, Polly, & Sherman, 1976). Such techniques alone are likely to be less effective in field studies with community fitness classes or exercise groups, or interventions to encourage the sedentary to adopt exercise. Field studies typically combine these techniques with others derived from social-learning and social psychological theories, and aim for relatively looser control over individuals' activity (e.g., Martin et al., 1984). Most, again, start with motivated individuals and do not address the issue of persuading people to begin exercising, only that of ensuring that they continue to do so.

Martin and his colleagues have recently begun experimenting systematically with a number of exercise class components which derive from cognitive behavioral and social-learning theories. Martin et al. (1984) compared the use of personalized feedback with that of standard feedback in a jogging class, and found the personalized feedback to increase attendance rates; they also compared distance goals with time goals, and found distance goals more effective. Both these differences held up when joggers were reassessed at a three-month follow-up. In a second study, they introduced an attendance lottery but found this to produce somewhat lower attendance; in this study, they also compared the use of flexible and of fixed goals and found flexible goals to be more effective in maintaining attendance. In a further investigation, Martin et al. (1984) examined the relative effectiveness of proximal and distal goal setting in a fitness class, but found, contrary to expectation and previous findings (e.g., Bandura & Schunk, 1981), that long-term goals resulted in better attendance than proximal goals. They suggested that the greater flexibility of distal goals made them more acceptable to joggers. It is probable that there is an ideal goal-setting interval which varies depending upon the activity and situation and which could be determined empirically.

Martin et al. (1984) found in a further study that class attendance and extra training were more frequent for joggers who had been taught realistic goal-setting and cognitive strategies to distract them from discomfort and deal with self-defeating thoughts than for a control group.

The combined findings of Martin and his colleagues suggested that a number of behavioral, cognitive-behavioral, and self-control techniques are useful in modifying exercise behaviors. Altering aspects of the setting and of the activity can make them more acceptable to individuals, and appropriate goals and feedback appear to provide information which helps the individual maintain a pattern of exercising.

Others have also found the use of such informational techniques to be more useful than cognitive-behavioral methods alone. For example, Goodrick (1979) used training in self-monitoring and stimulus control to increase adherence to independent exercising, but found them insufficient. Subjects appeared unwilling to use the techniques. Goodrick suggests that these strategies alone do not solve maintenance difficulties, and suggested that combining of cognitive and behavioral techniques with social support may add to their effectiveness.

Lee, Owen, and Innes (1981) conducted a set of trials of self-management techniques adapted for use in community exercise courses. Levels of maintenance following a self-management program tended to be higher than those following a standard exercise curriculum. However, these trials indicated that there could be major difficulties in convincing exercise class instructors of the value of self-management techniques and in training instructors to apply them. This problem was addressed through the development of instructor training protocols and a detailed behavioral curriculum manual (Owen, 1985; Sedgwick & Owen, 1982). It would seem that if behavioral self-management methods are to have a broad impact on exercise maintenance, they must be presented and packaged in a manner which is acceptable to, and readily applicable by, exercise instructors. Factors which influence instructor and trainee acceptance and use of behavioral self-management techniques will clearly be important in the development of such programmes, and require careful investigation.

An alternative approach might involve examining individual differences. Some people may fare better in some programs than in others. For example, a program package incorporating the matching of aspects of training settings to maintenance settings and the teaching of self-management skills was compared to a standard fitness course. Overall, the long-term effects were no better than for the standard fitness course, but there was an interaction effect, such that individuals exhibiting the Type A behavior pattern responded better to the "control" course, while those without this pattern showed greater maintenance with the treatment package (Lee, Owen, & Innes, 1981). This suggests that it may be possible to identify groups of people who will find particular approaches most useful, and tailor packages to suit these groups. Such an approach could use social-learning and social psychological approaches to identify or attempt to change relevant characteristics and behavior patterns, followed by the application of the behavioral techniques described earlier in a more discriminating fashion. This is not to suggest that only some individuals should be targeted for behavior change, but that a range of techniques be developed to deal with relevant individual differences. Choice of activity may be important in developing commitment, and there is some evidence (Thompson & Wankel, 1980) that a perception of choice in activities or an opportunity to reach a personal decision to exercise will enhance maintenance with that activity.

The social-learning theory emphasis on reciprocal interactions between situations, cognitions, and behavior is central to the approach maintenance developed by Marlatt and his associates (e.g., Marlatt, 1982; Marlatt & Gordon, 1980). They examined reported determinants of relapse following treatment for addictive behaviors and argued that a range of high-risk relapse situations could be identified, and that clients should be taught in advance how to deal with these situations if they arose. Teaching specific skills to cope with difficult situations was recommended, as well as teaching individuals to cope with a single relapse episode without returning immediately to pretreatment patterns of responding. They refer to the "abstinence violation effect," a phenomenon in which a single relapse episode is interpreted by the individual as inability to remain abstinent. This results in a dramatic lowering of self-efficacy, causing the individual to give up the newly learned abstinence behaviors and relapse into addiction. Marlatt suggested that a high level of self-efficacy is necessary to avoid such a self-defeating pattern of cognition.

Marlatt's model of relapse can readily be translated into a model of maintenance of behavior change. Individuals who are attempting to instate a new behavior should be instructed on how to cope with risky situations, and how to deal with occasional lapses without completely giving up the new behavior. This work on relapse prevention is related to Nation and Woods' (1980) proposals regarding intermittent reinforcement. Both attempt to prepare the individual to deal with specific events and settings which are likely to occur in the maintenance environment and which could increase the risk of recidivism.

It seems probable (e.g., Abrams et al., 1982) that a multiple approach using techniques derived from operant conditioning, cognitive behavior modification, behavioral self-control, and social-learning theory is likely to be superior to a singular approach. Because of the complexities of the individual's environment, both physical and social, and his or her work, family, and leisure commitments, no single approach is likely to provide comprehensive guidelines.

THE INTEGRATION OF BEHAVIORAL PERSPECTIVES ON EXERCISE PROMOTION

Given that the promotion of habits of regular, vigorous, physical activity on a community-wide basis requires a number of different levels of intervention (Abrams et al., 1982), it is unlikely that any one theoretical framework will itself provide a sufficient conceptual base for all aspects of intervention. Operant and instrumental conditioning theories will provide strong and useful guidelines for those conditions in which environmental cues and contingencies are highly salient and can be controlled. In circumstances where people are instructed, but take responsibility for arranging their exercise habits independently, cognitive-behavioral and social-learning theories also provide guidelines for mediated instructional formats, such as booklets, pamphlets, and kits. Social-psychological theories can also be used to guide the development of mass-media campaigns (Solomon, 1981). There are areas of overlap between these theories and areas of application. Frameworks which attempt to integrate theoretical points of view have been developed and applied. In particular, combinations of operant and cognitive behavioral approaches have been used, but more recently combinations have incorporated social-learning, social psychological, and other viewpoints as well.

A number of reviewers (e.g., Hanna & Owen, 1977; Karoly & Steffen, 1980; Marholin, Siegel, & Phillips, 1976; Owen, 1981) have listed techniques for enhancing the transfer and maintenance of newly learned behaviors to the natural environment. These approaches have combined operant techniques, cognitive behavioral methods, and self-management strategies. Generally, they use operant principles to support the argument that the training situation be made less discriminable from the maintenance environment. Suggested techniques include the training of family members in the contingent administration of reinforcement in the maintenance environment, by varying the conditions of training so that the trainee is less likely to discriminate between training and nontraining environments, the use of intermittent reinforcement and gradual fading of external reinforcers, and the provision of a wide range of credible models for the new behaviors. Reviewers recommend that these techniques be combined with cognitive and self-control methods. Specifically, they propose teaching clients goal-setting and planning strategies, skills in self-observation and self-recording, skills in identifying and altering cues in the environment, and the use of self-administered reinforcement on a predetermined schedule, as well as covert techniques such as self-talk (Meichenbaum, 1977).

A number of broader integrative approaches have been proposed. Dishman's (1982) review of exercise adherence research concluded that an integration of biological, psychological, sociodemographic, and environmental perspectives was most likely to result in generalizable findings. For example, although there is convincing evidence that exercise maintenance is strongly associated with convenience of exercise location and with family support (e.g., Andrew et al., 1981), it appears probable that other characteristics of the individual, the setting, and their interaction will be important.

Abrams et al. (1982) present an approach based on social-learning theory but integrated across levels of intervention. Abrams et al. argue that the principle of reciprocal causality between actions, cognitions, and the environment should be applied in understanding the workings of groups, of organizations, and of whole communities as well as the activities of individuals. Reciprocal action between individuals and larger groups, and between larger groups themselves, are the focus of this approach. They recommended that different strategies be applied at different levels of intervention: individual skills in problem solving and self-control; group processes of modeling and group support; organizational and community application of behavioral technologies. Such an approach is pluralistic, arguing that individuals and groups are influenced by activities at all levels, and that if changes are introduced simultaneously at several levels, the chances of general adoption are greatly increased.

A number of reviewers (e.g., Abrams et al., 1982; DiClemente & Prochaska, 1982; Dishman, 1982; Olson & Zanna, 1981) argue that techniques derived from different theoretical approaches will be maximally effective at different points in the change process. Educative and persuasive techniques designed to alter beliefs and attitudes, and derived from social psychological theories, might be most useful in developing awareness and motivation, while behavioral techniques may be more important in establishing and maintaining new behaviors.

Another, broader, approach integrates social-learning and economic theories in an attempt to influence community-wide patterns of behavior. Winkler and Winett (1982) pointed out that while specificity of target behaviors is important for interventions, any target behavior is part of a number of systems of behaviors and consequences, both at the individual level and in the interactions between the individual and society. Social-learning theory provides an account of the effect of cognitions and reinforcing contingencies on behavior, while the economic perspective accounts for the influence of changes in patterns of contingencies on social groups.

The processes of altering patterns of exercise for individuals and communities are complex, and encompass a number of stages of change and many interacting levels from the physiological and cognitive to the social and environmental (Sedgwick & Owen, 1981; Serfass & Gerberich, 1984). Within this complexity, however, it may be most effective to design a range of specific interventions aimed at particular changes in particular individuals and particular settings.

DIRECTIONS AND RESEARCH ISSUES

The development of effective applied programs from basic research requires a number of steps. In the development of exercise programs and strategies, these steps might be characterized as: basic theoretical research in laboratory situations; use of principles derived from laboratory work with structured and closely controlled exercise classes; the extension of this to exercise classes in community settings run by nonexperts; further extension to self-help and to minimal-intervention programs using print and broadcast media; coordination of media and face-to-face programs with environmental and social change to affect community-wide behavior patterns (see Lee & Owen, 1986b). A step beyond this, and one which is increasingly receiving attention, is the development of public policy which will influence health-related behaviors (Owen & Lee, 1984). Legislation has become a major tool for lifestyle change, and in recent years governments have begun to be more receptive to the recommendations of behavioral scientists (e.g., Olson & Zanna, 1981; Owen & Lee, 1984).

It is clear from this review that all of the links in the chain of development from theory to public policy have not yet received attention, and it has been suggested (e.g., Solomon, 1981) that there is a tendency within health promotion to move ahead to large-scale campaigns that lack a sufficient base of relevant research. This section examines some issues at each step of this chain of development, and suggests some topics for investigation.

Basic Theoretical Issues

Given that the promotion of regular vigorous activity is a large-scale social enterprise which can be dealt with from many perspectives, an approach involving aspects of learning theory, attribution theories, social-learning theory, and behavioral economics might be the most effective. Self-efficacy theory (Bandura, 1977b, 1982) and behavioral economics (Winkler, 1983) are relatively recent theoretical developments, and there is a need for continued research on some of the specific aspects of these theories. A detailed consideration of future developments at a theoretical level falls outside the scope of this review. However, it is clear that all subsequent steps depend heavily on the state of development of the theories on which they are based, and that there is a strong need for continuing development of theories of behavior change and maintenance.

Basic Behavioral Research on Exercise

Applications of theory need to be tested first in well-controlled situations which allow causal inferences to be made. A number of lines of research appear worth developing. For example, the relationship between perceived choice and persistence (e.g., Thompson & Wankel, 1980) is potentially useful in the exercise field. Evidence that internal attributions of success relate to high levels of motivation and enjoyment (e.g., Spink & Roberts, 1980) suggests that efforts to increase internal attributions for physical activity could enhance maintenance.

The work of Martin et al. (1984), which applies behavioral and cognitive self-management procedures in experimental exercise classes, is another promising recent development. Further investigations of the effects of goal setting and modeling may be useful in developing techniques for promoting maintenance.

Applications of other social-learning approaches in exercise settings could also be investigated. The enhancement of self-efficacy (e.g., Bandura, 1982) could be a powerful strategy for improving maintenance.

Strategies derived from Marlatt's (1982) relapse-prevention approach are also potentially useful. Both approaches need careful experimentation in controlled exercise-class settings in order to determine appropriate strategies for their application in community settings.

Community-Based Exercise Programs

Possibly the most important issue in the transfer of techniques from experimental classes to community-based programs is the training of instructors. Programs to train instructors in behavioral techniques and principles need development and validation (Oldridge, 1977) and there is a need for the provision of incentives for instructors to follow them.

The standard exercise class, involving a brief period of stretching, aerobic running or possibly games, and another brief warming-down period (Stoedefalke, 1974) may not provide sufficient interest or incentive to produce long-term adherence (cf. Fitness Ontario, 1981). Many fitness instructors appear to consider complex theoretical notions irrelevant. However, there have been developed a number of variations and addenda to standard programs which are theoretically based. These (e.g., Franklin, 1978; Oldridge, 1977) have been presented in a common-sense framework which appears more acceptable to trainers without a psychological background. These recommendations include: avoidance of heavy loads; emphasis on group games and noncompetitive activities rather than regimented calisthenics and running; involvement of family members and development of opportunities for socializing to enhance mutual support; the provision of regular feedback on improvement; the use of music and variety to increase enjoyment; and the encouragement of group cohesiveness through social events or clothing designed specifically for the exercise class group. It appears that the development of methods to encourage fitness instructors to use such techniques consistently might be a useful development in research and program development.

Self-Instructional and Minimal-Intervention Programs

Research in the smoking-cessation area, albeit almost 20 years old, suggests that most smokers prefer assistance which does not involve joining groups or having other face-to-face contact (Schwartz & Dubitzky, 1967). Similarly, it might be that many individuals would prefer to take up exercise on their own rather than join a class. Information on how to do so effectively and safely can be distributed in a number of forms, including self-help books (e.g., Cooper, 1970), kits, records and cassette tapes, and videotapes. With these methods there are general problems with the provision of accurate, up-to-date, information and techniques, and the validation of effectiveness under the conditions in which people will use them (Glasgow & Rosen, 1978, 1979; Owen, 1989).

However, there exists considerable potential for the use of self-instructional materials in closely supervised, sequential programs such as correspondence courses (e.g., Jeffrey, Danaher, Killen, Kinnear, & Farquhar, 1982). There is potential for the recruitment of large numbers of people to behavior change programmes which can be administered using modern information-management methods. Such programs also require careful development and assessment (Owen & Lee, 1986). The combination of self-instructional materials with face-to-face contact has also been investigated (Glasgow, Schafer, & O'Neill, 1981), and could result in guidelines for the development of effective self-instructional exercise programs.

A different minimal-intervention approach has been proposed by Brownell, Stunkard, and Albaum (1980). They argue that it was usually unrealistic and ineffective to attempt to add special programmed exercise to an otherwise sedentary lifestyle and expect it to be adopted without problems. A more effective approach, they suggested, would be to alter the environment so that the amount of incidental exercise required to carry out normal activities was increased. They have shown that displaying signs encouraging the use of stairs rather than escalators has been effective in public places (Brownell, Stunkard, & Albaum, 1980). Similarly, Epstein, Wing, Koeske, Ossip, and Beck (1982) have shown improved adherence to an exercise program for obese children when it was integrated into their daily routine as active play, rather than programmed as a separate exercise session.

Ways to increase incidental exercise through environmental manipulation require further research. By making the exercise instrumental in performing other activities, or by integrating it into existing leisure time, it could be possible to make use of naturally occurring reinforcers.

Exercise in Specific Environments

A potentially powerful technique for enhancing rates of exercise is the provision of opportunities and incentives to exercise in work or school environment.

Exercise promotion in the workplace has been proposed as an effective method of improving the health and productivity of workers (Corroll, 1980). While it has been stated by some (e.g., Everitt, 1979) that the costs of such endeavors will vastly outweigh the possible benefits, others (e.g., Shephard, 1983) have suggested that considerable financial benefit could accrue to companies promoting exercise. Employee fitness programs have been described in recent years (e.g., Wilbur, 1983), and the issues involved in the setting up of such programs and involvement of workers are beginning to be considered (Fitness Ontario, 1980; Pate & Blair, 1983). It is clear, however, that these are relatively early developments and that considerable work is necessary in order to assess the potential for health and financial benefits.

Social Marketing of Exercise

The development of sound principles for promoting exercise, and the application of these in a range of settings, has the potential to increase levels of exercise substantially; broader social and environmental interventions may be necessary to produce changes in social norms and expectancies regarding regular exercise. It has been pointed out that adding regular exercise to existing patterns of behavior can require major realignment of other activities (e.g., Briggs & Nettleton, 1979) and that such a realignment may require changes in social norms and in opportunities.

A method much favored for social intervention is the mass media campaign (e.g., Rice & Paisley, 1981). Campaigns using broadcast and print media have been favored because they make use of existing information networks, they have the potential to reach large numbers of people, and thus they do not require the development or implementation of additional delivery systems and organizational structures. However, mass-media behavior change programs are not always effective (Solomon, 1981). Some investigators have rejected the mass media as inappropriate channels for information, or have seen them as useful only in reinforcing change which has already occurred (Ben-Sira, 1982). However, Solomon (1981) argues that poor research and planning, low budgets, and lack of continuity in media campaigns have meant that such projects have not reached the potential for change of which they are capable. The Stanford Heart Disease Prevention Program (e.g., Maccoby & Alexander, 1980; McAlister, Farquhar, Thoresen, & Maccoby, 1976) has concentrated on social marketing, based on approaches derived from psychological theory, to develop a highly effective media campaign. The Stanford campaign preparation included physiological testing as well as self-reports concerning awareness, knowledge, motivation, presence of required skills, and the use of maintenance and self-management techniques that were specifically linked to particular behaviors. Through these preparation strategies, this media campaign was able to provide the most appropriate information for the population for which it was designed. Solomon (1981) stressed the need for highly specific information giving clear behavioral guidelines so that it is easy for people to act on messages. Olson and Zanna (1981) also recommended such a specific approach. They also proposed that campaigns should present a diversity of messages, some aimed to increase knowledge and motivation, some to teach skills required in making a behavioral change, and some to enhance maintenance. All three types of message, they argued, should have a variety of individual, specific, exemplars, so that the probability that at least one message will be appropriate to any one person is increased.

The effectiveness of media campaigns and comparisons with face-to-face, small-group programs requires careful examination (McAlister, Farquhar, Thoresen, & Maccoby, 1976). Examination of the relative or combined effectiveness of television, print, interactive, and face-to-face change programs in health areas seems an important direction for research. Such strategies applied to the promotion of physical activity require careful evaluation.

An alternative approach to large-scale changes in attitudes and behavior is a focus on environmental change, rather than on individual change. The economic benefits and costs of any action are relevant in individual choices to change behavior (Winkler, 1983), and changes in economic and social incentives may increase the extent to which they reinforce desirable behavior. However, work in the domain of social engineering must be tempered by an appreciation of the multiple constraints on individual choice, so that the victims of inequitable social arrangements are not blamed or unjustly penalized (Brown & Margo, 1978; Crawford, 1977). The ethical and social concerns raised by the emphasis on social engineering to promote health, and on individual responsibility, have been considered in detail by Winkler (in press). However, opportunities for behavioral scientists to be active in developing government policy on health issues are increasing (cf. Owen & Lee, 1984) and it is important that we are able to provide theoretically valid information in a form which is acceptable to politicians and decision makers.

CONCLUSION

Behavioral research on exercise promotion is a relatively new field, which shows considerable promise. Theory and experimental research are beginning to increase the scientific understanding of exercise as a behavior. However, exercise as a social innovation and as a vehicle for health promotion has such a widespread popularity that applications are moving far beyond the relatively limited psychological knowledge base so far developed. It is therefore crucial that good quality research, theoretically informed program development, and sound program evaluation methods be developed. This must happen at all levels of application, from public policy and mass media promotions, through print and audiovisual instructional formats, to face-to-face exercise counseling. Theories of, and methods for achieving, behavior change have been developed and applied to behavior disorders, and more recently to health-related behaviors such as cigarette smoking and overeating. The challenge is to continue to apply this knowledge in a rigorous and creative fashion to the adoption and maintenance of exercise habits.

REFERENCES

Abrams, D. B., Elder, J. P., Lasater, T. M., & Carleton, R. A. (1982, November). *Social learning theory principles for community health promotion: An integration across levels of intervention.* Paper presented at the 16th Annual Convention of the Association for Advancement of Behavior Therapy, Los Angeles.

Allen, D. W., & Quigley, B. M. (1977). The role of physical activity in the control of obesity. *Medical Journal of Australia, 2,* 434–438.

Allen, L. D., & Iwata, B. A. (1980). Reinforcing exercise maintenance using existing high-rate activities. *Behavior Modification, 4,* 337–354.

Allison, M. G., & Ayllon, T. (1980). Behavioral coaching in the development of skills in football, gymnastics and tennis. *Journal of Applied Behavior Analysis, 13,* 297–314.

Allison, K., & Coburn, D. (1981). *Blue collar workers and physical activity.* Ontario, Canada: Ministry of Culture and Recreation, Sports and Fitness Branch.

American College of Sports Medicine. (1978). The recommended quantity and quality of exercise for developing and maintaining fitness in healthy adults. *Medicine and Science in Sports, 10,* vii–viii.

Amsel, A., & Ward, J. S. (1965). Frustration and persistence: Resistance to discrimination following prior experience with the discriminanda. *Psychological Monographs,* Whole no. 597.

Andrew, G. M., Oldridge, N. B., Parker, J. O., Cunningham, D. A., Rechnitzer, P. A., Jones, N. L., Buck, C., Kavanaugh, T., Shephard, R. J., & Sutton, J. R. (1981). Reasons for drop-out from exercise programs in post-coronary patients. *Medicine and Science in Sports and Exercise, 13,* 164–168.

Australian Labor Party. (1982). *The ALP Sports and Recreation Policy.* Canberra, Australia: Author.

Baer, D. M., Wolf, M. M., & Risley, T. R. (1968). Some current dimensions of applied behavior analysis. *Journal of Applied Behavior Analysis, 1,* 91–97.

Bandura, A. (1969). *Principles of behavior modification.* New York: Holt Rinehart & Winston.

Bandura, A. (1977a). *Social learning theory.* Englewood Cliffs, NJ: Prentice-Hall.

Bandura, A. (1977b). Self-efficacy: Toward a unifying theory of behavioral change. *Psychological Review, 84,* 191–215.

Bandura, A. (1982). Self-efficacy mechanism in human agency. *American Psychologist, 37,* 122–147.

Bandura, A., & Schunk, D. H. (1981). Cultivating competence, self-efficacy, and intrinsic interest through proximal self-motivation. *Journal of Personality and Social Psychology, 41,* 586–598.

Ben-Sira, Z. (1982). The health promoting function of mass media and reference groups: Motivating or reinforcing of behavior change. *Social Science in Medicine, 16,* 825–834.

Blair, S. N. (1982). Exercise and coronary heart disease. *Behavioral Medicine Update, 4,* 13–16.

Blair, S. N., Cooper, K. H., Gibbons, L. W., Gettman, L. R., Lewis, S., & Goodyear, N. (1983). Changes in coronary heart disease risk factors associated with increased treadmill time in 753 men. *American Journal of Epidemiology, 118,* 352–359.

Briggs, C. A., & Nettleton, B. (1979). Lifestyle and activity patterns. *Australian Sports Medicine, 11,* 71–73.

Brown, E. R., & Margo, G. E. (1978). Health education: Can the reformers be reformed? *International Journal of Health Services, 8,* 3–126.

Brownell, K. D. (1982a). Exercise and obesity. *Behavioral Medicine Update, 4,* 7–12.

Brownell, K. D. (1982b). Obesity: Understanding and treating a serious, prevalent and refractory disorder. *Journal of Consulting and Clinical Psychology, 50,* 820–840.

Brownell, K. D., Stunkard, A. J., & Albaum, J. M. (1980). Evaluation and modification of exercise patterns in the natural environment. *American Journal of Psychiatry, 37,* 1540–1545.

Carleton, R. A., & Lasater, T. M. (1983). Coronary heart disease and human behavior. *Preventive Medicine, 12,* 610–618.

Carmody, T. P., Senner, J. W., Manilow, M. R., & Matarazzo, J. D. (1980). Physical exercise rehabilitation: Long-term dropout rate in cardiac patients. *Journal of Behavioral Medicine, 3,* 163–168.

Cooper, K. H. (1970). *The new aerobics.* New York: Bantam.

Corroll, V. J. (1980). Employee fitness programmes: An expanding concept. *International Journal of Public Health, 23,* 35–41.

Crawford, R. (1977). You are dangerous to your health: The ideology and politics of victim blaming. *International Journal of Health Services, 7,* 663–680.

DiClemente, C. C., & Prochaska, J. O. (1982). Self-change and therapy change of smoking behavior: A comparison of processes of change in cessation and maintenance. *Addictive Behaviors, 7,* 133–142.

Dishman, R. K., (1982). Compliance/adherence in health-related exercise. *Health Psychology, 1,* 237–267.

Donahue, J. A., Gillis, J. H., & King, K. (1980). Behavior modification in sport and physical education: A review. *Journal of Sport Psychology, 2,* 311–328.

Egger, G. (1979). *Running high: The inner spaces of jogging and how to get there.* Melbourne: Sun Books.

Epstein, L. H., & Wing, R. R. (1980). Aerobic exercise and weight. *Addictive Behaviors, 5,* 371–388.

Epstein, L. H., Wing, R. R., Koeske, R., Ossip, D., & Beck, S. (1982). A comparison of lifestyle change and programmed aerobic exercise on weight and fitness changes in obese children. *Behavior Therapy, 13,* 651–665.

Epstein, L. H., Wing, R. R., Thompson, J. K., & Griffin, W. (1980). Attendance and fitness in aerobics exercise: The effects of contracts and lottery procedures. *Behavior Modification, 4,* 465–479.

Everitt, M. D. (1979). Strategies for increasing employees' level of exercise and physical fitness. *Journal of Occupational Medicine, 21,* 463–467.

Fitness Ontario (1980). Employee fitness: "The how to . . ." *Proceedings of the Ontario Employee Fitness Workshop, March 1979,* Toronto, Ontario: Ministry of Culture and Recreation; Sports and Fitness Branch.

Fitness Ontario. (1981). *Low active adults: Who they are, how to reach them.* Toronto, Ontario: Ministry of Culture and Recreation.

Fitness Ontario. (1984). *Physical activity patterns in Ontario-IIa.* Ontario, Canada: Ministry of Tourism and Recreation.

Folkins, C. H., & Sime, W. E. (1981). Physical fitness training and mental health. *American Psychologist, 36,* 373–389.

Franklin, B. A. (1978). Motivating and educating adults to exercise. *Journal of Physical Education and Recreation, 49,* 13–17.

Glasgow, R. E., & Rosen, G. M. (1978). Behavioral bibliotherapy: A review of self-help behavior therapy manuals. *Psychological Bulletin, 85,* 1–23.

Glasgow, R. E., & Rosen, G. M. (1979). Self-help behavior therapy manuals: Recent developments and clinical usage. *Clinical Behavior Therapy Review, 1,* 1–20.

Glasgow, R. E., Schafer, L., & O'Neill, H. K. (1981). Self-help books and amount of therapist contact in smoking cessation programs. *Journal of Consulting and Clinical Psychology, 49,* 659–667.

Goodrick, G. K. (1979, December). *Maintenance of aerobic exercise behavior: A pilot study.* Paper presented to the Society for Behavioral Medicine, San Francisco.

Griest, J. H., Klein, M. H., Eischens, R. R., Faris, J., Gurman, A. S., & Morgan, W. S. (1978). Running through your mind. *Journal of Psychosomatic Research, 22,* 259–294.

Hanna, R. C., & Owen, N. (1977). Facilitating transfer and maintenance of fluency in stuttering therapy. *Journal of Speech and Hearing Disorders, 42,* 65–76.

Heinzelman, F., & Bagley, R. W. (1970). Response to physical activity programs and their effects on health behavior. *Public Health Reports, 85,* 905–911.

Hunt, W. A., Barnett, L. W., & Branch, L. A. (1971). Relapse rates in addiction programs. *Journal of Clinical Psychology, 27,* 455–456.

Iverson, D. C., Fielding, J. E., Crow, R. S., & Christenson, G. M. (1985). The promotion of physical activity—the United States population: The status of programs in medical, worksite, school and community settings. *Public Health Reports, 100,* 212–224.

Jasnoski, M. L., Holmes, D. S., Solomon, S., & Aguiar, C. (1981). Exercise, changes in aerobic capacity, and changes in self-perceptions: An experimental investigation. *Journal of Research in Personality, 15,* 460–466.

Jeffery, R. W., Danaher, B. G., Killen, J., Kinnier, R., & Farquhar, J (1982). Self-administered programs for health behavior change: Smoking cessation and weight reduction by mail. *Addictive Behaviors, 7,* 57–63.

Kaplan, R. M., Atkins, C. J., & Reinsch. (1984). Specific efficiency expectations mediate exercise compliance in patients with COPD. *Health Psychology, 3,* 223–242.

Karoly, P., & Steffen, J. (1980). *Improving the long-term effects of psychotherapy.* New York: Gardner Press.

Kazdin, A. E. (1979). Editorial: The scope of *Behavior Therapy. Behavior Therapy, 10,* 1–7.

Kazdin, A. E. (1980). Covert and overt rehearsal and elaboration during treatment in the development of assertive behavior. *Behaviour Research and Therapy, 18,* 191–201.

Keefe, F. J., & Blumenthal, J. A. (1980). The life fitness program: a behavioral approach to making exercise a habit. *Journal of Behaviour Therapy and Experimental Psychiatry, 11,* 31–34.

Ledwidge, B. (1978). Cognitive behavior modification: A step in the wrong direction? *Psychological Bulletin, 85,* 353–375.

Ledwidge, B. (1980). Run for your mind: Aerobic exercise as a means of alleviating anxiety and depression. *Canadian Journal of Behavioral Science, 12,* 126–140.

Lee, C., & Owen, N. (1986a). Community exercise programs: Follow-up difficulty and outcome. *Journal of Behavioral Medicine, 9,* 111–117.

Lee, C., & Owen, N. (1986b). Exercise persistence: Contributions of psychological theory to the promotion of regular physical activity. *Australian Psychologist, 21,* 427–466.

Lee, C., Owen, N., & Innes, J. M. (1981) Durability of risk factor change: Evidence, models and methods. In J. W. G. Tiller & P. Martin (Eds.), *Behavioral medicine* (pp. 221–230). Sydney, Australia: Ciba-Geigy.

Libb, J. W., & Clements, C. B. (1969). Token reinforcement in an exercise program for hospitalized geriatric patients. *Perceptual and Motor Skills, 28,* 957–958.

Luria, M. H., & Koepke, K. R. (1975). The physical conditioning effects of walking. *Journal of Sports Medicine and Physical Fitness, 15,* 272–274.

Maccoby, N., & Alexander, J. (1980). Use of media in lifestyle programs. In P. O. Davidson & S. M. Davidson (Eds.), *Behavioral medicine: Changing health lifestyles* (pp. 351–370). New York: Brunner/Mazel.

Mahoney, M. J. (1976). Terminal terminology: A self-regulated reply to Goldiamond. *Journal of Applied Behavior Analysis, 9,* 515–517.

Mahoney, M. J., & Thoresen, C. E. (1974). *Self-control: Power to the person.* Monterey, CA: Brooks/Cole.

Manuso, J. S. J. (1983). The equitable life assurance society program. *Preventive Medicine, 12,* 658–662.

Marholin, D., Siegel, L. J., & Phillips, D. (1976). Treatment and transfer: A search for empirical procedures. In M. Hersen, R. N. Eisler, & P. M. Miller (Eds.), *Progress in behavior modification* (pp. 293–342). New York: Academic Press.

Marlatt, G. A. (1982). Relapse prevention: A self-control program for the treatment of addictive behaviors. In R. B. Stuart (Ed.), *Adherence, compliance and generalization in behavioral medicine.* (pp. 329–378). New York: Brunner/Mazel.

Marlatt, G. A., & Gordon, J. R. (1980). Determinants of relapse: Implications for the maintenance of behavior change. In P. O. Davidson & S. M. Davidson (Eds.), *Behavioral medicine: Changing health lifestyles* (pp. 410–452). New York: Brunner/Mazel.

Martin, J. E., & Dubbert, P. M. (1982a). Exercise applications and promotion in behavioral medicine: Current status and future directions. *Journal of Consulting and Clinical Psychology, 50,* 1004–1017.

Martin, J. E., & Dubbert, P. M. (1982b). Exercise and health: The adherence problem. *Behavioral Medicine Update, 4,* 17–24.

Martin, J. E., Dubbert, P. M., Thompson, J. K., Raczynski, J. R., Lake, M., Smith, P. O., Webster, J. S., Sikora, T., & Cohen, R. E. (1984). The behavioral control of exercise in sedentary adults: Studies 1 through 6. *Journal of Consulting and Clinical Psychology, 52,* 795–811.

McAlister, A., Farquhar, J., Thoresen, C., & Maccoby, N. (1976). Applying behavioral sciences to cardiovascular health. *Health Education Monographs, 4,* 45–74.

McReynolds, W. T., Green, L., & Fisher, E. B. (1983). Self-control as choice management with reference to the behavioral treatment of obesity. *Health Psychology, 2,* 261–276.

Meichenbaum, D. (1977). *Cognitive behavior modification.* New York: Plenum Press.

Ministry of Tourism & Recreation, Ontario. (1983) *Physical activity patterns in Ontario II.* Toronto, Ontario: Author.

Morgan, W. P. (1982). Psychological effects of exercise. *Behavioral Medicine Update, 4,* 25–30.

Nation, J. R., & Woods, D. J. (1980). Persistence. The role of partial reinforcement in psychotherapy. *Journal of Experimental Psychology: General, 109,* 175–207.

National Heart Foundation of Australia. (1983). *Risk factor prevalence study.* Canberra, Australia: Author.

Oldridge, N. B. (1977). What to look for in an exercise class leader. *Physician and Sports Medicine, 5,* 85–88.

Oldridge, N. B. (1982). Compliance and exercise in primary and secondary prevention of coronary heart disease: A review. *Preventive Medicine, 11,* 56–70.

Oldridge, N. B., & Jones, N. L. (1983). Improving patient compliance in cardiac exercise rehabilitation: Effects of written agreement and self-monitoring. *Journal of Cardiac Rehabilitation, 3,* 257–262.

Olson, J. M., & Zanna, M. P. (1981). *Promoting physical activity: a social psychological perspective.* Toronto, Ontario: Ministry of Culture and Recreation.

Owen, N. (1981). Facilitating maintenance of behavior change. In E. Boberg (Ed.), *Maintenance of fluency* (pp. 31–70). New York: Elsevier.

Owen, N. (1985). Advising patients to stop smoking. *Medical Journal of Australia, 142,* 176–378.

Owen, N. (1989). Behavioural medicine: prospects and limits. In J. L. Sheppard (Ed.), *Advances in behavioural medicine, Volume 3.* Sydney, Australia: Cumberland College of Health Sciences.

Owen, N., & Lee, C. (1984). *Why people do and do not exercise.* Adelaide, Australia: Department of Recreation and Sport.

Owen, N., & Lee, C. (1986). Towards more rigorous evaluation of health promotion programmes. *Australian Psychologist, 21,* 79–91.

Pate, R. R., & Blair, S. N. (1983). Physical fitness programming health promotion at the worksite. *Preventive Medicine, 12,* 632–643.

Pollock, M. L., Gettman, L. W., Milesis, C. A., Bah, M. D., Durstine, L., & Johnson, R. B. (1977). Effects of frequency and duration of training on attrition and incidence of injury. *Medicine and Science in Sports, 9,* 31–36.

Rice, R. E., & Paisley, W. (Eds.). (1981). *Public communication campaigns.* Beverly Hills: Sage.

Richards, S. C., & Perri, M. G. (1978). Do self-control treatments last? An evaluation of behavioral problem solving and faded counselor contact as treatment maintenance strategies. *Journal of Counseling Psychology, 25,* 376–383.

Rushall, B. S. (1979). *Psyching in sport.* London: Pelham Books.

Rushall, B. S., & Pettinger, J. (1969). An evaluation of the effect of various reinforcers used as motivators in swimming. *Research Quarterly, 40,* 540–545.

Ryan, A. J. (1978). Don't overdo it. *Physician and Sports Medicine, 6,* 3.

Sacks, M. H., & Sachs, M. L. (1981). *Psychology of running.* Champaign, IL: Human Kinetics.

Schachter, S. (1982). Recidivism and self-cure of smoking and obesity. *American Psychologist, 37,* 436–444.

Schwartz, J. L., & Dubitzky, M. (1967). Expressed willingness of smokers to try ten smoking withdrawal methods. *Public Health Reports, 82,* 855–861.

Sedgwick, A. W., Brotherhood, J. R., Harris-Davidson, A., Taplin, R., & Thomas, O. W. (1980, July 5). Long-term effects of physical training program on risk factors for coronary heart disease in otherwise sedentary men. *British Medical Journal,* 7–10.

Sedgwick, A. W., & Owen, N. (1981). Integrating environmental, behavioural and organismic aspects of health promotion. In J. L. Sheppard (Ed.), *Advances in behavioural medicine, Volume 1* (pp. 143–158). Sydney, Australia: Cumberland College of Health Science.

Sedgwick, A. W., & Owen, N. (1982). *Lifelong fitness: Instructors' Manual.* Adelaide, Australia: Institute for Fitness Research and Training.

Serfass, R. C., & Gerberich, S. G. (1984). Exercise for optimal health: Strategies and motivational considerations. *Preventive Medicine, 13,* 79–99.

Shephard, R. J. (1979). Exercise prescription—North American experience. *British Journal of Sports Medicine, 12,* 227–234.

Shephard, R. J. (1983). Employee health and fitness: The state of the art. *Preventive Medicine, 12,* 644–653.

Shephard, R. J., & Cox, M. (1980). Some characteristics of participants in an industrial fitness program. *Canadian Journal of Applied Sport Science, 5,* 69–76.

Siscovick, D. S., LaPoste, R. E., & Newman, J. M. (1985). The disease-specific benefits and risks of physical activity and exercise. *Public Health Reports, 100,* 180–188.

Skinner, B. F. (1977). Why I am not a cognitive psychologist. *Behaviorism, 5,* 1–10.

Solomon, D. S. (1981). A social marketing perspective on campaigns. In R. E. Rice & W. J. Paisley (Eds.), *Public communication campaigns* (pp. 281–291). Beverly Hills: Sage.

Spevak, P. A. (1982). A multi-strategy approach to the maintenance of personal fitness programs. *Dissertation Abstracts International, 42,* 3445B. (University Microfilms No. 82 02668).

Spink, K. S., & Roberts, G. C. (1980). Ambiguity of outcome and causal attributions. *Journal of Sport Psychology, 2,* 237–244.

Stamler, J. (1981). Primary prevention of coronary heart disease: The last 20 years. *American Journal of Cardiology, 47,* 722–735.

Stephens, T., Jacobs, D. R., Jr., & White, C. C. (1985). A descriptive epidemology of leisure-time physical activity. *Public Health Reports, 100,* 147–157.

Stoedefalke, K. G. (1974). Physical fitness programs for adults. *American Journal of Cardiology, 33,* 787–790.

Stokes, T. F., & Baer, D. M. (1977). An implicit technology of generalization. *Journal of Applied Behavior Analysis, 10,* 349–367.

Stuart, R. B. (Ed.). (1977). *Behavioral self-management.* New York: Brunner/Mazel.

Stuart, R. B. (Ed.). (1982). *Adherence, compliance and generalization in behavioral medicine.* New York: Brunner/Mazel.

Taylor, C. B., Sallis, J. F., & Needle, R. (1985). The relation of physical activity and exercise to mental health. *Public Health Report, 100,* 195–201.

Thompson, C. E., & Wankel, L. M. (1980). The effects of perceived activity choice upon frequency of exercise behavior. *Journal of Applied Social Psychology, 10,* 436–443.

Thompson, J. K., Jarvie, G. J., Lahey, B., & Cureton, K. (1982). Exercise and obesity: Etiology, physiology and intervention. *Psychological Bulletin, 91,* 55–79.

Turner, R. D., Polly, S., & Sherman, A. R. (1976). A behavioral approach to individualized exercise programming. In J. D. Krumboltz & C. E. Thoresen (Eds.), *Counseling methods* (pp. 349–359). New York: Holt, Rinehart & Winston.

Vance, B. (1976). Using contracts to control weight and to improve cardiovascular fitness. In J. D. Krumboltz & C. C. Thoresen (Eds.), *Counseling methods* (pp. 527–540). New York: Holt, Rinehart & Winston.

Walker, W. J. (1983). Editorial—changing U.S. lifestyle and declining vascular mortality—a retrospective. *New England Journal of Medicine, 308,* 649–651.

Wilbur, C. S. (1983). The Johnson and Johnson program. *Preventive Medicine, 12,* 672–681.

Williams, R. L., & Long, J. D. (1975). *Towards a self-managed life style.* Boston: Houghton-Mifflin.

Wilson, G. T. (1980). Cognitive factors in life-style changes: A social learning perspective. In P. O. Davidson & S. M. Davidson (Eds.), *Behavioral medicine: Changing health lifestyles* (pp. 453–471). New York: Brunner/Mazel.

Wilson, G. T., & Franks, C. M. (Eds.). (1982). *Contemporary behavior therapy: Conceptual and empirical foundations.* New York: Guildford Press.

Winkler, R. C. (1983). *Rights versus duties in behavioral health care.* Unpublished manuscript, University of Western Australia.

Winkler, R. C. (in press). The contribution of behavioural economics to behaviour modification. In M. Rosenbaum, C. M. Franks, & T. Jaffe (Eds.), *Perspectives on behavior therapy in the eighties.* New York: Springer.

Winkler, R. C., & Winett, R. A. (1982). Behavioral interventions in resource conservation: A systems approach based on behavioral economics. *American Psychologist, 37,* 421–436.

Wysocki, T., Hall, G., Iwata, B., & Riordan, M. (1979). Behavioral management of exercise: contracting for aerobic points. *Journal of Applied Behavior Analysis, 12,* 55–64.

Author Index

A

Abel, G.G., 309, *325*
Abell, T., 301, *324*
Abramowitz, S., 242, *250*
Abrams, D.B., 47, 50, *55*, *60*, 404, 413, 414, *421*
Ackerman, S.H., 135, *148*
Adams, A., 244, *244*
Adams, D., 74 *85*
Adams, D., *85*
Adams, H.E., 200, *209*, 305, 306, 312, 315, *326*, *329*
Adams, R.O., 9, *28*
Adamson, J.D., 138, *145*
Addison, R.G., 360, *387*
Ader, R., 136, *143*
Addario, D.A., 151, *171*
Adler, C.S., 150, 156, *166*, 188, 189, *202*, 309, *325*
Adler, R., *207*
Agras, S., 161, *165*
Agudelo, C., 215, *248*
Aguiar, C., 401, *424*
Ahern, D.K., 199, *204*, 232, 244, *244*, 246, 261, *291*
Ahern, G.L., 316, *328*
Ahlborg, B., 300, *325*
Ahles, T., 227, *244*
Ahmed, S., 215, *251*
Akeson, W.H., 195, *208*, 216, 223, 227, *251*
Albaum, J.M., 418, *422*
Alexander, J., 404, 419, *425*
Alexander, P.T., 163, *165*
Alexison, N.G., 22, *24*
Allan, J.H., 278, *290*
Allen, D.W., 400, *421*
Allen, L.D., 406, *421*
Allison, K., 402, 406, *421*
Allison, M.G., *421*
Almes, M.J., 38, *63*
Almquist, M., 348, 349, 371, *390*
Alperson, B.L., 276, *291*
Amsel, A., 405, *421*
Anch, M., 351, 364, *391*
Ancoli-Isreal, S., 357, 362, 366, 367, 368, 369, 373, *387*, *390*, *391*, *392*
Anderson, C.D., 312, *323*
Anderson, G.D., 9, *24*, 109, *125*
Anderson, J.A., 189, *203*
Anderson, K.O., 133, 136, 139, *143*, *144*, 215, *248*
Anderson, J.A.D., 254, 279, *289*
Anderson, N.B., 307, *323*
Andersson, G.B.J., 254, 277, 278, 279, *289*, *290*
Andrasik, F., 38, *59*, 164, *168*, 299, 301, 302, 305, 307, 309, 312, 313, 314, 315, *323*, *324*, *326*, 329
Andreoli, K., 21, 22, *24*
Andrew, G.M., 414, *421*
Andrews, G., 214, *244*
Angelopoulos, N. 351, *389*
Apley, J., 179, *201*
Appelbaum, K.A., 313, *324*
Appenzeller, O., 156, *165*
Arand, D., 370, *388*
Arbetarskyddsfonden, 254, *289*
Arena, J.G., 299, 302, 305, 307, 313, 314, 315, *323*, *324*, *329*

Armentrout, D., 196, *201*, 221, 242, *244*
Armor, D.J., 15, *24*
Arnold, C.B., 21, *29*
Arnold, G.E., 158, *169*
Aronoff, G.M., 192, *201*, 261, *289*
Aronow, W.S., *24*
Arthur, R., 230, *250*
Artz. L., 50, *60*
Ascher, L.M., 344, 345, 381, 383, 384, *387*
Atkins, C.J., 410, *424*
Atkinson, J.H., 191, *206*, 216, 217, 218, 220, 229, 243, *244*, *247*, *251*
Attanasio, V., 314, *324*
Averasturi, L.G., 75, *85*
Ayllon, T., 406, *421*
Azevedo, E.S., 9, *27*

B
Bachrach, S., 132, *146*
Badia, P., 372, *287*
Badley, E.M., 274, 280, *294*
Baekelund, F., 154, *165*
Baer, D.M., 403, 405, *422*, *427*
Bagley, R.W., 404, *424*
Bagshaw, A., 135, *146*
Bah, M.D., 401, *426*
Baile, W.F., 51, *55*
Baily, M., 348, *395*
Bakal, D., 219, 221, 225, 226, 229, *245*, 299, 307, 312, 314, 315, 318, 321, *324*, *327*
Baker, B.L., 154, 161, *168*
Baker, C., 19, *26*, 40, *62*
Baker, M., *165*
Balaschak, B.A., 337, *345*
Balkin, T., 372, *387*
Ball, K.P., 40, *60*
Ball, S., 361, 363, *394*
Ballard, P., 162, *165*
Bali, L.T., 151, *170*
Ballick, L., 163, *165*
Balter, M.B., 348, 349, 351, 361, *387*, *392*
Bandura, A., 47, *56*, 407, 408, 409, 410, 416, *422*
Baragar, F.D., 138, *144*, *145*
Barberis, P., 300, *328*
Baric, L., 38, *56*
Barland, P., 135, *148*
Barlow, D.H., 161, *165*, 384, *390*
Bamard, K.E., 68, 79, *87*
Barnat, M., 237, *244*
Barnes, R.H., 157, 158, *169*
Barnett, L.W., 403, *424*
Barnett, J., *293*
Barrett, R., 216, *249*
Barrington, C.C., 163, *168*
Barris, R., 106, 107, *126*
Barron, K.D., 305, 313, 315, *324*
Bartlett, E.E., *64*
Basch, C.E., 53, *56*
Baskerville, J.C., 51, *61*
Basmajian, J.V., 161, *165*, 316, *324*
Bass, F., 53, *56*
Bassett, D., 216, 232, *249*
Batshaw, M.L., *165*
Batson, J.W., *145*
Batterman, R.C., *147*
Battié, M.C., 277, *289*
Battista, R.N., *56*
Batzel, L.W., 334, *344*
Bauer, M.L., 351, 361, *387*
Baurle, J.A., 278, *294*
Baum, J., 134, 135, *144*, *145*
Bauman, K. E., 38, 54, *56*
Baumann, L.J., 68, 79, *87*
Beaglehole, R., 11, *25*
Beals, R., 278, *289*
Bearpark, H.M., 359, *387*
Beck, A.T., 160, *165*
Beecher, H.K., 176, 193, *201*
Beck, S., 418, *423*
Beemsterboer, P., 159, 160, *166*, 269, 270, *290*
Behan, R.C., 181, *205*
Beitman, B., 238, *244*
Belar, C.D., 200, *209*, 318, *324*
Belloc, N.B., 7, 8, *24*, 32, *56*
Belmaker, R.H., 135, 136, *147*
Bendix, T., 278, *289*
Bennett, S., 216, *250*
Ben-Sira, Z., 419, *422*
Benson, D.F., 334, *344*
Benson, J.W., 137, *145*
Benya, A., 34, *63*
Berendes, H.W., 9, *26*
Berg, S., 278, *290*
Bergman, J.A., 285, *291*
Bergner, M., 199, *201*
Bergstrom, K.J., 194, *209*
Berk, S, 244, *249*
Berkman, L.E., 350, *395*
Berkman, L.F., 8, *29*, 138, *144*

Berkowitz, M., 183, *201*
Berman, P., 53, *56*
Berman, S.R., 388, *390*
Bernhardt, A.J., 161, *165*
Bernstein, D.A., *58*, 157, *165*
Berrenberg, J.D., 164, *171*
Berry, D.T.R., 370, *387*
Bertelson, A.D., 381, 383, 384, *392*
Besner, H.F., 154, *165*, *169*
Best, J.A., 34, 35, 37, 43, 44, 45, 50, 51, 53, 54, *56*, *61*, *62*
Bigelow, G.E., 36, 51, 52, *55*, *62*, *63*
Biering-Sörensen, F., 256, 278, 279, 280, 289
Bigos, S.J., 277, *289*
Billė, B., 301, *324*
Billings, A., 214, *244*
Birk, L., *85*
Bischoff, D.P., 278, *290*
Bishop, D.B., 42, *56*
Bixler, E.O., 348, *349*, *350*, *356*, *364*, *373*, *387*, *391*
Bjorkqvist, S., 44, *62*
Bjurstrom, L.A., 22, *24*
Black, R., *245*
Blackburn, H., 50, *56*
Blackwell, B., 179, *209*
Blair, G., 352, *289*
Blair, S.N., *25*, 400, *419*, *422*, *426*
Blanchard, E.B., 299, 302, 305, 307, 313, 314, 315, *323*, *324*, *329*
Bland, J.S., 12, *24*
Blaszcynski, A.P., 302, *324*
Blidner, I.N., 9, *24*
Bliwise, D.L., 372, 373, *389*
Bloch, M., 54, *56*
Block, A.J., 178, 193, *206*, 215, 216, *244*, *247*, *387*
Block, A.R., 139, *145*, 189, 192, 193, *202*, *205*
Block, F., 219, 243, *247*
Block, J., 370, *387*
Blom, G.E., 134, *144*
Blouin, D.C., 312, *330*
Blume, H.G., 312, *328*
Blumenthal, J.A., 410, *424*
Blumer, B., *202*
Blumer, D., 177, *202*, 334, *344*
Bobey, M.J., 176, *202*
Bobbitt, R.A., 199, *201*
Bober, H., 159, *165*
Bodner, A.J., 5, *28*
Bolis, L., 300, *328*
Bomar, G., 371, *390*
Bombardier, C., 109, *125*
Bond, M., 238, 242, *244*, *250*
Bonebakker, A., 233, *249*, 265, 266, *291*
Bonica, J.J., 195, *203*, 239, *245*
Bonnett, M.H., 367, 370, *388*
Boomkamp, A., 372, 373, *389*
Booth, C.L., 68, 79, *87*
Booth, G.L. 364, *391*
Bootzin, R.A., 154, *170*, 363, 375, 381, 382, *388*
Bootzin, R.R., 376, 379, 383, *389*, *393*
Borgeat, F., 307, *324*
Borkovec, T.D., 154, 157, *165*, 375, 376, 377, 378, 381, 384, 385, *388*, *394*
Bornstein, P.H., 381, *393*
Boudewyns, P.A., 303, *324*
Bowersox, S.S., 340, *345*
Bowman, G., 224, 229, 241, *251*, 302, *329*
Boyd, D., 241, *249*
Boylan, M.B., *393*
Boysen, P., 370, *387*
Bracht, N., 50, *56*
Bradford, L.A., 192, *203*
Bradley, L.A., 133, 134, 136, 139, *143*, *144*, 191, 194, 195, 196, *202*, *205*, *207*, 215, 217, 242, *245*, 248, *250*, 254, 261, 284, *289*, *292*
Bradner, M.N., 142, *147*
Brady, J.P., 8, 23, *24*, 66, *87*
Brady, J.V., 179, *202*
Braff, D., 216, 220, *251*
Braithwaite, G.H., 280, *289*
Branch, L.A., 403, *424*
Branco, J.A., 189, *203*
Brand, L., 240, *245*
Brand, R.J., 8, 29, *350*, *395*
Brandsma, J.M., 15, *24*
Brandt, K.D., 141, *145*
Brantmark, B., 44, *57*
Bratlid, T., 375, *392*
Braubard, B.I., 9, *26*
Brauer, E., 199, *205*
Bray, G.A., 10, *24*
Brena, S.F., 178, 182, 192, 195, *202*, *203*, *204*, 218, 226, 228, 230, *245*, *246*
Brengelmann, J., 39, *57*, 75, *85*
Brent, R.J., 70, 74, *86*
Breslow, L., 7, *24*, 32, *57*, 278, *289*
Brezinova, V., 364, *388*

Bridges, A., 352, *389*
Briggs, C.A., 419, *422*
Brockway, J., 285, *291*
Brodwin, M.G., 194, *209*
Brodwin, S.K., 194, *209*
Brook, R.H., 42, *63*, 269, *294*
Brooks, A.L., 138, *146*
Broste, S.K., 52, *61*
Brotherhood, J.R., 400, *427*
Broughton, R., 360, 364, 371, *388*
Brown, A., 224, 229, *249*
Brown, B.W., *146*
Brown, C., 269, 270, 275, *291*
Brown, E.N., 381, *389*
Brown, E.R., 420, *422*
Brown, G., 214, *245*
Brown, J., 224, 229, *249, 388*
Brown, K.S., 43, *57*
Brown, L.L., 134, 135, *144*
Brown, P.E., 138, *144*
Brown, R.A., 14, 21, *26*, 47, *55*
Brown, S.L., 316, 328
Browne, G., 270, 279, *290*
Brownell, K.D., 17, *29*, 400, 401, 418, *422*
Bruce, D.W., 348, 375, *391*
Brudny, J., 162, *165*
Bruhn, J.G., 138, *144*
Bruhn, P., 308, *325*
Buchanan, W.W., 109, *125*
Buckenmaier, C.C., 19, *27*
Buchsbaum, M., 154, *166*
Buck, C., 414, *421*
Buckingham, B., 189, *208*
Buckle, P.W., 280, *290*
Buckley, M.F., 162, *168*
Budzynski, T.H., 150, 151, 156, 162, *166, 167*, 188, *202*, 308, 309, *325*
Burchhardt, C., 217, *245*
Burgess, P.L., 40, *58*
Burish, T.G., 178, *205*, 308, *326*
Burke, J.P., 105, *125*
Burnis, S.M., 74, *85*
Burrows, G.D., 189, *204*
Burt, A., 38, *57*
Bush, C., 269, *293*, 305, 306, 307, 308, *325*
Byrne, M., 191, *202, 207*, 217, *245, 250*

C

Cady, L.D., 278, *290*
Caddy, G.R., 14, 15, *24, 26*
Cadieux, R.J., 348, 364, *391*
Cailliet, R., 96, *101*
Caine, T., 215, *246*
Cairns, D., 178, 180, 192, 193, *202, 208*, 262, 264, *290*
Caldwell, A.B., 154, *168*
Califano, J.A., 8, 13, 22, *24*, 32, *57*
Calimlim, J.F., 189, *208*
Callahan, L.F., 134, 138, *146*
Callen, K.E., 272, *293*
Calsyn, D.A., 195, *202, 204*, 218, 220, 226, 227, 236, *246, 252*
Cameron, D.E., 99, *101*
Camic, P.M., 13, *27*
Cantrell, P., 372, *387*
Cape, J., 216, *250*
Caplan, B., 231, *245*
Capra, P., 284, *293*
Carlaw, R., 50, *56*
Carleton, R.A., 11, *28*, 400, 413, 414, *421, 422*
Carlsson, A.M., 190, *203*
Carman, W.J., 7, *26*
Carmody, T.P., 402, 403, *422*
Carnahan, C., 163, *171*
Carr-Kaffashan, L., 380, 384, *388, 395*
Carron, H., 235, *245*
Carskadon, M.A., 348, 350, 357, 360, 369, *388, 389*
Carter, W.B., 199, *201*
Cartwright, R., 372, *389, 392*
Casas, J.M., 159, *166*, 269, 270, *290*
Cassileth, B.R., 134, 135, *144*
Catchlove, R., 235, *245*, 276, 284, *290*
Catterall, J.R., 370, *394*
Chambliss, C., 52, *57*
Chaney, E.F., 271, 273, *293*
Chapman, C.R., 189, 192, *203, 245, 246, 252*, 261, 269, 274, *294*
Chapman, S.L., 178, 182, 192, 195, *202, 203*, 221, 226, 230, 235, 239, *245*
Charter, R.A., 192, *203*
Chave, S.P.W., 11, *26*
Chayes, C.M., 159, *171*
Cheers, Y., 364, *390*
Chembtob, C.M., 74, *85*
Chesney, M.A., 157, *166*, 310, *325*
Chila, A.G., 309, 310, *326*
Chöler, V., 256, 285, *290*
Christian, J.J., 137, *144*
Christenson, G.J., 53, *60*
Christenson, G.M., 402, *424*

Christie, D.G.S., 37, 40, *62*
Chyatte, S., 226, 230, *245*
Cinciripini, P.M., 192, 193, *203*, 215, *245*, 276, *290*
Cirignotta, F., 348, 364, *392*
Clancy, S., 243, *252*
Clark, G.T., 159, 160, *166*, 269, 270, *290*
Clark, M., 372, *393*
Clarke, P., 217, *245*
Clayman, K.K., 163, *166*
Cleary, P.J., 163, *166*
Cleeland, C.S., 143, *148*, 12, *166*, 189, *203*
Clements, C.B., 406, *424*
Clouser, R.A., 154, *167*
Coates, T.C., *60*
Coates, T.J., 42, 52, *58*, 160, *170*, 378, *389*
Cobb, J., 216, *250*
Coburn, D., 402, *421*
Coccagna, G., 348, 364, *392*
Cogswell, J.J., 38, *57*
Cohen, K., 233, 235, *245*, 265, 266, 276, 284, *290*
Cohen, M.J., *207*
Cohen, M.S., 276, *291*
Cohen, N., 136, *143*
Cohen, M., 241, *249*
Cohen, R.A., 305, 312, *325, 329*
Cohen, R.E., 410, 411, 416, *425*
Cohen, S., 361, 363, *394*
Cohen, W.S., 21, 22, *24*
Cole, A., 195, *209*
Cole, P.V., *62*
Coleman, R.M., 372, 373, *389*
Colletti, G., 52, *57*
Colligan, R.C., 333, *344*
Collins, F.L., 189, *203*
Collins, G.A., 265, 266, *291*
Collins, G.H., 9, *28*
Collins, K.J., 355, *390*
Colman, A., *248*
Colwell, L., 37, *62*
Comrey, A., 216, *245*
Connors, L., 161, *171*
Cook, W.A., 193, *205*, 224, 225, 226, 240, *247*
Cooper, K.H., 400, 418, *422*
Cooperstock, R., 51, *57*
Cope, D., 243, *251*
Corbisiero, R., 305, 306, 307, 308, *325*
Corey, P., 22, *25*
Correa, P., 9, *25*
Corroll, V.J., 419, *422*
Cory, D.T., 273, *290*
Costas, R., 11, *25*
Costell, S., 164, *168*, 312, *327*
Coursey, R., 154, *166*, 375, 378, 279, *389*
Coyne, J., 163, *166*, 214, 230, *247*
Cox, D.J., 157, *166*, 309, 310, *325*
Cox, G.B., 195, *203, 245*
Cox, M., 22, *25, 427*
Craig, A. R., 163, *166*
Craig, K.D., 178, 180, 192, *203*, 278, *290*
Crawford, G.G., 15, *25*
Crawford, R., *422*
Creasy, M., 215, *246*
Creetenden, I., 233, *250*
Crippa, D., 371, *389*
Crisp, A., 215, *245*
Criqui, M.H., 46, *59*
Crocker, M., 178, *203*, 262, 264, *290*
Crockett, D.J., 191, *203*
Cromwell, L., 150, *166*
Crook, J., 279, *290*
Cross, P., 134, 135, *144*
Crow, R.S., 402, *424*
Crown, J.M., 135, *144*
Crown, S., 135, *144*, 215, *245*
Cruz, M., 300, *328*
Cruz-Vidal, M., 11, *25*
Cuevas, J., 305, 307, 317, *326*
Cullen, J.W., 33, *59*
Culver, D., 163, *170*
Cummings, N.A., 74, *85*
Cunningham, D.A., 414, *421*
Cureton, K., 400, *428*
Czeisler, C.A., 360, 361, *389*

D

Dalessio, D., 224, 229, 241, *251, 302*, 308, *325, 329*
Dalessio, J., 156, *166*
Dalton, E.R., 38, *57*
Daly, E.J., 158, *166*, 312, *325*
Damkot, D.K., 280, *290*
Danaher, B.G., 39, 42, *57, 59*, 418, *424*
Daniels, M., 140, *147*
Daube, J.R., 338, *344*
Daughton, D.M., 51, *57*
Daut, R.L., 189, *203*
d'Avernas, J., 35, *62*
David, H.P., 75, *85, 87*
Davidson, P.O., 176, *202*

Davidson, R.J., *167*
Davies, D.F., *25*
Davis, A.L., 39, 48, 53, *57*
Davis, B., 17, *28*
Davis, R., 40, *60*
Davison, G., 51, *57*
Dawson, E., 195, *207*, 218, 227, 243, *348*
Dazzi, H., 362, *392*
DeBacker, G., 37, 40, 52, *59*
DeBoer, K.F., 162, *171*
De Bruyn, L., 372, 373, *389*
Decker, J.L., 127, *144*
Deering, W.M., 341, *344*
DeGood, D., 221, 235, *245, 251*, 278, *294*
Dehlin, O., 278, *290*
DeLateur, B., 178, 195, *204*, 218, 228, 230, *246*
DeLeon, P.H., 66, 69, 74, 78, *85, 86*
DeLuca, J.R., 10, *25*
Dement, W.C., 348, 350, 357, 358, 360, 361, 363, 369, 372, 373, *388, 389, 394, 395*
Demjen, S., 219, 221, 225, 226, 229, *245*, 312, 314, 315, *324*
Denney, D.R., *170*
Dessonville, C.L., 177, *203*
Deutscher, S., 9, *25*
Denson, R., 38, *57*
Dent, C.W., 38, 54, *56*
Derksen, H., 75, 80, *86*
De Rogatis, L., 215, *245*
Deveno, T., 314, 315, *325*
De Vivo, D.C., 336, *344*
Dexter, J.R., 370, *388*
Deyo, R., 232, *245*
Diamond, S., 314, 315, *325*
Diamond-Falk, J., 314, 315, *325*
Dickel, M.J., 370, *389*
DiClemente, C.C., 403, 414, *423*
Di Clemente, C.O., 35, 47, 50, *57, 62*
Dietvorst, T.F., 163, *167*
Dikmen, S., 333, *344*
Dishman, R.K., 404, *414*
DiTecco, D., 52, *58*
Ditman, K.S., 15, *25*
Dodds, S.A., 337, *345*
Dodrill, C.B., 332, 333, 334, 338, *344, 346*
Doerhring, D.G., 333, *344*
Doerr, H., 162, *165*
Dohrmann, R., 269, 270, *290*
Dok, C., 109, *125*
Doleys, D.M., 178, *203*, 262, 264, *290*
Domino, E., 316, *325*
Domino, G., 352, *389*
Donahue, J., 74, *85*, 406, *423*
Donn, P.A., 158, *166*, 312, *325*
Donovan, J.V., 40, *58*
Dore, C., 355, *391*
Dorfman, S., 42, 52, *60*
Dorken, H., 74, 80, *86*
Dorsey, C., 363, *389*
Downie, W.W., 189, *203*
Dramaix, M., 37, 40, 52, *59*
Drummond, P.D., 303, *325*
Dubey, D., 137, *147*
Dubbert, P.M., 20, 23, *26*, 400–404, 410, 411, 416, *425*
Dubitzky, M., 417, *426*
Dubner, R., 190, 191, *205*
Dubuisson, D., 191, *203*
Dudek, B.C., 299, *324*
Duffy, M., 51, *57*
Dunn, B.E., 299, *327*
Durstine, L., 401, *426*
Duthie, J.J.R., 138, *144*
Dworkin, R., 240, *245*
Dwyer, J., 9, *25*
Dzubay, B., 242, *247*

E

Eastop, J.J., *101*
Eaton, H.M., 134, 135, *145*
Ebstein, R., *147*
Edelstein, C., 140, *147*
Edlund, S.R., 314, *324*
Edwards, A.R., 37, *62*
Efran, J.S., *387*
Efron, R., 337, *344*
Egan, P., 349, *391*
Egger, G., 401, *423*
Ehlhardt, J., 134, 140, *147*
Ehrisman, W.J., 157, 158, *169*
Eidelman, B.H., 314, 315, *327*
Eischens, R.R., 401, *423*
Ekbom, K., 300, *325*
Elder, J.P., 47, *55*, 404, 413, 414, *421*
Eldrod, E., 97, *101*
Elfner, L., 163, *165*
Elie, R., 307, *324*
Ellertsen, B., 339, *344*
Elliott, G.R., 37, *59*, 68, 79, *86*
Elliot, M.L., 32, 44, *63*
Ellis, B.W., 351, *389*

Elton, D., 189, *204*
Emanuel, I., 38, *60*
Enders, P.L., 192, *201*
Emrick, C.D., 15, *25*
Enders, P.L., 261, *289*
Enstrom, J.E., 32, *57*
Epstein, L.F., 38, *59*, 157, 158, *167*
Epstein, L.H., 308, 309, *325*, 400, 418, *423*
Epstein, W., 135, 136, *148*
Eriksson, G., 371, *390*
Ettlin, D., 273, *290*
Evans, D.D., 313, *324*
Evans, W.O., 192, *201*, 261, *289*
Everitt, B.S., 191, *208*
Everitt, M.D., 419, *423*
Everitt, M.G., 11, *26*
Ewart, C.K., 42, 52, *58*, 60
Ewins, A., 48, 54, *61*
Ewrlich, G.E., *147*
Ewy, H.W., 153, *171*
Exton-Smith, A.N., 355, *390*
Eysenck, H.J., 197, *206*, 215, *246*, 302, *325*
Eysenck, S., 215, *246*, 302, *325*

F

Fager, C., *246*
Fagerstrom, K.A., 37, 44, *58*
Fairchild, M.D., 340, *345*
Falke, R., 140, *147*
Farquhar, J.D., 39, 47, *59*
Farquhar, J.W., 22, *26*, 50, *58, 424*
Fagerweather, W.E., 17, 23, *27*
Faris, J., 401, *423*
Farquhar, J., 408, 419, 420, *425*
Faust, R., 39, 41, 48, *57*
Featherstone, H., 238, *244*
Fedoravicius, A.S., 179, *209*
Feinlaub, M., 7, *25*
Feltin, M., 132, *146*
Felton, B.J., 138, *144*
Feltz, C., 196, *201*, 242, *244*
Fenton, C.H., 142, *147*
Ferini-Strambi, L., 371, *389*
Feuerstein, M., 231, 235, 244, *246*, 305, 306, 307, 308, *325*
Feyerabend, C., 37, *59, 62*
Fielding, J.E., 34, 49, *58*, 402, *424*
Figueroa, J.L., 303, 312, *326, 329*
Fineberg, H.V., 48, *60*
Finley, W.W., 161, *167*
Finneson, B., 278, *290*
Fiocco, V., 134, *147*
Fireman, B.H., 140, *147*
Fishbain, D., 242, *246*
Fisher, E.B., 34, 42, *56, 58*, 408, *424*
Fisher, L., 277, *289*
Fishgood, H., 154, *171*
Fitzpatrick, R., 237, *246*
Fix, A.J., 51, *57*
Fixley, M.F., 372, *393*
Flanery, R.C., 189, *203*
Flay, B.R., 33, 40, 41, 50, 52, 53, 54, *58*
Fleming, A., *144*
Flenley, D.C., 371, *394*
Flor, H., 178, *209*, 261, 269, 271, *290, 294*
Floreen, A., 192, 193, *203*, 215, *245*, 276, *290*
Folkins, C.H., 19, *25*, 401, *423*
Folkman, S., 214, *246*
Follick, M.J., 199, *204*, 232, 244, *244, 246*, 261, *291*
Fontham, E., 9, *25*
Fordyce, W.E., 178, 192, 195, 196, 199, *204, 205*, 218, 220, 226, 228,230, 235, 236, *246, 252*, 255, 259, 261, 262, 272, 285, *291, 326*
Forgy, E.W., 15, *25*
Forster, F.M., 338, *344*
Forsythe, A.B., 37, 44, *63*
Fortmann, S.P., 47, 50, *58*
Foulds, G., 215, *246*
Fowler, J.E., 162, *167*
Fowler, R., 178, *204*
Fowles, D.C., 376, 377, 378, *388*
Fox, R.E., 70, 74, *86*
France, R.D., 177, *204*
Franceschi, M., *389*
Franchi, J., 99, *101*
Frank, R.G., 272, *293*
Frankel, B.L., 154, *166*, 375, 378, 379, *389*
Franklin, B.A., 417, *423*
Franks, C.M., 405, 407, *428*
Franks, R.D., 307, *323*
Freedman, R.R., 134, *144*, 375, 377, 378, *389, 390*
Freeman, C.W., 195, 196, *202, 204, 206*, 227, *246*
Freese, A., 278, *290*
Freidberg, S., *246*
Freundlich, A., 157, *166*, 309, 310, *325*

Friar, L., 342, *345*
Fricton, J.R., 254, *291*
Frye, R.A., 180, *209*
Frymoyer, J.W., 280, *290*
Friedman, L.W., 153, *166*
Friedman, R., *167*
Froedb, H.F., 9, *28*
Fuchs, V.R., 53, *58*
Funk, E.J., 11, *28*
Funk, G.A., 137, *144*
Furst, G.P., 121, *125*

G

Gaarder, K.B., 378, 379, *389*
Gaebe, G., *172*
Galiher, M.J., 158, *166*, 312, *325*
Gallagher, D., 177, *203*
Gannik, D., 280, *291*
Gannon, L.R., 200, *204*, 305, 307, 317, *326*
Gans, L., 381, 382, 384, *392*
Garcia-Palmieri, M.R., 11, *25*
Gardiner, J., 137, *145*
Garfinkel, L., 20, *25*, 349, *392*
Garfinkel, R., *390*
Garron, D.C., 191, 196, *206*, 217, 224, 227, *246, 247*
Gatchel, R.J., 284, *293*
Gaulier, B., 227, *244*
Gay, T.J.A., 348, 349, 375, *391*
Gaylor, M., 178, 180, 192, 193, *202, 206*, 216, 244, 247
Gegelman, R., 56, *58*
Geisinger, K., 191, *207*, 217, *245, 250*
Genest, M., 133, *145*, 176, 185, 188, 193, *204, 209*, 274, *294*
Gentry, W.D., 179, 196, *202, 204*, 242, *245*, 278, *291*
George, B., 373, *390*
George, J.M., 160, *170*
Gerard, P., 355, *390*
Gerber, L.H., 109, 121, *125*
Gerherich, S.G., 400, *427*
Gergen,K.J., 71, *86*
Gerrity, E.T., 39, *63*
Gershman, L., 154, *167*
Getchell, B., 17, 20, *25*
Gettman, L.R., 401, *422*
Gettman, L.W., 400, *426*
Getto, C.J., 199, *205*
Gewanter, H.L., *145*
Giblin, E., 369, 370, *393, 394*
Gibbons, L.W., 400, *422*
Gibson, C., 231, *245*
Gilbert, A., 139, *148*
Gillis, J.H., 406, *423*
Gilson, B.S., 199, *201*
Gislason, T., 371, *390*
Giurgea, D., *294*
Giurgen, D., 179, *209*
Glasgow, R.E., 34, 36, 42, 46, 51, 53, 54, *58, 59*, 418, *423*
Glass, D., 134, *147*
Glickman, I., 159, *167*
Gloor, P., 341, *344*
Goedert, J.J., 5, *28*
Goldberg, D., 215, *246*
Goldberg, M., 242, *246*
Golden, C.J., 312, *328*
Goldfoot, D.A., 176, *205*
Goldfried, M.R., 160, *167*
Goldney, R., 239, *246*
Goldstein, I.B., 99, *101*
Godding, P.R., 54, *58*
Goldenthal, P.A., *28*
Goodell, H., 189, *205*
Goodrick, G.K., 411, *423*
Goodyear, N., 400, *422*
Gordon, A., 229, 239, *246, 250*
Gordon, J.R., 412, *425*
Gordon, R., 140, *147*
Gorsuch, R., 215, *251*
Götestan, K.G., 139, *145*, 254, 255, 257, 260, 263, 265, 272, *292*
Gottlieb, H., 192, *204*, 276, *291*
Gottlieb, J., 305, *325*
Gottfried, B., 137,*147*
Gottheil, E., 15, *24*
Gottlieb, S.H., 51, *55*
Gover, V., 221, 222, *252*
Gozman, N.O., 92, *101*
Gracely, R.H., 190, 191, *204, 205*
Grant, J.P., 70, *86*
Grant, P.S., 153, *171*
Grayson, J.B., 377, *388*
Grayzel, A.I., 135, *148*
Green, C.J., 198, *207*
Green, D.E., 42, *59*
Green, L., 408, *425*
Greenhalgh, R.M., 51, *59*
Greenwald, P., 33, *59*
Gregory, V.R., 54, *60*
Griest, J.H., 401, *423*
Griffin, P., 157, *167*, 306, 309, 310, *326*

Griffin, W., 410, *423*
Grimby, G., 278, *290*
Grinker, R.R., 99, *101*
Groban, S.E., 199, *205*
Gross, M., 141, *145*
Grossman, J., 82, *87*
Grove, D.A., 42, *59*
Grynbaum, B.B., 162, *165*
Gucer, P., 194, *205*
Guilbaud, G., 154, *171*
Guilleminault, C., 348, 350, 358, 371, *388, 393, 395*
Guillory, M.M., 21, 22, *24*
Guitar, B., 163, *167*
Gunnerson, D., *58*
Gurman, A.S., 401, *423*
Guy, W.B., 137, *145*

H

Haag, G., 269, 271, *290*
Haber, J., 182, *205*, 306, *326*
Hade, B., 307, *324*
Haenszel, W., 9, *25*
Hagberg, M., 287, *291*
Hale, W.E., 11, *27*
Haley, W., 220, *246*
Hall, G., 409, *428*
Hall, J.R., 309, 310, *326*
Hall, W., 221, *246*
Hallstrom, A.P., 11, *28*
Hamburg, D.A., 32, *59*, 68, 79, *86*
Hamilton, J., 200, *204*, 305, *326*
Hamilton, M., 215, *251*
Hamilton, P.J.S., 37, 41, *62*
Hammond, E.C., 20, *25*, 348, 349, 351, *390, 392*
Handel, S., 37, *59*
Handlin, D., 240, *245*
Hanna, R., 163, *167*, 413, *424*
Hansen, T., 375, *392*
Hansson, T.H., 277, *289, 291*
Hanvik, L.J., 195, *205*, 227, *246*
Hardy, J., 189, *205*
Harley, E.E., 9, *26*
Harley, J.P., 333, *344*
Harper, R.G., 306, 313, *326, 329*
Harris, E.D., 108, *125*
Harris, J.E., 42, *59*
Harris, R., 188, *205*
Harris, T., 214, *245*
Harris-Davidson, A., 400, *427*
Harrison, R.H., 301, *326*
Hart, R., 243, *246*
Hartmann, E., 155, *167*, 379, *390*
Harsh, J., 372, *387*
Hasan, J., 349, *395*
Hasenfeld, R., 154, *171*
Haskell, W.L., 19, *25*
Haslam, R.H., *165*
Hassanein, K., 298, *330*
Hassanein, R., 298, *330*
Hatch, J.P., 163, *167*
Hauri, P., 155, *167*, 377, 378, 379, *390*
Havlik, R.J., 11, *25*
Haynes, R.B., 5, *27*
Haynes, S.G., 7, *25*
Haynes, S.N., 157, *167*, 200, *204*, 305, 307, 309, 310, 317, *326*, 375, 378, 383, 384, *390*
Hayward, L., 221, *246*
Healey, S., 154, *168*, 348, 349, 375, *387, 391*
Heath, H.A., 99, *101*
Heaton, R.K., 199, *205*
Hebel, R., 40, *63*
Heczey, M., 163, *171*
Heffler, D., 378, *392*
Heft, M.W., 188, *205*
Heilbronn, M., 177, *202*
Heiman, E., 243, *251*
Heinrich, R.L., 265, 266, *291*
Heinzelman, F., 404, *424*
Heiser, P., *326*
Hellekson, C., 155, *167, 390*
Heller, R.F., 37, 40, *62*
Hemphill, D.P., 157, 158, *167*, 308, *325*
Henderson, J.B., 38, *60*
Hendler, N., 194, *205*
Hendrie, H.C., 138, *145*
Henkle, C., 140, *145*
Hennings, B.L., 378, *388*
Henoch, M.J., *145*
Henryk-Gutt, R., 301, *326*
Henschel, A., 359, *390*
Herd, J.A., *60*
Hersen, M., 157, 158, 161, *165, 167*, 308, *325*, 384, *390*
Hess, D.W., *146*
Hester, R.K., 15, *26*
Hetta, J., 348, 349, 371, *390*
Hettinger, T., 254, *291*
Hewett, J., 196, *201*, 242, *244*
Hewson, D., 214, *244*
Hickman, N., 278, *289*

Hicks, G.J., 364, *390*
Hicks, R.A., 364, *390*
Hill, E., 161, *169*
Hill, R., 219, 226, 240, *247*
Hillier, V., 215, *246*
Hindi, L., 140, *147*
Hinkle, J.E., 154, 157, *168, 171*
Hirshfeld, A.H., 181, *205*, 231, 237, 242, *247*
Hirschfield, M., 231, 237, 242, *247*
Hitchcock, E., 229, *246*
Hoch, C.C., 356, 357, 358, 363, *390, 394*
Hochstim, J., 7, *24*
Hodes, R., 143, *148*
Hockersmith, V., 192, *204*
Hoelscher, T.J., 313, *326*
Hikkanen, E., 300, 304, *327*
Holcombe, R., 218, 228, 230, *246*
Holcombe, S., 195, *204*
Holm, J., 305, 309, 310, *326*
Holman, H.R., *146*
Holmes, D.S., 178, *205*, 308, *326*, 401, *424*
Holmes, T., 231, *246*
Holroyd, K., 157, 163, 164, *166, 168, 170*, 301, 305, 309, 311, 312, *324, 326*
Holzer, C.E., 351, *391*
Holzman, A.D., 273, *291*
Hopkins, A., 237, *246*
Hopson, L., 191, 195, *202, 207*, 217, *250*
Horn, D., 42, *59*
Hossack, 40, *58*
Hotchin, J., 137, *145*
Houck, P.R., 358, *390*
Houle, M., 231, 235, 244, *246*
House, J., 7, *26*, 151, *171*
Hoy, P., 154, *165*
Hrubes, V., 189, *205*
Hudson, M.P., 280, *294*
Hughes, C.A., 35, *57*
Hughes, H.H., 383, *390*
Hughes, R.C., 383, *390*
Hughes, J.R., 37, 38, *59*
Hultman, G., 281, *291*
Humphry, M., 277, 278, 279, *291*
Hunt, L., 370, *387*
Hunt, P.T., 53, *59*
Hunt, W.A., 403, *424*
Hunter, J.E., 300, *328*
Hunter, M.S., 200, *207*, 215, 217, 219, *247, 249, 328*
Hursey, K.G., 305, 309, 310, *326*
Hursch, C.J., *395*
Huskisson, E.C., 189, 190, *205, 208*
Hussaini, G., 70, *87*
Huster, W.J., 42, 52, *60*
Hutchings, D.F., 156, 157, 158, *168, 170*, 309, 310, 315, *327, 328*
Hutchinson, P.C., 305, *325*
Hymowitz, N., 52, *61*
Hyde, R.T., 20, *27*

I

Ianni, P., *144*
Ignelzi, R., 229, *247*
Illaria, R., 348, *391*
Illingworth, D., 38, *57*
Ilstrue, D., 216, *248*
Ingram, R., 243, *244*
Innes, J.M., 411, 412, *424*
Inouye, D.K., 69, 74, *87*
Inui, T.S., 11, *28*, 232, *245*
Iverson, D.C., 402, *424*
Ivnik, R., 216, *248*
Iwata, B.A., 406, 409, *421*, *428*

J

Jackson, R.T., 11, *25*
Jacob, R.G., 314, *327*
Jacobs, D., 47, 50, *56*, 403, *427*
Jacobson, A.M., 142, *145*
Jacobson, E., 21, *25*, 376, *391*
Jacobus, S., *55*
Jacoby, J.A., 356, 373, *387*
Jacox, R.F., *146*
Jahanshahi, M., 220, 229, *249*
Jainchill, J., 132, *146*
James, S.A., *146*
Jamieson, A., 371, *393*
Jankel, W.R., 162, *168*
Janowsky, J.S., 338, *344*
Janssen, K., 157, 158, *168*
Jarrell, H.P., 312, *329*
Jarvie, G.J., 400, *428*
Jarvik, M.E., 37, 44, *63*
Jarris, M.J., 37, *59, 62*
Jaski, M., 372, *389*
Jasnoski, M.L., 401, *424*
Jeans, M., 240, *248*
Jeffery, R.W., 39, *59*, 418, *424*
Jensen, I., 284, *292*
Jenson, M.M., 137, *144*
Jespersen, M., 280, *291*

Johns, M.W., 348, 349, 351, 375, *389, 391*
Johnson, G., 157, *170*
Johnson, J.J., 21, *26*
Johnson, R., 161, *169*, 401, *426*
Johnson, W., *201*
Johnston, N., 37, *64*
Jones, B., 221, 243, *252*
Jones, G.E., 162, *168*
Jones, J.S., 9, *26*, 222, *251*
Jones, M.E., 277, *289*
Jones, N.L., 409, 414, *421, 426*
Jones, R.K., 372, *393*
Joyce, C.R., 189, *205*
Jurish, S.E., 313, 314, 315, *324, 329*

K

Kaganov, J.A., 299, 307, 312, 314, 315, *324, 327*
Kahn, M., 154, *168*
Kalandidi, A., 9, *28*
Kales, A., 154, *168*, 348, 349, 350, 356, 364, 366, 373, 375, *387, 391*
Kales, J.D., 348, 364, 366, *391*
Kaloupek, D.G., 154, *165*, 378, *388*
Kamarck, T.W., 14, *16*
Kamwendo, K., 283, 287, *292*
Kane, R.L., 42, *63*
Kanfer, F.H., 176, *205*
Kannell, W.B., 7, 8, 20, *25, 26*
Kanner, A., 214, 230, *247*
Kaplan, O., 368, 369, *392*
Kaplan, R.M., 46, *59*, 410, *424*
Kaprio, J., 351, 361, *393*
Karacan, I., 153, *168*, 348, 351, 356, 364, *391, 395*
Karoly, P., 402, 403, 407, 413, *424*
Karzmark, P., 160, *170*
Kashurba, G.J., 364, *391*
Kasinoff, B., 348, *395*
Kass, I, 51, *57*
Katell, A.D., 20, 23, *26*
Katon, W., 238, *244*
Katranides, M., *326*
Katsikitis, M., 216, *250*
Katz, J., 240, *248*
Kavanaugh, T., 414, 421
Kavesh, W., 132, *146*
Kazdin, A.E., 376, *391*, 403, 408, *424*
Keeler, E., 226, 236, 238, *250*
Keenan, D.M., 313, *329*
Keller, M.L., 68, 79, *87*
Keefe, F.J., 139, 142, *145*, 178, 193, 194, *205*, 215, 219, 224, 225, 226, 240, 243, *248, 252*, 269, 270, 275, *291*, 410, *424*
Keeley, J., 284, *293*
Kellgren, J.H., *145*
Kelley, W.N., 108, *125*
Kelly, J.L., 200, *210*
Kelsey, J.L., 278, *291*
Kelvie, W., 199, *208*
Kember, P.A., 280, *290*
Kennedy, S., 75, *87*
Kerns, R.D., 199, *206*, 273, *291*
Kidson, M., 219, 220, 223, *249*
Kielhofner, G., 104, 105, 106, 107, 113, *125, 126*
Kilburn, P., 216, *250*
Killen, J., 37, 39, *59*, 418, *424*
King, K., 406, *423*
Kinnier, R., 39, *59*, 418, *424*
Kirk, C.J.C., 51, *59*
Kirkland, J.A., 34, 35, 50, *56*
Kirkpatrick, M., 19, *26, 27*
Kischt, J.P., 276, *292*
Kishino, N., 284, *293*
Kittel, F., 37, 40, 52, *59*
Kjervik, D.K., 69, 74, *86*
Kleeman, M., 192, *204*
Klein, M.H., 401, *423*
Klemport, A., 372, *387*
Klesges, R.C., 34, 42, 46, 54, *58, 59*
Klesges, L.M., 36, 42, 51, 53, 54, *58*
Kline, E.G., 50, *56*
Klove, H., 333, 335, 336, 339, *344, 345*
Knafl, K., 244, *251*
Knight, R.G., 300, *328*
Koch, G.G., 38, 54, *56*
Kochanowicz, N.A., 164, *168*, 312, *327*
Koehler, H., 269, 271, *290*
Koeple, K.R., 401, *425*
Koeske, R., 418, *423*
Kohl, J.S., 19, *26*
Kohn, R., 35, *59*
Koller, R., 192, *204*, 276, *291*
Kopel, S.A., 52, *57, 391*
Korein, J., 162, *165*
Kornitzer, M., 37, 40, 52, *59*
Koskela, K., 44, *62*
Koskenvuo, M., 351, 361, *393*
Kostopoulus, G.K., 341, *344*
Kowalesky, R.A., 341, *345*
Kowirokko, K.J., 92, *101*

Kraft, G.H., 259, *292*, 308, *328*
Kraft, J.K., 137, *147*
Kraines, R.G., *146*
Kramer, M., 154, *170*, 375, *394*
Kranz, H., 219, 220, 223, *249*
Kraus, H., 277, *292*
Kraut, A.G., 69, 74, *86*
Kravitz, H., 372, *392*
Kremer, A., 218, *247*
Kremer, E., 178, 180, 190, 192, 193, *202, 206*, 216, 217, 229, 243, 244, *244, 247*
Kremsdorf, R.B., 164, *168*, 312, *327*
Kreuter, M.W., 53, *60*
Kribbs, N., 362, *394*
Krieger, J., 370, *391*
Kripke, D.F., 349, 357, 362, 366, 367, 368, 369, 373, *387, 390, 391, 392*
Krishman, K.R., 177, *204*
Krishnaswami, 9, *25*
Kuczmierczyk, A.R., 306, *326*
Kudrow, L., 182, *206*, 229, *247*, 302, *327*
Kukulka, C.G., 161, *165*
Kunkel, J., 381, 383, 384, *392*
Kunzel, M., 224, 229, 241, *251*, 302, *329*
Kupfer, D.J., 356, 357, 358, 363, *390, 394*
Kurke, D.S., 19, *27*
Kurland, S., 134, *147*
Kurtz, D., 370, *391*

L

Lack, L., 355, 357, 358, 359, 360, 361, 375, 385, *390, 392, 393, 394*
Lacks, P., 381, 383, 385, *392*
Lahey, B., 400, *428*
Lake, A.E., 185, *206*, 237, *244, 303, 327*
Lake, M., 20, 23, *26*, 410, 411, 416, *425*
Lalonde, M., 32, *60*
Lancaster, R., 351, *389*
Lance, J., *325*
Landesman-Dwyer, S., 38, *60*
Lando, H.A., 54, *60*
Landsverk, J., 140, *147*
Langinvainio, H., 351, 361, *393*
Lansky, D., 218, *246*
Lantz, D., 342, *344*
Lanyon, R.I., 163, *168*
Laporte, W., 287, *292*
LaPoste, R.E., 400, *427*
Large, R.G., 200, *206*
Larouche, L.M., 307, *324*
Larson, A., 238, *247*
Larson, M., 134, 135, *145*
Larsson, R., 256, 285, *290*
Lasagna, L., 189, *208*
Lasater, T., 47, 50, *60*, 400, 404, 413, 414, *421, 422*
Laskin, D., 269, 270, *290*
Lavie, P., 360, *392*
Lawlis, G.F., 195, 196, *207*, 242, *248*
Lawrie, A.J., 138, *144*
Laxer, K.D., 338, *344*
Lazarus, R., 214, 230, *246*
Lazarus, R.S., 153, 163, *168, 169*, 214, *247*
Leaf, A., 20, *27*
Leavitt, F., 217, 227, *246, 247*
Leatham, P.A., 189, *203*
Leavitt, F., 194, *206*
LeBoeuf, A., 152, *169*
Ledwidge, B., 401, *424*
Lee, C., 399, 402, 404, 409, 411, 412, 418, 420, *424, 426*
Lee, K.H., 161, *169*, 370, *394*
Lefebvre, M.F., 185, *206*, 216, 220, *247*
Lehman, R.A.W., 199, *205*
Lehmann, J., 178, *204*
Lehrer, P.M., 380, *395*
Leiberman, M., *249*
Leininger, J., 232, *245*
Lelieuvre, R.B., 264, *293*
Lellouch, J., 9, *27*
Lenzi, P.L., 348, 364, *392*
Leo, L.A., 350, *387*
Lenox, S., 132, *146*
Lerner, D.J., 8, *26*
Lerner, T., 338, *345*
Levenson, H., 231, 237, 242, *247*
Levidow, L., *165*
Levine, B.A., 315, *327*
Levine, S., 7, *25*, 137, *147*
Levitt, S.R., 191, 199, *206*
Levy, L.M., 300, 304, *327*
Lewis, S., 400, *422*
Li, V.C., 42, 52, *58, 60*
Liang, M.D., 134, 135, *145*
Libb, J.W., 406, *424*
Libo, L.M., 158, *169*
Lichstein, K.L., 313, *326*
Lichtenstein, E., 14, *26*, 34, 42, 50, 51, 54, *57, 60*
Lick, J., 378, *392*
Lieberman, A., *165*

Lieberskind, J.C., 195, *206*
Liljenberg, B., 348, 349, 371, *390*
Lin, Y., 9, *25*
Lindquist, B., 159, *169*
Lingiaerde, O., 375, *392*
Linnoila, M., 362, *393*
Linton, S.J., 139, *145*, 190, *206*, 220, *247*, 254, 255, 259, 260, 261, 263, 265, 266, 269, 272, 274, 281, 283, 284, 287, *292, 293*
Lipton, J., 216, 219, 222, 223, 228, 234, 236, 237, *247, 248*
Lisansky, E.T., 134, *147*
Lisman, S.A., 382, 383, 384, *395*
Littell, R., 153, *168*
Lloyd, J., 239, *248*
Lloyd, S., 372, *389, 392*
Lockwood, G., 378, *390*
Lodge, J., 152, *169*
Loeser, J.D., *206*, 218, 228, 230, *246*
Loeser, V., 177, 195, *204*
Loh, T., 219, 220, 223, *249*
Long, D., 194, *205*
Long, J.D., 408, *428*
LoPresti, R.W., 339, *345*
Lord, J., 280, *290*
Lorig, K., 141, *146*
Louis, T.A., 418, *60*
Louks, J., 195, 196, *202, 204, 206*, 227, *246*
Lowe, J.D., 349, *394*
Lubar, J.F., 341, *344*
Lubeck, D., *146*
Ludwig, A.O., 134, *146*
Luepker, R.V., 50, *56*
Lugaresi, E., 348, 364, *392*
Lund, P., 228, *248*
Lund, V.J., 51, *59*
LuPolover, R., *392*
Luria, M.H., 401, *425*
Lushene, R., 215, *251*
Lusk, E.J., 134, 135, *144*
Luthe, W., 21, *27*, 151, 157, *171, 394*
Lutker, E.R., 154, *168*
Lutz, R.W., 275, *293*
Lutz, T., 154, *170*, 375, *394*
Lynn, A., 197, *206*
Lyttle, D., 237, *252*

M

MacAndrew, C., 15, *25*
MacArthur, C., 38, *56*
MacCoby, N., 17, 22, *26*, 37, 47, 50, *58, 59*, 404, 408, 419, 420, *425*
MacConall, M.A., 92, 96, *101*
MacMahon, B., 9, *28*
Madorsky, A., 192, *204*
Magyary, D.L., 68, 79, *87*
Mahoney, M.J., *425*
Main, C.J., 196, *207*, 233, *248*
Malcolm, R.E., 44, *60*
Malhotra, L., 224, *249*
Malmo, R.B., 150, *169*
Malone, T.B., 19, *26*
Manilow, M.R., 402, 403, *422*
Manschreck, T.C., 142, *145*
Manske, S.R., 37, 48, 53, *62*
Manuso, J.S.J., *425*
Marbach, J., 216, 219, 222, 223, 228, 234, 236, 237, *247, 248*
Marcer, D., 238, *247*
Marchisello, P.J., 191, *202*, 217, *245, 250*
Marcille, P., 309, 310, *326*
Marcus, R., 140, *147*
Margo, G.E., *422*
Margolis, R., 196, *202*, 242, *245*
Marholin, D., 405, 423, *425*
Mark, R., 132, *146*
Marlatt, G.A., 412, 417, *425*
Marshall, C., 161, *165*
Martin, J.E., 20, 23, 26, *238*, 251, 400–404, 410, 411, 416, *425*
Martin, M.J., 156, *169*, 297, *301, 306, 327*
Martin, P.R., 301, 303, 304, 305, 307, 308, 309, 310, 320, *327*
Maruta, T., 191, *209*, 216, 241, 243, *251, 252*
Masi, A., 227, *244*
Massey, J.D., 9, *26*
Masi, A.T., *146*
Mason, R.M., 189, *205*
Mason, W., 362, 368, 369, 373, *387, 391, 392*
Massong, S.R., *168*
Master, R.J., 132, *146*
Masterson, J.P., 348, 349, 375, *391*
Matarazzo, J.D., 32, 46, 49, *60*, 402, 403, *422*
Mathers, C.D., 364, *394*
Mathew, R.J., 152, *172*
Mathews, A.M., 305, 306, 307, 308, 309, 310, *327*

Mathews, C.G., 333, 335, 336, *344, 345*
Matsuoka, H., 364, *393*
Matsue, Y., *393*
Matsutsuyo, J., 114, *125*
Maultsby, M.C., 15, *24*
Mausner, J.S., 37, *60*
Mausner, R., 37, *60*
May, J., 163, *165*
Mayer, H., 284, *293*
Mayer, T.G., 284, *293*
McAlister, A.L., 17, 22, *26*, 408, 419, 420, *425*
McArthur, D., 233, *249*
McCabe, T.G., *393*
McCauley, J.P., 272, *293*
McClemont, S., 9, *24*
McCoy, C.E., 195, 196, *207*
McCreary, C., 195, *207, 209*, 218, 227, 242, 243, *248*
McCullough, J.A., 54, *60*
McDaniel, L.K., 133, 136, 139, *143, 144*, 215, *248*
McGhie, A., 360, *392*
McGill, J.C., 195, 196, *207*, 242, *248*
McGinnis, J.M., 21, *26*
McGrath, P., 189, 191, *205, 208*
McLean, S., 335, *345*
McKenzie, R.E., 157, 158, *169*
McNeill, B., 163, *167*
McNulty, T.F., *395*
McNulty, T.J., 380, *395*
McPhee, B., 254, *293*
McPhee, M., 192, *209*
McPherson, F.M., *87*
McPherson, M.P., 69, 75, *87*
McReynolds, W.T., 408, *425*
McWaters, M.D., 38, *57*
Mead, A., 36, 52, *62*
Meagher, R.B., 198, *207*, 242, *246*
Meares, R., 161, *169*
Medina, J., 314, 315, *325*
Medsger, T.A., *146*
Meenan, R., *148*
Mehta, G., 189, *208*
Mehta, S., 215, *251*
Meichenbaum, D., 153, 160, *169*, 176, 185, 188, 193, *204, 209*, 274, *294*, 312, *327*, 414, *425*
Meinert, C.L., 41, *60*
Meklas, J.F., 159, *169*
Melgaard, B., 308, *325*
Melin, L., 254, 255, 259, 263, 265, 266, 271, 272, *292, 293*
Mellinger, G.D., 348, 349, *392*
Melzack, R., 176, 188, 190, 191, *203, 207*, 217, 240, *248*, 255, *293*
Menaghan, E., 214, *249*
Mendelson, G., 219, 220, 223, 240, *248, 249*
Mermelstein, R.J., 50, *60*
Merriman, R., 37, *62*
Mersky, H., 176, 189, 195, 197, *210*, 220, 224, 228, 229, 232, 236, 240, 241, *249*, 252, *303, 327*
Messin, S., 362, 368, 369, *387, 391*
Mettrop, P.J., 137, *146*
Metzler, F., 254, *293*
Metzner, H.L., 7, *26*
Meon, M.E., 372, 373, *389*
Meyer, A.J., 17, 22, *26*, 38, *60*
Meyer, R.G., 157, *166*, 309, 310, *325*
Meyerwitz, S., 133, 136, *146*
Michael, J.M., 32, *60*, 82, *87*
Michelacci, S., 99, *101*
Michie, P.T., *387*
Midax, D., 191, *207*, 217, *250*
Middaugh, S., 161, *169*
Milesis, C.A., 401, *426*
Miller, C., 264, 273, *293*
Miller, D.S., 134, 135, *144*
Miller, L.C., *59*
Miller, N.E., *60*
Miller, P.C., *290*
Miller, R.C., 153, *171*
Miller, S.A., 35, 37, 42, *59*
Miller, W.R., 14, 15, *26*, 355, 360, 361, *392*
Millingen, K.S., 335, *345*
Millon, T., 198, *207*
Mills, D.E., 34, 35, 50, *56*
Mills, W.R., 9, *26*
Milstein, V.M., 337, *345*
Mindham, R.H.S., 135, *146*
Minniti, R., 216, *249*
Mintz, M., 338, *345*
Mirmiran, M., 361, *395*
Mitchell, S.K., 68, 79, *87*
Mitler, M.M., 348, 350, 358, *388, 395*
Mittelmark, M., 50, *56*
Moffett, A.M., 304, *327*
Mohamed, S., 243, *249*, 279, *293*
Mohr, E.M., 278, *294*
Mohr, J.P., 161, *171*
Molomut, N., 137, *147*
Monaco, G., 188, 205
Mondine, S., 348, 364, *392*

Monguillot, J.E., 305, 312, *325, 329*
Montoe, L.J., 153, *169*, 375, *393*
Monroe, S., *249*
Montgomery, D.D., 154, *169*
Montgomery, I., 154, *169*, 375, *393*
Montgomery, P.S., 157, 158, *169*
Monti, P.M., 47, *55*
Mooney, D., 157, *167*, 309, 310, *326*
Mooney, N.E., 139, *146*
Mooney, V., 192, 193, 195, 196, *202, 207, 208*, 242, *248*, 284, *293*
Moore, G.F., 9, *26*
Moore, J.D., 163, *165*, 196, *201*, 242, 244, *244*
Moore, J.E., 271, 273, *293*
Moore, M., *249*
Moos, R.H., 134, 136, *146*, 214, *244*
Morgan, W.P., 401, *425*
Morgan, W.S., 401, *423*
Morris, J.N., 11, *26*
Morris, M., 375, 385, *393*
Morrison, D., 224, *249*
Mosko, S., 370, *389*
Moskowitz, H., 15, *25*, 362, *393*
Mosteller, F., 48, *60*
Mostofsky, D.I., 331, 332, 334, 337, 338, *345, 346*
Mothersill, K., 269, 270, *294*
Mott, E.E., 378, 379, *389*
Mullan, J., 214, *249*
Mullaney, D.J., 150, 156, *166*, 188, *202*, 309, *325*
Mungas, D.M., *393*
Murawski, B.J., 134, 135, *145*
Murphy, E., 195, *201*
Murphy, R.W., 183, *208*, 216, 223, 227, *251*
Murray, E.J., 52, *57*
Murrell, T., 239, *250*
Myslobodsky, M.S., 338, *345*

N

Nachemson, A., 254, 256, 259, 279, 285, *290, 293*
Nacht, M., 200, *210*
Nagi, S., 130, *146*
Naliboff, B.D., 196, *207*, 233, 241, *249*, 265, 266, *291*
Nanson, J.L., 38, *57*
Narayan, M.G., 161, *165*
Nash, J.D., 17, 22, *26*
Nathan, P.R., 301, 303, 304, *327*
Nation, J.R., 405, 413, *425*
Nau, S.D., 154, *165*
Needle, R., 401, *427*
Neff, D.F., 313, 314, 315, *324, 329*
Nehemkis, A.M., 192, *203*
Nentwig, C.G., 53, *61*
Nepomuceno, C., 192, *208*, 215, 219, *250*
Nettleton, B., 419, *422*
Newman, A.C., 163, *168*
Newman, J.M., 400, *427*
Newton, K.M., 38, *63*
Nevitt, M., *148*
Nicassio, P., 154, *170*, 375, 376, 379, 382, 383, *388, 393*
Nicholls, G., 134, *145*
Nielson, W.R., *328*
Nikiforow, R., 300, 304, *327*
Niman, C.A., 161, *167*
Noble, J., 309, *326*
Norton, G.R., 303, *328*
Norton, R., 216, *250*
Noskin, D.E., 279, *294*
Nossal, G.J.V., 70, *87*
Nouwen, A., 269, 270, 271, *293*
Nuechterlein, K.H., 157, *170*
Nunn, K., 238, *251*
Nypaver, A., 244, *249*

O

Oakley, F., 106, 107, *125, 126*
O'Brien, G.T., 377, *388*
O'Brien, M.D., 307, *388*
O'Connell, E.R., 278, *20*
Ockene, J.K., 13, *27*, 52, *61*
Offord, K., 333, *344*
Ogunyemi, A.O., 304, *328*
Ohlin, P., 44, *57*
Ohlson, N., 275, *293*
Ohnhaus, E.E., 189, *207*
Okawa, M., 364, *391*
Oken, D., 99, *101*
Okudaira, N., 366, 367, 373, *392*
Okuma, T., 364, *393*
Oldridge, N.B., 409, 414, 417, *421, 426*
Olesen, J., 308, *325*
Olmstead, E., 377, *390*
Olson, J.M., 404, 415, 420, *426*
Olson, T.W., 312, *323*
Omran, A.R., *61*
O'Neill, H.K., *423*
Ordentlich, M., 39, 41, 48, *57*
Orlebeke, J.F., 302, *328*
O'Rourke, D., 372, *387*
Orr, W.C., 372, *393*

Osborne, D., 163, *167*, 333, *344*
Ossip, D., 418, *423*
Ossip-Klein, D.J., 39, 46, 51, *56, 61, 63*
Ostfeld, A.M., 307, *328*
Oswald, I., 362, 370, *393, 394*
Overman, S., 232, *245*
Owen, L.E., 48, 53, *56*
Owen, N., 54, *61*, 399, 402–405, 407, 411, 412, 413, 415, 418, 420, *424, 426, 427*

P

Pace, J., 192, *202*
Packard, R., 236, 237, *249*
Packer, M.J., 48, *61*
Paffenbarger, R.S., 11, 20, *27*
Page, A.R., 37, 44, 45, *61*
Paisley, W., 419, *426*
Pallak, M.S., 78, *86*
Pallmeyer, T.P., 314, 315, *324*
Palmer, J.A., 22, *27*
Paockop, D.J., 92, *101*
Papsdorf, J.D., 377, 378, *389*
Papsdorf, L., 153, 154, *167*
Paraskevas, F., 138, *145*
Parise, M., 157, *167*, 308, *326*
Parker, J., 188, *201*, 242, *244*, 414, *421*
Parker, S.R., 196, *205*
Parise, M., 306, 310, *327*
Parron, D.L., 32, *59*, 68, 79, *86*
Partinen, M., 349, 351, 361, 371, *393, 395*
Pasino, J.A., 178, 180, 192, 193, *202*, 262, 264, *290*
Passchier, M.S., 302, *329*
Pate, R.R., 419, *426*
Patil, K.D., 51, *57*
Patois, E., 9, *27*
Patterson, N., 361, 363, *394*
Patton, D., 178, *203*, 262, 264, *290*
Paul, G.L., 376, *393*
Paul, I.L., 97, *101*
Paul, L.A., 195, *206*
Paulin, J.M., 300, *328*
Pauly, J.T., 22, *27*
Paynes, L.E., 138, *146*
Pearce, S., 268, *293*
Pearlin, L., 214, 243, *249*
Pearne, D.H., 163, *170*
Peck, C.L., 308, *328*
Peck, D.F., 162, *170*
Pederson, L.L., 51, *61*
Pedoe, H.T., 37, 40, *62*
Pedraza, E., 177, *202*
Peeke, H.V., 151, *170*
Peled, R., 360, *392*
Pell, S., *27*
Pellegrini, A., 341, *344*
Pelletier, K.R., 12, 21, *27*
Pelz, M., 232, 236, 240, *249*
Pemberton, J.S., 195, *207*
Penzien, D.B., 305, 309, 310, *326*
Percy, L., 155, *167*, 379, *390*
Perkin, G., 154, *169*
Perri, M.G., 408, *426*
Perry, M.G., 35, *61*
Pesch, R., 226, 236, 238, *250*
Peterson, A.V., 43, *57*
Peterson, D.R., 11, *28*
Peterson, G.M., 335, *345*
Peterson, L.E., 256, 285, *290*
Petrovic, L., 216, *249*
Pettinger, J., 406, *426*
Peyser, W.P., 163, *170*
Pfeiffer, E.A., 150, *166*
Pfeiffer, G.J., 22, *27*
Phillips, B.U., 138, *144*
Phillips, C., 156, *170*, 178, 190, 200, *207*, 215, 216, 219, 220, 229, *247*, *249*, 300, 302, 306, 309, *328*
Phillips, D., 405, 413, *425*
Philips, H.C., 273, *293*
Pickle, L.W., 9, *25*
Piccione, A., 160, *170*
Pikoff, H., 305, *328*
Pilon, R.N., 142, *145*, *147*
Pilowsky, J., 198, 199, *207*, 215, 216, 223, 228, 232, 233, 236, 237, 238, 239, *249*, *250*
Pincherle, G., 37, *61*
Pincus, T., 134, 138, *146*
Pinsky, J.J., 177, *207*
Pinto, R.P., 47, *55*
Pitkin, D.H., 137, *146*
Polich, J.M., 15, *24*
Pollard, R., 11, *26*
Pollock, R., 11, *26*
Pollock, M.L., 401, *426*
Polly, S., 410, *428*
Pomerleau, C.S., 54, *61*
Pomerleau, OLF., 54, *61*, 66, *87*
Pope, M., 134, *147*, 280, *290*

Pratt, J.M., 312, *329*
Preston, T.A., 154, *168*, 348, 349, 375, *391*
Price, D.D., 189, *208*
Priest, R.G., 351, *389*
Prieto, E.J., 191, 195, *202*, *207*, 217, *245*, *250*
Prinz, P., *393*
Pritchard, D.W., 305, *328*
Prkachin, K.M., 180, 191, *203*
Prochaska, J.O., 35, 47, 50, 51, *57*, *62*, 403, 414, *423*
Prokop, C.K., 195, 196, *202*, 242, *245*
Puska, P.M, 44, *62*

Q

Queisser, H.R., 334, *344*
Quigley, B.M., 400, *421*

R

Rabkin, M., 132, *146*
Rachlin, H., 255, *293*
Rachman, S.J., 262, *294*
Raczynski, J.M., 315, *328*
Raczynski, J.R., 20, 23, *26*, 410, 411, 416, *425*
Radin, E.L., 97, *101*
Rafii, A., 189, *208*
Rahe, R., 230, 231, *246*, *250*
Ralph, D., 369, *393*
Rand, C., 36, 52, *62*
Ransford, A.O., 193, *208*
Raptopoulos, R., 351, *389*
Raskin, M., 151, 157, *170*
Rausch, A., 19, *27*
Raw, M., 37, *59*, *62*
Ray, O.S., 16, *27*
Read, L.L., 37, *63*
Reading, A.E., 191, *208*, 217, *250*
Reding, G.R., 159, *170*
Ready, L.B., 192, *208*, 216, 220, 226, 236, *250*, *252*
Rechnitzer, P.A., 414, *421*
Redington, D., 358, *395*
Rees, W., 301, *326*
Reeves, J.L., 177, *203*
Regenos, E., 161, *165*
Regestein, Q.R., 348, *393*
Reich, J., 242, *250*
Reich, P., 137, *147*, 348, *393*
Reichler, R., *126*
Reed, R.W., 42, 44, *59*
Reilly, R.E., 19, *27*
Reimherr, F., 195, *209*
Reinking, R.H., 156, 157, 158, *168*, *170*, 309, 314, 315, *327*, *328*
Reinsch, 410, *424*
Relinger, H., 381, *393*
Reynolds, M.D., 131, *146*
Revenson, T.A., 138, *144*
Reyes, J.R., 364, *390*
Reynolds, C.F., 356, 357, 358, 363, *390*, *394*
Rhind, V.M., 189, *203*
Rhodes, G.G., 9, *26*
Rial, W.Y., 37, *60*
Rice, R.E., 419, *426*
Richards, C.S., 35, *61*
Richards, S.C., 408, *426*
Ribordy, S.C., *170*
Richards, J.S., 192, *208*, 215, 219, *250*
Richardson, G.S., *389*
Richlin, D., 219, 222, 223, 240, *245*, *248*
Richmond, J.B., 32, *62*
Rickels, K., 215, *245*
Rickles, W., 162, *170*
Rideout, E., 279, *290*
Rigotti, N.A., 20, *27*
Riles, M., 192, *208*, 215, 219, *250*
Riley, S., 227, *244*
Rimon, R., 135, 136, *147*
Riordan, M., 409, *428*
Rios, C.D., 360, 361, *389*
Ripley, C., 224, *249*
Risley, T.R., 403, *422*
Ristanovic, R., 372, *389*, *392*
Ritzler, B.A., 349, *394*
Rivers, P.M., 280, *294*
Robbins, C.A., 338, *346*
Roberts, G.C., 416, *427*
Roberts, J., 360, 364, 371, *388*
Roberts, N., 216, *250*
Roberts, W.C., 11, *28*
Robertson, L.S., 19, *27*
Robinson, C.E., 134, *147*
Robinson, J., 195, *209*
Robinson, T., 153, *170*
Rock, A., 215, *245*
Rock, D., 218, *246*
Rockette, H.E., 9, *25*
Rodgers, D.A., 74, *87*

Rodichok, L.D., 302, 307, 313, 314, 315, *323*, *324*
Roehrs, T., 362, *394*
Rogacz, S., 360, 361, *389*
Rogers, L., 309, 310, *326*
Rogers, M., 134, 135, 137, *145*, *147*
Roghmann, K.J., *145*
Romano, J., 220, *246*
Rondestvedt, S.W., 157, *170*
Rodman, G., 108, *126*
Romero, M., 352, *389*
Rock, J., 226, 236, 238, *250*
Ronda, J.M., *389*
Roos, B., 371, *390*
Roos, C., 182, *205*
Rose, G., 37, 40, 41, *62*
Rose, R.M., 97, *101*
Rosen, G.M., 49, *62*, 418, *423*
Rosenbaum, J.F., 177, *208*
Rosenstiel, A., 243, *250*
Rosenthal, R., 160, *170*
Rosner, B., 9, *28*
Rosomoff, H., 242, *246*
Rosser, W.W., 37, 40, *62*, *63*
Roth, B., 360, 366, *394*
Roth, S., *345*, 364, 375, *387*
Roth, T., 154, *170*, 362, *394*
Rowat, K., 244, *251*
Rowlingson, J., 278, *294*
Rubin, A.H., 360, *392*
Rubinstein, A., 239, *251*
Rubright, W.C., 159, *170*
Ruddy, S., 108, *125*
Rudy, T., 217, *252*
Rudy, T.E., 191, 199, *206*, *209*, 273, *291*
RoyByrne, P., 140, *147*
Ruler, A., 357, 358, 361, *394*
Rugh, J.D., 160, *166*
Rundell, OLH., 372, *393*
Rushall, B.S., 406, 407, *426*
Rushmer, D.S., 338, *344*
Russ, D., 155, *167*
Russ, K.L., 162, *170*
Russe, D., 379, *390*
Russell, G., 161, *172*
Russell, M.A.H., 37, 40, 44, *59*, *62*
Russell, S., 195, *209*, 360, *392*
Ryan, A.J., 401, *426*
Ryan, E.S., 38, 54, *56*

S

Saccuzzo, D., 216, 220, 243, *244*, *251*
Sachs, H., 300, *328*
Sackett, D.L., 5, *27*
Sacks, M.H., 402, *426*
Sachs, M.L., 402, *426*
Sacktor, J.D., 51, *55*
Safranek, R., 200, *204*, 305, *326*
Said, G., 9, *27*
Sajben, N., 372, 373, *389*
Sale, W.G., 138, *146*
Salis, P., 153, *168*, 364, *391*
Sallis, J.F., 401, *427*
Salovey, P., 217, *252*
Sambuc, R., 300, *329*
Sanchez, R., 360, 361, *389*
Sanders, S.H., 178, 179, 185, 192, 194, 197, *208*, 209, *263*, 265, 267, 279, *294*
Sanders, S., 216, *251*
Saper, J.R., 182, *208*
Salovey, P., 177, 191, *209*
Samuels, R.M., 74, *87*
Sargent, J.D., 300, 313, *329*
Sarkis, E., 192, *208*, 216, *250*
Sarngadharan, M.G., 5, *28*
Sassin, J., 370, *389*
Satler, J., 163 *171*
Sattler, H.L., 375, *390*
Saunders, N.L., 305, 314, 315, *325*
Sanders, W.B., 4, *27*
Sausa, D.G.F., 9, *27*
Schachter, S., 402, *426*
Schaefer, C., 214, 230, *247*
Schafer, L., 418, *423*
Schandler, S., 162, *170*
Schapira, B., 269, 270, 275, *291*
Scharer, P., 159, *170*
Scarone, S., 373, *387*
Schele, R., *325*
Schlegel, R.P., 35, 37, 44, 45, 48, 52, 53, *58*, 61, *62*
Schneider, C., 163, *170*
Schneider, N.G., 34, 44, *63*
Schneider, S.J., 37, *63*
Schoen, L., 372, *387*
Schoenberg, B., 300, *328*
Schooler, C., 214, 243, *249*
Schlutter, L.S., 312, *328*

Schnarch, D.M., 300, *328*
Schwartz, G.E., *328*
Schwartz, J.L., *426*
Scott, J., 189, *208*
Scott, D., 219, 220, 223, *249*
Scott, L.P., *323*
Schubart, A.F., 134, *147*
Schulthies, K.R., 35, *61*
Schultz, J., 21, *27*, 151, 157, *171*, *394*
Schmacher, M.D., *126*
Schunk, D.H., 409, *422*
Schur, P.H., 134, 135, *145*
Schwab, J., *391*
Schwartz, B., 154, 159, *171*
Schwartz, D., 221, *251*, 278, *294*
Schwartz, L., *171*
Schwartz, G.E., 66, 67, *87*, 152, *167*
Schwartz, J.H., 140, *147*
Schweiger, A., 37, 44, *63*
Scotch, N., 7, *25*
Scott, D.F., 303, 312, *327*
Scott, D.S., 304, *329*
Sedwick, A.W., 400, 411, 415, *427*
Sedlacek, K., 163, *171*
Sedlmayr, E., 39, *57*
Seeburg, K.N., 162, *171*
Seidel, W.F., 361, 363, *394*
Selby, D., 195, 197, *207*, 242, *248*
Seleznick, M., *146*
Sell, G., 137, *147*
Selwood, T., 218, 220, 223, *249*
Semchuk, K.M., 152, *172*
Senner, J.W., 402, 403, *422*
Serbanesco, F., 300, *329*
Serfass, R.C., 400, *427*
Serratrice, E., *329*
Sevilla, F., 300, *328*
Sexton, M., 40, 52, *61*, *63*
Shahani, B.T., 161, *171*
Shanfield, S., 243, *251*
Shannon, M.E., 37, 48, 53, *62*
Shapiro, C.M., 370, *394*
Shapiro, R.M., 39, 46, *61*, *63*
Sharpe, N., 11, *25*
Shaw, T.R.D., 38, *57*
Shealy, R.C., 349, 384, *394*
Shealy, C., 192, *208*
Shealy, M., 192, *208*
Shearn, M.A., 140, *147*
Sheinkop, M.B., 191, 194, *206*, 217, *247*
Shelton, J.L., 157, *166*, 218, *246*, 310, *325*
Shephard, R.J., 22, *25*, 414, 419, *421*, *427*
Sherman, A.R., 410, *428*
Sherwood, M., 38, *56*
Shipley, M.J., 37, *62*
Shipman, W.G., 99, *101*
Shirley, R.J., 54, *60*
Shirlow, M.J., 364, *394*
Shochet, B.R., 134, *147*
Shouse, M.N., 341, *345*
Shows, W.D., 179, *204*, *291*
Sicurella, J., 37, *64*
Sicuteri, F., 99, *101*
Sides, H., 378, *390*
Siegel, L.J., 405, 413, *425*
Sikora, T., 410, 411, 416, *425*
Silbert, M., 275, *293*
Sillanpaa, M., 300, *329*
Sillett, R.W., 44, *60*
Silverberg, E., 142, *145*
Sime, W.E., 19, *25*, 401, *423*
Simkins, L., 163, *166*
Simons, R., 349, 384, *392*
Simpson, F.O., 300, *328*
Sinclair, A., 109, *125*
Singer, H., 34, 43, *63*
Singh, B., 238, *251*
Sintonen, H., 6, *27*
Siscovick, D.S., 11, *28*, 400, *427*
Sivarajan, E.S., 38, *63*
Skevington, S., 218, 219, 234, 238, *251*
Skinner, B.F., 407, *427*
Slama, K.M., 154, *165*, 378, *388*
Sledge, C.B., 108, *125*
Sledmere, C.M., *208*
Slye, T., 350, *387*
Smallwood, R., *393*
Smiehorowski, T., 161, *169*
Smirne, S., 371, *389*
Smith, C.B., 121, *125*
Smith, D.W., 9, *26*
Smith, L.W., 137, *147*
Smith, P.O., 20, 23, *26*, 410, 411, 416, *425*
Smith, R., 216, *250*
Smith, T.W., 195, *204*, 232, *246*

Smythe, H.A., 134, *147*
Smyth, M., 370, *394*
Snaith, R., 215, *251*
Sobell, L.C., 15, *28*
Sobell, M.C., 15, *28*
Sola, A., 239, *245*
Soldatos, C.R., 348, 349, 356, 364, 366, 373, *387*, *391*
Solinger, J., 269, 270, *293*
Solomon, D.S., 401, *427*
Solomon, G.F., 134, 136, 137, *146*, *147*
Sobmonis, 413, 416, 419, 420, *424*
Sommer, A., 70, *87*
Sorman, K., 36, *63*
Sortie, P.D., 11, 20, *25*, *26*
Sours, J.A., 366, *394*
Spalding, D., 215, *250*
Spangfort, E., 284, *292*
Sparros, L., 9, *28*
Spear, F., 217, *245*
Speizer, F.E., 9, *28*
Spence, N.D., 198, 199, *207*, 216, 223, 228, 237, 238, *250*
Spengler, D., 285, *291*
Spergel, P., 134, *147*
Spevak, P.A., 409, *427*
Spiegel, J.S., 140, *147*
Spiegel, R., 348, 350, *388*, *394*
Spiegel, T., 140, *147*
Spieker, S.J., 68, 79, *87*
Spielberg, L.A., 42, 52, *60*
Speilberger, C., 215, *251*
Spiker, D.G., 356, 357, *394*
Spink, K.S., 416, *427*
Spirduso, W.W., 19, *28*
Sprock, J., 216, 220, *251*
Sriwatanakul, K., 189, *208*
Stachnik, T., 36, 42, *63*
Stack, J.A., 358, *390*
Stagoll, B., 239, *248*
Stambul, H.B., 15, *24*
Stamler, J., 23, *28*, 400, *427*
Stanley, G.V., 189, *204*
Standley, J., 161, *167*
Stapp, J., 74, 80, *86*
Starker, S., 154, *171*
Stauffer, L., 50, *56*
Steele, K., 242, *246*
Steffen, J., 402, 403, 407, 413, *424*
Stegall, P., 226, 230, *245*
Steger, J.C., 306, 313, *326*, *329*
Steinbrocker, O., 138, *147*
Steinmark, S.W., 376, 381, 384, *394*
Stenn, P.G., 269, 270, *294*
Stephens, R., 316, *329*
Stephens, T., 403, *427*
Stephenson, N.L., 162, *171*
Sterman, M.B., 339, 340, 341, 342, *344*, *345*
Stern, G.S., 153, 164, *171*
Sternbach, R.A., 193, 195, *208*, *209*, 216, 218, 223, 224, 227, 229, 237, 238, 241, 242, *251*, 302, 303, *329*
Stevens, J.R., 337, *345*
Stewart, A.L., 42, *63*
Stewart, P.J., 40, *63*
Steinmark, S.W., *165*
Stiggins, J., 39, 46, *61*
Stinson, W., *87*
Stitzer, M.L., 36, 51, 52, *55*, *62*, *63*
Stjernlöf, K., 265, 271, *292*
Stoedefalke, K.G., 417, *427*
Stoffelmayr, B., 36, 42, *63*
Stokes, T.F., 405, *427*
Stolov, W., 218, *246*
Stoyva, J.M., 150, 156, *166*, 188, *202*, 308, 309, *325*
Strassberg, D.S, 195, *209*
Strauss, G.B., 140, *147*
Strite, L., 192, *204*
Strouse, T.B., 134, 135, *144*
Stuart, R.B., 17, *28*, 403, 408, *427*
Stubbs, D.A., 280, *294*
Stunkard, A.J., 418, *422*
Sturner, W.Q., 11, *28*
Suer, Z., 192, *208*, 215, 219, *250*
Suhel, P., 163, *171*
Sullivan, P., 215, *251*
Sult, S., 231, 235, 244, *246*
Sundell, L., 284, *292*
Sundstrom, W.R., 143, *148*
Suriano, T., 352, *389*
Surwit, R.S., 139, *147*, 269, 270, 275, *295*
Susanto, D., 70, *87*
Sutkus, B.J., *327*
Sutton, E.P., 200, *209*, 318, *324*
Surwit, R.S., 142, *145*, *291*
Sutkus, B., 229, *243*
Sulton, J.R., 414, *421*
Swafford, J., 134, 135, *145*
Swannell, A.J., *146*
Swanson, D., 192, *209*, 217, 241, 243, *248*, *251*, *252*

Swanson, G., 216, 233, *249*
Swash, M., 304, *327*
Swenson, W., 192, *209*, 241, *252*, 333, *344*
Syme, S.L., 138, *144*
Szekely, B.C., 314, *327*

T

Tager, I.B., 9, *28*
Tait, R., 235, *245*
Takebe, K., 161, *165*
Taplin, R., *427*
Tapp, J.T., *28*
Tarwotjo, I., 70, *87*
Taska, L.S., 357, *394*
Tasto, D.L., 157, *171*
Taube, A., 371, *390*
Taylor, C.B., 40, 43, *59*, *62*, 401, *427*
Taylor, H.L., 37, 50, *56*
Taylor, J., 134, 135, *145*
Teders, S.J., 302, 307, 313, 314, 315, *323*, *324*, *329*
Teevan, R.C., 302, 307, *323*
Temkin, N.R., 334, *344*
Tenaglia, A.N., 134, 135, *144*
Tennant, C., 214, *244*
Terborg, J.R., 53, *63*
Thaller, J.L., 159, *171*
Thelen, M.H., 180, *209*, 272, *293*
Thom, B., 51, *57*
Thomas, G.S., 20, *27*
Thomas, L., 179, *202*
Thomas, M., 192, *204*, 237, *252*, *291*
Thomas, O.W., 400, *427*
Thomas, P.C., 278, *290*
Thompson, C.E., 400, 410, 411, *428*
Thompson, J.K., 303, 305, 315, *329*, 410, 416, *423*, *428*
Thompson, L.W., 177, 200, *203*
Thompson, J.K., 11, 20, 23, *26*, 189, *203*, 209, *328*, 412, *425*
Thompson, P.D., 11, *28*
Thompson, P.M., 334, *346*
Thompson, S., 225, *252*
Thoresen, C.E., 48, *63*, 378, *39*, 408, 419, 420, *435*
Thornby, J.I., 348, 351, 364, *391*
Thornley, P., 38, *57*
Thorpy, M.J., 360, *387*
Timmermans, G., 242, *251*, 303, *329*
Tobin, D.L., 309, 310, *326*
Toderman, L., 92, *101*
Toomey, T., 221, 222, *252*
Torgerson, W.S., 190, *207*
Townley, M., 233, *250*
Townsend, R.E., 151, *171*
Toyomura, K., 364, *393*
Traeger, C.H., 138, *147*
Trichopoulos, D., 9, *28*
Trief, P.M., 195, *209*, 216, *252*
Trimble, R.W., 376, *393*
Trinder, J., 375, *393*
Troy, A., 191, *202*, *245*
Truelove, L.H., 138, *144*
Tubbs, W., 163, *171*
Tugwell, P., 109, *125*
Tunis, M.M., 156, *171*, 308, *329*
Tunks, E., 261, *294*
Tupin, J., 242, *250*
Turk, D.C., 176, 177, 178, 185, 188, 191, 193, 199, *204*, *206*, *209*, 217, *252*, 261, 269, 271, 273, 274, *290*, *291*, *294*
Turkat, I.D., 279, *294*, *329*
Turner, B., 132, *146*
Turner, D., 355, 381, 383, 384, *392*
Turner, J.A.M., 44, *60*, 192, 195, *207*, *208*, *209*, 215, 216, 218, 220, 226, 227, 235, 236, 243, *246*, *248*, *250*, *252*, 261, 269, 271, 273, 274, *294*
Turner, R., 38, *57*, 139, *144*, *248*, 361, 383, *387*
Turner, R.D., 410, *428*
Turner, R.M., 360, 381, *394*, *395*
Turner, S.M., 314, *327*
Tursky, B., 193, *209*
Ty, T., 217, *248*

U

Udelman, D.L., 140, *147*
Udellman, H., 140, *147*
Unikel, I.P., 192, *202*
Unlenhuth, E.H., 348, 349, *392*
Urponen, H., 349, *395*
Usselman, L.B., 150, *166*

V

Vaillant, G., 214, *244*
Vällfors, B., 281, *294*
van Boxtel, A., 156, *172*
Vance, B., 410, *428*
Vandenbergh, R.L., 162, *167*
Vanden Bos, G.R., 52, *641*, 66, 69, 74, 78, 80, *85*, *86*

Van Den Hoed, J., 360, *389*
Van der Heide, L., *245*
Van der Helm-Hyllkema, H., 302, *328*
Van der Keide, L.H., 191, *202*
Van der Ven J.R., 156, *172*
Vandiver, F.E., *87*
Van Gool, W.A., 361, *395*
Van Keppel, M., 303, 304, *327*
Vannucci, C., 240, *245*
Varni, J.W., 139, *147*, *148*, 162, *165*
Vasey, M., 54, *58*
Vaughn, W.K., 134, 138, *146*
Vela-Bueno, A., 348, 364, 373, *387*, *391*
Vernallis, F.F., 159, *172*
Vestergaard, C.L., 159, *172*
Victor, M., 9, *28*
Viernstein, M., 194, *205*
Villa Lobos, S., 352, *389*
Viney, L., 214, *252*
Vinterberg, H., 278, *289*
Violon, A., 179, *209*, 279, *294*
Visser, P., 137, *146*
Vitello, M., 369, *393*
Vollhardt, B.R., 125, *148*
Von Baeyer, C.L., 194, *209*
Vyori, I., 349, *395*

W

Waal-Manning, H.J., 300, *328*
Waddell, G., 233, *248*
Wagner, D.A., 75, *87*
Wagner, J., 192, *204*
Wainwright, P.E., 34, 35, 50, *56*
Walker, W.J., 400, *428*
Wall, P., 176, *207*, 217, *248*, *252*, 255, *293*
Waller, B.F., 11, *28*
Wallston, B.S., 199, *209*
Wallston, K.A., 199, *209*
Walsh, D.C., 49, *64*
Walters, D., 37, 44, 45, *61*
Wankel, L.M., 412, *428*
Wansley, R.A., 161, *167*
Waranch, H.R., 313, *329*
Ward, J., 362, *392*, 405, *421*
Ward, M., 195, *209*
Ware, J.C., 348, *391*
Warheit, G.J., 351, *391*
Warren, L.W., 333, *345*
Waters, W.E., 299, 305, *325*, *329*
Watson, D., 220, 241, *252*
Watson, G., *249*
Waring, E., 243, *249*
Waving, E.M., 279, *293*
Webb, W.B., 347, 356, 358, 370, *387*, *395*
Webster, J.S., 20, 23, *26*, 410, 411, 416, *425*
Weerts, T.C., 377, *388*
Weibell, F.J., 150, *166*
Weibell, F.G., 150, *166*
Weiner, H., *64*
Weinman, M.L., 152, *172*
Weis, O.F., 189, *208*
Weisenberg, M., 185, *209*
Weiss, D.J., 333, *345*
Weiss, H., 348, *395*
Weiss, J.M., 154, *168*
Weiss, N.S., 9, *28*
Weiss, R., 231, *245*
Weiss, S.H., 5, *28*
Weiss, S.M., 32, *60*, *64*, 66, 67, *87*
Weiss, S.T., 11, *28*
Weisz, G., 243, *249*, 279, *293*
Welsch, B.L., 74, *85*
Welsh, G., 215, *251*
Welsh, R.J., 15, *24*
Welstein, L., 358, *395*
Wenig, P., *144*
Werder, D.S., 300, 313, *329*
Westbrook, M., 214, *252*
Westbrook, T., 312, *326*
Westling, H., 44, *57*
Whisler, W.W., 191, 194, *206*, 217, *247*
White, B., 179, *209*, 265, 267, *294*
White, C.C., 403, *427*
White, J.R., 9, *28*
White, K.L., *59*
White, P., 35, 38, *57*
Whitehead, W.E., 179, *209*
Wickramasekera, I., 157, 158, *172*
Wiener, C., 225, *252*
Wilbur, C.S., 419, *428*
Wilfling, F., 163, *167*
Wilkins, R.H., 193, *205*, 224, 225, 226, 240, *247*
Wilkus, R.J., 334, *346*
Willard, R.R., 272, *293*
Williams, A.F., 12, *29*
Williams, C.L., 21, *29*
Williams, R.T., 344, *346*
Williams, R.B., 139, *145*, 153, *168*, 269, 270, 275, *291*

Williams, R.L., 351, 356, 364, *391*, *395*, 408, *428*
Williamson, D.A., 305, 308, 312, *325*, *329*
Williamson, H.O., 137, *144*
Williamson, P., 238, *244*
Wilson, C., *62*
Wilson, D., 37, 40, 43, *64*
Wilson, E., 318, *324*
Wilson, G.T., 17, *29*, 262, *294*, 405, 407, 408, *428*
Wilson, J., 9, *29*
Windsor, R.A., *64*
Winefield, H.R., 278, *294*
Wing, A.L., 20, *27*
Wing, R.R., 400, 410, 418, *423*
Wingard, D.L., 8, *29*, 350, *395*
Winkler, R.C., 312, *330*, 415, 416, 420, *428*
Winett, R.A., 415, *428*
Wise, C., 133, *143*
Wise, D., 154, *169*
Wittchen, H.V., 75, *85*
Wolf, M.M., 403, *422*
Wolf, S.L., 161, *165*, *210*
Wolf, S.R., 195, 200, *208*, 216, 223, 227, *251*
Wolfe, F., 134, *146*
Wolff, H.G., 156, *171*, 189, *205*, *328*
Wolff, B., 217, *252*
Wolff, H.G., 307, 308, *329*
Wood, A.B., *290*
Wood, M.M., 305, *328*
Wood, P.H.N., 280, *294*
Wood, S.N., 280, *290*
Woods, D.J., 405, 413, *425*
Woodforde, J., 176, 195, 197, *210*, 228, *252*
Wooley, S., *209*
Woolfolk, R.L., 380, 384, *388*, *395*
Wong, J., 19, *27*
Wood, P.H.N., 130, *148*
Wood, G., 37, *64*
Woolcock, N.E., 51, *59*
Wooldridge, C.P., 161, *172*
Wooringham, C.J., 280, *294*
Wortley, M.D., 277, *289*
Wortman, P.M., 41, *64*
Wright, C.C., 22, *27*
Wright, H.B., 37, *61*
Wright, V., 189, *203*
Wyler, A.R., 338, *346*
Wyler, D.J., 70, *88*
Wynder, E.L., 21, *29*
Wynne, J., 370, *387*
Wyrwicka, W., 339, *345*
Wysocki, T., 409, *428*

Y

Yates, J., 238, *251*
Yelin, E., 138, *148*
Yellen, A.N., 196, *207*
Yost, D., 361, 363, *394*
Yuan, H.A., 195, *209*
Yucum, D.E., 143, *148*
Yonkers, A.J., 9, *26*
Young, L.D., 133, 136, 139, *143*, *144*, 215, *248*
Yudkin, G.D., 40, *58*
Yunus, M., 227, *244*

Z

Zackler, L., 140, *147*
Zamproni, P., 371, *389*
Zanna, M.P., 415, 420, *426*
Zarcone, U., 348, 350, *388*
Zborowski, M., 179, *210*
Zeitlin, D.J., 136, *148*
Zepelin, H., 360, *395*
Ziegler, D.K., 298, *320*
Zigelbaum, S.D., 163, *170*
Zimmerman, J.S., *166*
Zimmerman, J.S., 312, *325*
Zimmerman, S.O., 158, 159, *170*
Zitter, R.E., 261, *291*
Zomer, J., 360, *392*
Zorick, F., 177, *202*, 362, *394*
Zucconi, M., 348, 364, *392*
Zuidema, H., 254, *294*
Zung, W., 215, *252*
Zutish, D.W., 189, *205*
Zvaifler, N.J., 108, *126*
Zwart, S.A., 382, 384, *395*

Subject Index

A
Aids, 4–5
Alcohol, 9–10

B
Biofeedback
  anxiety disorders, 150
  relaxation, 150–153
Bruxism, 159–160

D
Diseases of lifestyle, 5
Drugs 9–10, 14

E
Exercise,
  and heart attack, ii
  as prevention, 400–401
  cognitive theories, 407–413
  persistence, 402–403
  psychological effects, 401–402
  operant theories, 405–407
  reversal issues, 415–420

H
Health
  changing perspectives, 4–6
  definitions, 4
  epidemiology, 7
  lifestyle changes, 33–34
  policy, 3–4
  promotion, 3–4, 22
  risk factor intervention, 12
  risk factors, 7–12
  status assessment, 6–7

I
Inflammatory disease, 128–130
Insomnia, 153–155

M
Musculoskeletal disabilities,
  dysfunction, 91
  evaluation tools, 112
  physician evaluation, 108–110
Musculoskeletal system
  cartilage, 96
  muscle 97–100
  pain, 91
  soft tissue, 92–96

N
Neuromuscular rehabilitation, 160
Nutrition, 10–16

O
Occupation, 105

P
Pain,
  assessment, 180–185
  biofeedback, 269

clinical characteristics, 217–230
cognitive techniques, 268–269
density, 190
development, 255–261
disruption to daily tasks, 230
McGill pain questionnaire/MPPI, 190–192, 194–197
measures of intensity, 188–189
operant techniques, 261–268
prevention, 275, 282–288
psychological factors, 176–180
relaxation, 269
visual analogy scaling, 189–190
Physical fitness
aerobic exercises, 21
training, 19
Prevention,
of disease, 3–4
education, 21
health promotion, 21

R
Raynaud's disease 141–142
Rheumatic disability,
types, 131–133
Rheumatoid Arthritis, 118

S
Safety,
habits, 17
in work place, 18
practices, 10
Seizure disorders,
assessments, 332–336
treatment, 336–343
Sleep disorders, 347–395
age effects, 356–360
behavioral treatment, 374–385
gender differences, 355–356
health problems, 348–349
hypnotic drugs, 361–362
laboratory studies, 356–358
measuring sleep, 350–352
narcolepsy, 364–366
nocturnal myclonus, 372–373
prevalence, 352
sleep apnea, 366–372
Smoking, 8–9
cessation, 13
evaluation studies, 39–40
high risk populations, 38
nicotine gum, 37
program development research 49–52
self help, 39
Spasmodic Torticollis, 113
Spondylitis, 132–133
Stress, 11
reduction, 20
Systemic Rheumatic disease,
behavioral treatment, 138–141
etiology, 133

T
Tension headache, 156
assessment, 319–321
EMG feedback, 309
functional aspects, 303–304
nature, 297–300
personality, 301–303
physiological mechanisms, 304–308
prevalence, 300–301
prognostic indicators, 314
relaxation, 310
research issues, 315–318
treatment of children, 313
Tobacco, 8–9

W
Weight loss, 17

www.ingramcontent.com/pod-product-compliance
Ingram Content Group UK Ltd.
Pitfield, Milton Keynes, MK11 3LW, UK
UKHW022254060626
471939UK00003B/307

9 780893 916800